The Student's Guide to Becoming a Midwife

Second edition

Edited by

Ian Peate

Visiting Professor of Nursing, University of West London
Editor-in-Chief, *British Journal of Nursing*

Cathy Hamilton

Senior Lecturer of Midwifery, University of Hertfordshire
Supervisor of Midwives, West Herts Hospitals NHS Trust

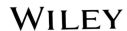

D1209258

This edition first published 2014 © 2014 by John Wiley & Sons, Ltd
First edition published 2008 © 2008 by John Wiley & Sons, Ltd

Registered Office
John Wiley & Sons, Ltd, The Atrium, Southern Gate, Chichester, West Sussex, PO19 8SQ, UK

Editorial Offices
9600 Garsington Road, Oxford, OX4 2DQ, UK
The Atrium, Southern Gate, Chichester, West Sussex, PO19 8SQ, UK
111 River Street, Hoboken, NJ 07030-5774, USA

For details of our global editorial offices, for customer services and for information about how to apply for permission to reuse the copyright material in this book please see our website at www.wiley.com/wiley-blackwell.

Library of Congress Cataloging-in-Publication Data

Becoming a midwife in the 21st century.
   The student's guide to becoming a midwife / edited by Ian Peate, Cathy Hamilton. – 2e
     p. ; cm.
   Preceded by Becoming a midwife in the 21st century / edited by Ian Peate, Cathy Hamilton. c2008.
   Includes bibliographical references and index.
   ISBN 978-1-118-41093-6 (pbk. : alk. paper) – ISBN 978-1-118-41094-3 (epub) – ISBN 978-1-118-41589-4 (epdf) –
ISBN 978-1-118-41629-7 (emobi) – ISBN 978-1-118-41638-9 – ISBN 978-1-118-41643-3
   I. Peate, Ian, editor of compilation.   II. Hamilton, Cathy, 1962– editor of compilation.   III. Title.
   [DNLM: 1. Midwifery.   2. Nurse Midwives–organization & administration.   3. Nurse Midwives–standards.
4. Perinatal Care–methods. WQ 160]
   RG950
   618.2′0233–dc23
2013026501

A catalogue record for this book is available from the British Library.

Wiley also publishes its books in a variety of electronic formats. Some content that appears in print may not be available in electronic books.

Cover image: Photo of a moments-old baby being handed to his mother. © iStockphoto / Yarinca.
Cover design by Steve Thompson

Set in 10/12pt Calibri by SPi Publishers Services, Pondicherry, India
Printed and bound in Malaysia by Vivar Printing Sdn Bhd

1   2014

Contents

Contributors

Laura Abbott MSc BA, BSc(Hons), RGN, RM, is a Senior Lecturer and Admissions Tutor for Pre-Registration Midwifery at The University of Hertfordshire. She is a supervisor of midwives for the East of England Local Supervisory Authority and is linked with the team of supervisors at East and North Herts NHS Trust. Laura has written on a variety of topics for midwifery and nursing journals. Her midwifery practice involved working independently for 6 years. Laura has been a guest speaker at conferences around the UK and internationally and is currently undertaking a Doctorate in Health Research.

Carmel Bagness MA, PGCEA, ADM, RM, RGN is the Midwifery and Women's Health Adviser at the Royal College of Nursing. The role enables her to develop UK-wide health and social care policy and practice, in both midwifery and various aspects of women's health. She is a practising midwife who has extensive experience in midwifery education, and worked at the Department of Health on the Midwifery 2020 programme. She uses her experience to channel knowledge and resources to make best use of evidence to influence contemporary practice to contribute to the healthcare requirements of the 21st century.

Emma Dawson-Goodey MA, DipHE, RM, RGN is a Senior Midwifery Lecturer at the University of Hertfordshire. She has worked in midwifery education since 2003 and her key interests have continued to be midwifery and sexual health, health law and professional regulation.

Tandy Deane-Gray MA, BSc, PGCEA, ADM, RM, RGN is a Senior Lecturer Midwifery at the University of Hertfordshire. She has worked in Midwifery Education since 1988. She has attended home births in Bermuda. Her key interests have continued to be midwifery, parenting and communication. She facilitates baby massage, as she is particularly interested in parent infant attachment, and also works as a psychotherapist.

Lyn Dolby BSc(Hons) RGN, DPSM, PGCert is a Senior Midwifery Lecturer at the University of Hertfordshire. She began working in midwifery education at Nottingham University and then joined the University of Hertfordshire in 1996. She is the lead on the Physical Examination of the Newborn and her Masters dissertation relates to this area of her expertise. Her present doctoral research is exploring the experience of student midwives as they complete the Physical Examination of the Newborn module during their pre-registration midwifery programme.

Caroline Duncombe MSc, BSc(Hons), RGN, RM, DipHE Midwifery, PGCert is Midwife, Supervisor of midwives. She is currently an instructor on the ALSO (Advanced Life Saving in Obstetrics) Course. She works as a Diabetes Specialist midwife. Her interests include supporting women with medical complications through their pregnancy and birth and clinical risk management.

Cathy Hamilton MSc, BSc(Hons) RGN, RM, PGDip, PGCert is a Principal Lecturer at the University of Hertfordshire and is also a Supervisor of Midwives working with the supervisory team at West Herts NHS Trust. Her current research interests focus on midwifery care during the second stage of labour.

Annabel Jay BA(Hons), MA, FHEA, DipHE, RM, PGDip(HE) is a Senior Lecturer in Midwifery and is currently the admissions tutor for the pre-registration midwifery programme at the University of Hertfordshire. Annabel has published research into the Objective Structural Clinical Examination (OSCE) and has presented at various conferences. She is currently undertaking doctoral studies, exploring women's experiences of undergoing induction of labour. Annabel has a particular interest in the involvement of service users in midwifery education and continues to lead parent education classes in Hertfordshire.

Patricia Lindsay RN, RM, MSc, PGCEA, DHC did her nurse training in London then trained as a midwife. She has been a practising midwife since 1974 and a midwifery teacher since 1991. She has worked in the UK and in the Sultanate of Oman. She is currently Lead Midwife for Education at Anglia Ruskin University. Her doctoral thesis was on incident reporting in maternity care and she had presented posters on this topic at national and international conferences. Her interests are patient safety in maternity care, women's mental health and support worker training.

Jenny Lorimer MA, HDCR is a Senior Lecturer in diagnostic radiography and Lead for Interprofessional Education (IPE) at the University of Hertfordshire. The role at Hertfordshire involves students from 12 different disciplines, in very large cohorts, working and learning together. Jenny's research interest is the effect of IPE on students' attitudes.

Kath Mannion BSc Midwifery, MSc Midwifery, RM, RN, ADM is LSA Midwifery Officer for the North East Strategic Health Authority. Kath's current appointment includes investigating cases of alleged suboptimal practice by midwives and determining the appropriate supervisory action. She is an Advanced Life Support in Obstetrics (ALSO) Advisory Faculty and serves as a trustee on the executive team within that organisation. She regularly teaches on ALSO Provider and Instructor courses throughout the UK and Ireland.

Lisa Nash BSc (Hons), MBA (Herts), RM, PGDip (Learning and teaching), Dip HE Midwifery is Senior Lecturer in Midwifery at the University of Hertfordshire. Lisa has been in midwifery education since 2000 and works at the University of Hertfordshire in the school of Allied Health Professionals and Midwifery.

Maxine Offredy PhD is Reader in Primary Healthcare at the Centre for Research in Primary and Community Care, University of Hertfordshire. She is an editorial board member and book review editor for the journal *Primary Health Care Research and Development*. Key areas of interest include clinical decision making and qualitative research methodologies.

Marianne Peace MA, BSc(Hons), DipHE, RM, RN is a Senior Midwifery Lecturer at the University of Hertfordshire. Marianne qualified as a midwife in 1997 and has worked both in the UK and internationally, gaining experience as a midwife in the United Arab Emirates. She has been involved in midwifery education since 2005 whilst working as a midwife and she subsequently joined the university as a lecturer in 2007. Marianne's key interests include learning & teaching, midwifery care, female genital mutilation in relation to childbirth and safeguarding children, health promotion, inequalities in health and breastfeeding.

Ian Peate EN(G) RN DipN (Lond) RNT BEd(Hons) MA(Lond) LLM is Editor-in-Chief of the *British Journal of Nursing*, Visiting Professor of Nursing with University of West London and Independent Consultant. Ian began his nursing a career in 1981 at Central Middlesex Hospital, becoming an Enrolled Nurse working in an intensive care unit. He later undertook three years student nurse training at Central Middlesex and Northwick Park Hospitals, becoming a Staff Nurse then a Charge Nurse. He has worked in nurse education since 1989. He has published widely. His key areas of interest are nursing practice and theory, sexual health and HIV/AIDS.

Cathy Rogers MA, RN, RMN, RM, ADM, PGCEA, Supervisor of Midwives qualified as a midwife in 1984 and she has worked in all areas of midwifery practice. She is currently employed as a consultant midwife at Barnet and Chase Farm NHS Trust where she is responsible for leading midwifery-led services. She is also an honorary lecturer at the University of Hertfordshire and is specifically involved in the development and delivery of the postgraduate course for the preparation of supervisors of midwives and Newborn infant physical examination.

Celia Wildeman SCM, DipNS, ADM, BEd (Hons), PGDC, PGDSPCF, Supervisor of Midwives is a Senior Lecturer in the Department of Nursing and Midwifery at the University of Hertfordshire. Her special interests include women's sexual health, teenage pregnancy, domestic violence and abuse, equal opportunities and cultural diversity.

Sandy Wong MSc, ADM, RM, RGN, PGCert(HE), FHEA is a Senior Midwifery Lecturer at the University of Hertfordshire and a Fellow of the Higher Education Academy. Prior to joining the University of Hertfordshire, she was a clinical midwife for many years, largely in the community. Her previous role as a community clinical manager also involved her with child protection at a strategic level. Sandy undertook a qualitative research project on perinatal mental health for her MSc degree. She sees herself as an expert in normality in pregnancy and childbirth, with special interests in diversity and public health.

Carole Yearley MSc, RN, RM, ADM, PGCEA, PGCert, Supervisor of Midwives is a Principal Lecturer in Midwifery. She is part of the team of supervisors of midwives at Barnet, Enfield and Haringey Strategic Health Authority and currently is the Programme Tutor for the Postgraduate Certificate in the Supervision of Midwives at the University of Hertfordshire.

Preface to the Second Edition

In the UK, maternity services have developed significantly with an increasing recognition that midwives should take the lead role in the care of normal pregnancy and labour (DH 2007, 2010). Midwifery-led care has been seen to have good outcomes such as shared care, reports of greater satisfaction from women and a reduction in obstetric intervention rates (Devane et al. 2010).

The first edition of *Becoming a Midwife in the 21st Century* was published in 2008. Since then the world has changed and the practice of midwifery continues to evolve. This second edition reflects the changes that have occurred but maintains its central aim of helping to prepare the next generation of midwives who are fit for purpose and fit for practice.

Feedback from students and lecturers alike has been instrumental in ensuring that this edition will be as popular as the first one. There are now 20 chapters in this edition arranged around the new pre-registration midwifery standards. The five essential skills clusters have been interlinked within each of the chapters where appropriate.

The new edition builds upon the positive comments made by the reviewers and anecdotal comments concerning the current text's 'student friendliness'. Each chapter commences with an aim and a set of 4–6 objectives which will help you to pre-plan learning and understand the rationale for the discrete yet intertwined chapters.

We have reviewed the various elements of pedagogy, developing this further to make it stronger and more engaging. Readers will note that the text layout has been prepared in such a way as to make it more appealing.

Chapter order has been rearranged and we have retained the popular case studies and extended them further. Each chapter has review questions using a variety of formats with answers provided at the end of the book. The aim is to improve retention and enhance learning.

As appropriate, midwifery pearls of wisdom have been provided throughout the text, providing the reader with practical hints and tips. There is a glossary of terms at the end of the book.

Updated evidence to support discussion has been provided. Reference and referral to organisations such as National Institute for Health and a Care Excellence (NICE) and other appropriate government organisations have been retained. Throughout, referral to the *Code of Conduct* and *Guidance on Professional Conduct for Nursing and Midwifery Students* has been included.

Various White Papers that have had and will have an impact on the practice of midwifery and the care of women produced by the government have been included. An additional chapter has been included focusing upon public health and the role of the midwife.

We have sincerely enjoyed being able to provide you with an updated version of the first edition. We hope that you will enjoy reading it with the primary intention of providing safe and effective care based upon the best available evidence to those women and their families for whom you have the privilege to care.

Ian Peate and Cathy Hamilton

References

Department of Health (DH) (2007) *Maternity Matters: choice, access and continuity of care in a safe service*. London: Department of Health.
Department of Health (DH) (2010) *Midwifery 2020: delivering expectations*. London: Department of Health.
Devane D, Brennan M, Begley C et al. (2010) *A Systematic Review, Meta-analysis, Meta-synthesis and Economic Analysis of Midwife-led Models of Care*. London: Royal College of Midwives.

Acknowledgements

We would like to thank all of our colleagues for their help, support, comments and suggestions.

Cathy would like to thank her friends and family for their patience and encouragement.

Ian would like to thank his partner Jussi Lahtinen and Frances Cohen for their continued support and encouragement.

Introduction

Ian Peate and Cathy Hamilton

This text is primarily intended for midwifery students, midwifery support workers, healthcare assistants, those undertaking Scottish Vocational Qualifications/National Qualifications Framework level of study or anyone who intends to undertake a programme of study leading to registration as a midwife. Throughout the text, the terms midwife, student and midwifery are used. These terms and the principles applied to this book can be transferred to a number of healthcare workers at various levels and in various settings in order to develop their skills for caring for women and their families throughout childbirth.

The unique role and function of the midwife

Midwives provide individual care to women and their families, encouraging them to participate in their pregnancy and determine how they want it to progress. Each year, over 700,000 women in the UK will give birth, nearly all of whom will have had the majority of their care from a midwife. In women's homes, birth centres and hospitals, midwives co-ordinate a woman's journey through her pregnancy, offering her continuity with the aim of ensuring that she experiences safe, compassionate care in an appropriate environment.

Midwife means 'with woman' and this highlights the empowering/partnership role of the midwife – the midwife works with the woman rather than telling her what to do. The underpinning philosophy of midwifery care is articulated by Page and McCandlish (2006) who suggest the following:

> The essence of being a midwife is the assistance of a woman around the time of childbirth in a way that recognises that the physical, emotional and spiritual aspects of pregnancy and birth are equally important. The midwife provides competent and safe physical care without sacrificing these other aspects.

The support the midwife offers is established by assessing the woman's individual needs and by working in partnership with her and other healthcare workers. The midwife is usually the lead healthcare professional involved in caring for pregnant women. There will be occasions when you will need to work on your own as a midwife and times when you will be working as a member of the wider team. It is

The Student's Guide to Becoming a Midwife, Second Edition. Edited by Ian Peate and Cathy Hamilton.
© 2014 John Wiley & Sons, Ltd. Published 2014 by John Wiley & Sons, Ltd.

2

important that midwives work collaboratively with other healthcare professionals, including obstetricians, paediatricians, specialist community public health nurses and paramedics, in order to ensure a high quality of care for women and their families.

Medforth et al. (2011) note that the definition of a midwife was first officially formulated in 1972. This was after discussions and debates among various organisations and committees and is as follows:

> *A midwife is a person who, having been regularly admitted to a midwifery educational programme, duly recognised in the country in which it is located, has successfully completed the prescribed course of studies in midwifery and has acquired the requisite qualifications to be registered and/or legally licensed to practise midwifery.*

The midwife is the senior professional attending over 75% of births in the UK, providing total care to mother and baby from early pregnancy onwards, throughout childbirth and beyond. The role of the midwife is thus multifaceted.

The midwife's role in public health

Another important aspect of that role is within the context of public health. Public health can be defined as improving the health of the population, as opposed to treating the diseases of individuals. This is particularly appropriate in midwifery as you will be caring for healthy individuals going through the physiological process of childbirth. Public health functions (DH 2004) include:

- health surveillance, monitoring and analysis
- investigation of disease outbreaks, epidemics and risks to health
- establishing, designing and empowering communities
- creating and sustaining cross-government and intersectoral partnerships to improve health and reduce inequalities
- ensuring compliance with regulations and laws to protect and promote health
- developing and maintaining a well-educated and trained, multidisciplinary public health workforce
- ensuring the effective performance of NHS services to meet goals in improving health, preventing disease and reducing inequalities
- research, development, evaluation and innovation
- quality assuring the public health function.

The Department of Health (2012a) defines public health as: 'about helping people to stay healthy and avoid getting ill'. Within this definition specific areas are included such as nutrition, recreational substance use, sexual health, pregnancy, immunisation and children's health. The key concerns of public health are dual: the health of populations and the health of individuals or groups within a population. The health needs of populations are embraced within overarching measures such as food and water safety, road safety and the provision of health services which are free at point of care.

A great deal of public health activity in the UK is derived from government; the drivers are political and economical, as the burden of disease is costly to a nation in which the state subsidises health and social care. Public Health England, introduced in April 2013, has been charged with protecting public health by delivering on the objectives of the Public Health Outcomes Framework (DH 2011, 2012b). The legislation responsible for this is the Health and Social Care Act 2012. At a national level in England, Public Health England will be the executive agency that delivers the wider agenda and at local level, the move of public health services into local authorities aims to create a multiprofessional approach to delivering local strategy and supporting better healthcare for the population.

Public health activities can take place with individuals, their families or communities, on a national or international level. The midwife is ideally placed to influence and enact public health policy when working with women and their families as well as being able to develop a population perspective within midwifery.

All the chapters in this text are concerned with midwifery practice, and as such are rooted in public health. Midwives make a substantial contribution to public health by promoting the long-term well-being of women, their babies and their families. They provide information and advice regarding screening and testing, sexual health, nutrition, exercise and healthy lifestyles. The midwife promotes breastfeeding, offering support and advice, as well as providing guidance to women and their families in relation to immunisation. Public health in midwifery is not new; midwives have always provided care that has a public health focus. Public health is at the heart of all aspects of midwifery practice.

Terminology

There are a variety of terms that can be used to describe women who use maternity services. 'Patient', 'woman', 'person' and 'client' are used throughout this text and refer to all groups and individuals who have direct or indirect contact with healthcare workers and in particular registered midwives, registered nurses and specialist community public health nurses.

'Patient' is the term commonly used within the NHS. It is acknowledged that not everyone approves of the passive concept associated with it or the way in which it can emphasise a medical focus. The term is used in this text in the knowledge that it is widely understood. The other two commonly used terms – 'woman' and 'client' – are also used to reflect changes in the way midwives and other care providers are considering their relationships with users of maternity services. The term 'client' emphasises the professional nature of the relationship that the midwife has with the women she cares for. The term 'consumer' is taken from the marketplace and highlights the concept of service users as consumers of products such as medications or care services. Client and consumer have their roots in healthcare provision during the 1980s and 1990s when, particularly in the health service, market forces and consumerism were in vogue. Another term used is 'expert'. Experts are said to be on an equal footing with expert care providers (for example, midwives and obstetricians). They are often patients who live with long-term health conditions.

There are 35,305 midwives on the midwives' part of the professional register (spring 2013) (see Table I.1). The majority of midwives in the UK are women and whilst it is acknowledged that the number of men entering the midwifery profession is increasing, for the sake of brevity this text uses the pronoun 'she'.

Table I.1   Number of midwives on the midwives' part of the professional register

	Number of midwives
Male	132
Female	35,169
Total	35,305 (four forms not filled)

Source: NMC 2008b.

4 The Nursing and Midwifery Council and Quality Assurance Agency (Education)

The primary aim of the Nursing and Midwifery Council (NMC), an organisation established by Parliament, is to protect the public by ensuring that midwives and nurses provide a high standard of care to their patients and clients.

The NMC is the regulatory body responsible for promoting best practice amongst the midwives and nurses registered with it. The key role of the NMC is to ensure that women receive the best possible care. It is the responsibility of the NMC to set and monitor standards in training (Nursing and Midwifery Order 2001). The NMC has produced a framework for quality assurance of education programmes which relates to all programmes that lead to registration or to the recording of a qualification on the professional register.

The programme you have embarked on, or are going to embark on, must meet certain standards. These include the standards set by your educational institution – for example, your university's policies and procedures relating to quality assurance and external influences. The NMC and the Quality Assurance Agency (QAA) standards must be satisfied before a programme of study can be validated and deemed fit for purpose. Other external factors that must be given due consideration are the European Directives. Two European Directives – 77/453/EEC and 89/595/EEC.

The Nursing and Midwifery Order 2001 provides the NMC with powers in relation to quality assurance and, as a result of this, the production of a framework that education providers (for example, universities) that offer, or intend to offer, NMC-approved programmes leading to registration or recording on the register have to adhere to. There are many provisions in place in the UK that ensure the quality of education programmes.

The NMC has to be satisfied that its standards for granting a licence to practise are being met as required and in association with the law. It does so by setting standards to maintain public confidence, as well as to protect the public. By appointing representatives, it can be satisfied that it is represented during the quality assurance process in relation to the approval, reapproval and annual monitoring activities associated with programmes of study.

Each programme of study for pre-registration midwifery must demonstrate explicitly and robustly that it has included the rules and standards of the NMC so that those who complete a recognised programme of study are eligible for registration. The *Standards for Pre-registration Midwifery Education* (NMC 2009) are examples of standards that must be achieved prior to registration.

Midwives' Rules and Standards

The Nursing and Midwifery Order 2001 demands that the NMC sets rules and standards for midwifery and local supervising authorities (LSAs) for the function of statutory supervision of midwives. *The Midwives' Rules and Standards* (NMC 2012) replace those produced in 2004. The current *Rules and Standards* came into force on 1 January 2013 (see Table I.2).

The NMC's Midwifery Committee undertook a full public consultation exercise when revising the *Midwives' Rules* (NMC 2012). As this second edition of this text goes to press the new rules are included in the content. The rules are set to have the most far-reaching changes since the establishment of the NMC. The changes ensure that the rules are streamlined, clear and relevant, and the NMC will continue to maintain a statutory framework for the practice and supervision of midwives that aims to protect the well-being of mothers and babies.

Major changes to the *Midwives' Rules and Standards* include the following:

- Some rules were simplified and clarified, and rules which are already covered by other standards or legislation have been removed.
- Local supervising authorities will be required to publish guidelines for the annual review of midwives' practice to ensure a standardised approach across the UK.

Table I.2   The 15 midwifery rules

Rule	Description
1.	Citation and commencement
2.	Interpretation
3.	Notification of intention to practise
4.	Notification by local supervising authority
5.	Scope of practice
6.	Records
7.	The local supervising authority midwifery officer
8.	Supervisor of midwives
9.	Local supervising authority's responsibilities for supervision of midwives
10.	Publication of local supervising authority procedures
11.	Visits and inspections
12.	Exercise by local supervising authority of its function
13.	Local supervising authority reports
14.	Suspension from practice by a local supervising authority
15.	Revocation

Source: NMC 2012.

- Guidance has been added to outline how best to deal with issues arising from a midwife's practice.

The rules will continue to state the requirements for practice and the accompanying standards offer extra guidance on what standard would reasonably be expected from a practising midwife.

Becoming a competent midwife

Those who wish to study to become a midwife, and then go on to register with the NMC and afterwards practise as a midwife must undertake a 3-year (or equivalent) programme of study. The number of hours to be studied by student midwives can vary. Each programme must comprise 2300 practice hours as a minimum and the programme must be at least 50% practice based (the total theory and practice combined must be a minimum of 4600 hours). The NMC, for example, allows for programmes to comprise 60% practice and 40% theory. This flexibility must be NMC approved.

The title 'registered midwife' is protected in law. This means it can only be used by a person who is registered with the NMC and her name must appear on the national register. There are three parts to the professional register:

1. Nurses
2. Midwives
3. Specialist community public health nurses

Table I.3   Summary of the standards for pre-registration midwifery education

Standard	Summary
Standard 1	Appointment of the LME
Standard 2	Development, delivery and management of midwifery education programmes
Standard 3	Signing the supporting declaration of good health and good character
Standard 4	General requirements relating to selection for and continued participation in approved programmes, and entry to the register
Standard 5	Interruptions to pre-registration midwifery education programmes
Standard 6	Admission with advanced standing
Standard 7	Transfer between approved education institutions
Standard 8	Stepping off and stepping on to pre-registration midwifery education programmes
Standard 9	Academic standard of programme
Standard 10	Length of programme
Standard 11	Student support
Standard 12	Balance between clinical practice and theory
Standard 13	Scope of practice experience
Standard 14	Supernumerary status during clinical placements
Standard 15	Assessment strategy
Standard 16	Ongoing record of achievement

Source: NMC 2009.
LME, lead midwife for education.

The student who wishes to undertake midwifery education must meet the NMC's requirements as well as any specific requirements the higher education institution may have. How these requirements are set is the prerogative of the individual educational institution; however, the NMC must agree to and permit these requirements and there must also be evidence of literacy and numeracy. Those wishing to practise in Wales must also be able to demonstrate proficiency in the Welsh language where this is required. On entry, during and on completion of their programme, all applicants must demonstrate that they have good health and good character sufficient for safe and effective practice. It is the responsibility of educational institutions to have procedures to ensure assessment of health and character. Any convictions, cautions or bind-overs related to criminal offences must be declared. There are several ways in which this can be achieved – for example, self-disclosure and/or criminal record checks conducted by accredited organisations.

   Completion of the programme and achievement of the standards mean that the student will graduate with both a professional qualification (registered midwife (RM)) and an academic qualification at degree level. The good character and good health declaration is made on an approved form provided by the NMC. This must be supported by the registered midwife whose name has been notified to the NMC, who is responsible for directing the educational programme at the university, or her designated registered midwife substitute. This midwife is known as the lead midwife for education (LME).

Once registered with the NMC, the midwife is accountable for her actions or omissions and is bound by the tenets enshrined in the *Code of Professional Conduct* (NMC 2008a). Legal requirements, such as participating in continuing professional development and maintaining a personal professional portfolio, must be addressed. This text provides you with insight into how to become a competent midwife.

There are 16 standards associated with pre-registration midwifery education. These range from the appointment of the LME to standards for the structure and nature of a pre-registration midwifery programme (see Table I.3). This text will address the standards for entry to the register for midwives. Currently, no other texts describe in the same detail the levels of education required to achieve the NMC standards for pre-registration midwifery education proficiency.

Case notes and activities

Most of the chapters provide the reader with case notes to consider and activities to carry out. They are included to encourage and motivate you, as well as for you to assess your learning and progress. It is also anticipated that they will enable you to link theoretical concepts with what is occurring in the clinical setting. There are a variety of review questions provided for you to attempt so you can test your understanding and learning. You are encouraged to delve deeper and seek other sources – both human and material – to help with your responses.

In most chapters you will find useful snippets of midwifery knowledge, gathered and honed as a result of many years of midwifery practice, called midwifery wisdom.

The aim of this text is to encourage, inspire and stimulate you, as well as instilling in you the desire, confidence and competence to become a registered midwife. What is required from you is an interest in women and their families through all stages of pregnancy. Becoming a member of the midwifery profession places many demands on you, the key demand being the desire to care with compassion and understanding for the women and families you will have the privilege to work with.

References

Department of Health (DH) (2004) *Standards for Better Health*. London: Department of Health.

Department of Health (DH) (2011) *Public Health England's Operating Model*. Available at: www.dh.gov.uk/prod_consum_dh/groups/dh_digitalassets/documents/digitalasset/dh_131892.pdf (accessed May 2013).

Department of Health (DH) (2012a) *Public Health, Adult Social Care and the NHS*. Available at: www.dh.gov.uk/health/category/policy-areas/public-health/ (accessed May 2013).

Department of Health (DH) (2012b) *Structure of Public Health England*. Available at: www.wp.dh.gov.uk/healthand-care/files/2012/07/PHE-structure.pdf (accessed October 2012).

Medforth J, Battersby S, Evans M et al. (2011) *Oxford Handbook of Midwifery*, 2nd edn. Oxford: Oxford University Press.

Nursing and Midwifery Council (NMC) (2008a) *The Code: standards, conduct, performance and ethics for nurses and midwives*. London: Nursing and Midwifery Council.

Nursing and Midwifery Council (NMC) (2008b) *Statistical Analysis of the Register: 1 April 2007 to 31 March 2008*. London: Nursing and Midwifery Council.

Nursing and Midwifery Council (NMC) (2009) *The Standards for Pre-registration Midwifery Education*. London: Nursing and Midwifery Council.

Nursing and Midwifery Council (NMC) (2012) *The Midwives' Rules and Standards*. Available at: www.nmc-uk.org/Documents/NMC-Publications/Midwives%20Rules%20and%20Standards%202012.pdf (accessed May 2013).

Page L, McCandlish R (eds) (2006) *The New Midwifery: sensitivity in practice*, 2nd edn. Edinburgh: Churchill Livingstone.

1

Effective Communication
Tandy Deane-Gray

Aim

This chapter aims to relate and understand how the development of communication from infancy can influence and inform our skills as adults in order to enhance your work-based experience to meet the needs of clients in your care.

Learning outcomes

By the end of this chapter you will be able to:

1. appreciate that development of interpersonal skills is co-dependent on key concepts from parent–infant interaction
2. analyse the needs of infants which parallel the needs of adults to enhance the care of mothers and babies
3. enhance communication skills to overcome common barriers to communication and building relationships in practice
4. develop strategies in practice that meet essential skills clusters for pre-registration midwifery education.

Introduction

This chapter will highlight the unique abilities of babies to communicate from birth, and how their optimal development relies on contingent responses, which are part of the parent–infant attachment process. These qualities in interpersonal skills are fundamental to building relationships, and the lessons from

The Student's Guide to Becoming a Midwife, Second Edition. Edited by Ian Peate and Cathy Hamilton.
© 2014 John Wiley & Sons, Ltd. Published 2014 by John Wiley & Sons, Ltd.

infancy influence our adult ability to communicate. Thus, by enhancing early relationships between parents and babies, midwives can reapply these principles in everyday communication. The common errors that inhibit midwifery communication will be outlined and skills of listening and empathy will be analysed.

Midwives are in a unique position to observe how humans learn to communicate. When time is taken to observe infants, it can be noticed that babies are 'pre-programmed' to interact with adults (Stern 1998). This is due to their preference for the sound, sight and movement of adults to other comparable stimuli and they are especially attracted to their mother. This interaction is probably a biological instinct, as humans depend on mother and other adults to care for them to ensure survival.

The work of MacFarlane (1977) clearly highlighted the ability of babies, and dispelled many myths around infants, such as the idea that babies cannot see. Not only can they see (and focus well at about 30 cm) but they like to look at contrast and contours found in the human face. They turn to sound, particularly the mother's voice; they will turn to the smell of their own mother's breast pad in preference to another. So they develop recognition of their mother very quickly through their senses, and communicate their needs through behaviours (RCM 1999). As adults, we also communicate through voice and behaviours.

The behaviours of a human baby are social and communicative; they mimic adults, most noticeably by facial changes. So if you smile, open your mouth wide or stick out your tongue, the baby will watch carefully and then copy (Murray & Andrews 2010), which is quite remarkable when you consider how they know that they even have a mouth. Indeed, this mimicking can be observed in the first hour after birth. This response to adults demonstrates babies turn taking in their non-verbal responses and vocalisations, provided the adult is sensitive to them (Brazelton et al. 1974).

Being sensitive to interaction in this dance of communication requires that the other is responding to that baby (or indeed an adult) and does not ignore or overwhelm with intrusive responses. The critical aspects of building relationships is engagement but its absence gives the message of indifference, which indicates lack of importance, and possibly feeling unwanted by the other or even a feeling of non-existence (McFarlane 2012). This indifference can readily be recognised when a mother is suffering with postnatal depression (RCM 2012). 'Insensitive mothers' may be overintrusive in communicating with their baby, and base their responses on their own needs and wishes, or general ideas about infants' needs. The same dynamic is easily replicated by midwives when they have an agenda which differs from the client's needs, for example during a booking history.

Midwifery wisdom

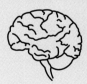 You cannot feel indifferent towards clients in your care. If you find yourself feeling this way, then think 'how can I love this person?'. And 'who can help me feel cared for?'.

Care taking and our sensitivity to infants are normally based on how we were cared for as infants. If we formed a good enough attachment to our parents and they were in tune with our needs, if they were 'baby centred', then we become secure adults (Steele 2002) and naturally become 'woman centred' in midwifery care. Sensitivity also comes from our attitudes and behaviours. Thus, every time babies are changed in a loving way or sympathetically responded to when lonely, tired, hungry or frightened, they take in the experience of being loved in the quality of care received. For a baby, physical discomfort is the same as mental discomfort and vice versa (Stern 1998).

The key aspects of early parenting and building a sensitive relationship are described clearly in the RCM's *Maternal Emotional Wellbeing and Infant Development* (RCM 2012). It is the parental attunement to the needs of the infant (which midwives have a role in fostering) that leads to loved individuals who do not become antisocial adults. Through our early relationships and communication from conception to 3 years of life, Sinclair (2007) suggests that we develop our emotional brain and our capacity for forming relationships. Fundamentally, human beings at any age respond and feel understood when an attuned warm, positive and sensitive other interacts with them. As a professional responding as a sensitive mother would, you too can communicate in this way with clients in your care, which can enhance how you build relationships and improve communication.

Sensitive responsiveness is one of the key constructs of attachment theory (Bowlby 1980, RCM 2012). The early infant–mother relationship has far-reaching consequences for the developing child's later social and mental health. It is the underpinning theory in national agendas and frameworks interventions (e.g. DfES 2006, DH 2004, 2009, RCM 2012, Sinclair 2007), recommended for effective practice in the promotion of family health and parenting skills, which are now a priority politically and professionally.

The concept of sensitive responsiveness includes the ability to accurately perceive and respond to infant signals, with contingent responses because the person is able to see things from the baby's point of view. These key concepts (in italics below), that mothers who are sensitively responsive seem to demonstrate, are fundamental to all our interactive relationships.

- An observer who *listens* and sees their strengths and helps them with their difficulties.
- Warm and responsive interactions with caretakers. The mother's task is to respond *empathically* – to mind read. The baby has no control or bad intent; they learn that they can self-regulate through maternal containment. They then learn to self-soothe, for example, by sucking.
- Structure and routine, flexible, and age appropriate, that give *boundaries*. Providing psychological and physical holding; holding also relieves anxiety the baby feels 'held together'.
- Maintains interest by providing things to look at and do through play and touch, but *in tune*, e.g. recognises that a yawn means 'leave me to sleep'.
- Vocalisation reinforced by response-dialogue. Hearing and *being heard* – responds to familiar parent voice, giving a sense of security. Babies need to hear talking in order to develop speech (DfES 2006, DH 2004, Paavola 2006, Ponsford 2006, RCM 2012).

Sensitive responsiveness can be facilitated, and when mothers' sensitivity and responsiveness are enhanced, this results in dramatic increases in secure attachments with fussy infants (Steele 2002).

Our infant–parent attachment patterns are largely acquired, rather than determined by genetic or biological make-up (Steele 2002), so with support we can all improve our ability to relate to others. For midwives, this means relating to clients and colleagues but also facilitating parent–infant relationships. This can be done by praising the sensitivity you observe in the parents, and helping them see and understand their baby. Using the questions in Box 1.1 with parents might enable them to realise that they can understand their baby. The RCM's *Maternal Emotional Wellbeing and Infant Development* (RCM 2012) also has many suggestions to develop your skills in this area.

Box 1.1   Helping parents to know their baby

- Ask them to tell you about their baby.
- What does he/she like?
- What does he/she like to hear, look at, feel and smell in particular?
- How does he/she get your attention?
- How does he/she tell you he/she is content?
- What does he/she like when going to sleep? What do you notice about sleep? Or crying?

The basic methods of improving relationships are those that mothers ideally use with their infants. This is primarily non-verbal so it is not surprising that over 65% of our communication is non-verbal (Pease & Pease 2006), observing bodily and facial cues, and being in touch with what the person might be feeling. This is truly listening and being with another person, and because we are listening and empathising, we provide a safe environment. Sometimes midwives demonstrate this by holding women physically, which seems to help contain the labouring women in their pain, and at birth by encouraging skin-to-skin contact, thus giving the baby safe framework after having been contained in the womb. But we also provide holding psychologically, by being with women and trying to understand what the experience is like for them; this is demonstrating empathy. When we reflect back what the client says and feels, by our actions, sometimes by touch or words, then the client feels held and heard.

Humans become socialised, and learn that they should not say this or that or that they should not upset another person or that they should not argue. We often learn to hide our feelings and not say clearly what we mean, which in turn leads to a lack of communication. Dissatisfaction in midwifery care and family life is often due to lack of communication. It is recognised that communication is one of the key elements for a compassionate workforce.

> *Communication is central to successful caring relationships and to effective team working. Listening is as important as what we say and do and essential for "no decision about me without me". Communication is the key to a good workplace with benefits for those in our care and staff alike.*
> (Commissioning Board Chief Nursing Officer and DH Chief Nursing Adviser 2012)

Our early skills in relation to communication become fixed into patterns, and the stamped foot of a temper tantrum in a toddler can still be apparent in the adult. Nichols (2009) summarises the four early stages of the development of self, described by Stern (1998), which helps inform us of how we adopt patterns of acting and reacting that become unconscious responses in adult life. This partly explains why, when we are in an anxious state, we cannot find the words to describe it because we have returned to a developmental stage which was preverbal.

Effective communication can be hard to achieve. Sometimes it seems that no matter how carefully we try to phrase the things we say, the listener either doesn't understand us or they misunderstand us. In verbal communication, we often add emphasis through body language or the intonation of our voice. We may adopt defensive or intimidating postures to reinforce the intended messages and, of course, we may raise or lower our voices. These techniques are used subconsciously, having developed through our socialisation from childhood.

Some common problems in communication

Bolton (1997) suggests that there are six common problems of human communication. These are mainly to do with understanding and listening:

1. Use of unclear meaning as words can have a different meaning.
2. Failing to understand because a message is 'coded'.
3. Failure to receive the message as another agenda clouded the issue.
4. Being distracted, and not hearing the message.
5. Not understanding because the message was distorted by perception or other filters.
6. Not handling emotions during a conversation.

The first problem is poor understanding, which is often due to an unclear message or unclear words, because words can have different meanings for different people. As Ralston (1998) points out, terms such as 'incompetent cervix' or 'inadequate pelvis' are open to very different interpretation for the non-professional listener. But even a straightforward term, such as 'mayonnaise' when it is not differentiated into 'home made' (with raw eggs, to be avoided in pregnancy) and the commercial product, can lead to women misunderstanding the information given (Stapleton et al. 2002).

When the message is 'coded', the real meaning is masked; for example, the client asks you to put her flowers in water but she could really be asking you to keep her company. It can also often be observed that clients present with one agenda but really have a different problem; for example, they present with backache but they are really concerned that the pregnancy is normal. Midwives also miss conversational codes for more information from clients (Kirkham et al. 2002a). 'I don't know' and 'What would you do?' are both tactics women use to elicit more information, which unfortunately are generally not very successful.

The way a sentence is spoken can also indicate an underlying message. Most speech has an obvious and a hidden meaning (Kagan et al. 1989). For example, 'What did you say?' has the obvious meaning of 'please say that again' but the hidden meaning could be 'you are so boring, I was not listening'. But if we said what was meant, we may hurt someone's feelings so we try to act in a professional way, thus creating barriers to communication, because we are not clear in our message. Indeed, as professionals there are times when we are acutely aware of appropriate interactions and needing to maintain a professional face. For example, it is inappropriate to look cheerful or go into a long explanation of care during life-threatening emergencies (Mapp and Hudson 2005).

Clients also do not hear or take in what we say because they are distracted, by the environment or physical symptoms. The disruption of a child needing attention during a conversation is an example of distraction, or a client may be in pain and can consequently miss the information given. However, what is tragic is that midwives often miss the non-verbal cues and often carry on with their own conversation, neglecting the woman. This could end up with the midwife thinking 'I know I have given the information', even if the client 'could not hear'. It is interesting to observe that mothers will say 'look at me when I am talking to you' when addressing their children, thus ensuring the non-verbal feedback that tells us we are being heard (Yearwood-Grazette 1978). Midwives need to ensure that they respond to non-verbal cues with their clients, particularly eye contact.

Midwifery wisdom

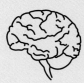 Reflect on your interactions with clients. If you are doing most of the talking, then you are not listening, and the client probably has switched off too!

Midwives and clients often filter information because of perception, emotions or simply hearing what they wish to hear. A midwife may say 'you can go home after the paediatrician has discharged the baby' but the client hears only the 'go home' part and so phones her partner to collect her immediately. Midwives filter information by avoiding discussion. They may emphasise physical tasks, giving the message that discussion, particularly on how women feel, is less important. Indeed, discussion if often avoided, for example by filling the time with asking for urine samples and ignoring possible anxiety, even when the last pregnancy was a stillbirth (Kirkham et al. 2002a). In essence, filters become blocks to communication.

Another block to communication is the phrase 'don't worry', used frequently to reassure (Stapleton et al. 2002). However, it has the effect of causing anxiety. The client is denied expression of how they really feel, and as such the words 'don't worry' should be avoided (Mapp and Hudson 2005) as this blocks the client from disclosing further concerns or feelings (Stapleton et al. 2002). A smile and touch are more helpful in allowing the client to feel human and reassured (Mapp and Hudson 2005).

It is not just what we say and do; it is also how we listen. It is rare for midwives to explore topics such as what foods a client eats, to invite discussion (Stapleton et al. 2002). This would enable the client to say what they know, but the midwife then needs to listen for the relevant missing information. This is harder work, so instead there is a tendency to tell clients what to do, things they often already know, such as the advantages and disadvantages of breastfeeding, but not what the client is seeking, for example how it feels to breastfeed (Stapleton et al. 2002).

Finally, people who have difficulty with emotional issues may deny their emotions or become blinded by them (Bolton 1997). Blinded because anxiety and fear or any high levels of emotional arousal lock the brain into one-dimensional thinking (Griffin & Tyrrell 2004). Our emotions are then affecting our physiology, hijacking the brain's capacity for rational thinking. This inhibits our ability to rationalise or entertain different perspectives, because these traumatic and distressing experiences, big and small, cause imbalance in the nervous system, thus creating a block or incomplete information processing. This is why it is difficult to take in medical or other information or advice when upset, frightened, angry or in pain. This dysfunctional information is then stored in its unprocessed state both in the mind (neural networks) and in the body (cellular memory) (Pert 1999). Certainly, during emergencies poor communication can compound the stress. Careful sensitive communication that is congruent, i.e. the non-verbal matches the verbal communication, is what is required (Mapp and Hudson 2005).

Non-emergency situations can also involve high emotional states. Emotional arousal, for example, as a consequence of a power struggle, will evoke a defensive response. The thinking part of the brain becomes inhibited in emotional arousal, so it follows that learning and taking in information cannot be effective when the client feels conflict or stress (Griffin & Tyrrell 2004). When a midwife says 'I want to tell you about breastfeeding', the emotional arousal in the client may come from the unsaid 'who are you to tell me how to bring up my family?'. It would be more useful to first reduce the emotional arousal, and reframe or present the information another way: 'It's good you have decided on your method of feeding and I would like to hear more about how you are going to feed your baby'. Nichols (2009) points out that 'It isn't exuberance or any other emotion that conveys loving appreciation; it's being noticed, understood and taken seriously'.

However, midwives may perceive that the use of open questions in this way will take up too much time. When information becomes blocked, then misunderstanding is increased which leads to spending more time correcting the problem at a later date. Midwives also limit their emotional effort, and they may stereotype in order to increase control over work situations (Kirkham et al. 2002b), although if they were able to increase their sensitive responsiveness, clients would be able to find out the information they need, understand and feel understood.

Midwives need to give emotional care to their clients, particularly those in labour, and this is draining for them. Many midwives realise they do not have time for their own emotional feelings so they pull down the shutters to look calm. It is this that can give the impression of 'aloofness', whereas others are perceived as naturally friendly (John & Parsons 2005). As John and Parsons (2005) suggest, support mechanisms need to be developed and implemented in order to reduce stress in practice. According to Nichols (2009): 'If you see a parent with blunted emotions ignoring a bright-eyed baby, you're witnessing the beginning of a long, sad process by which unresponsive parents wither the enthusiasm of their children like unwatered flowers'.

Midwifery wisdom

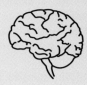 Blunted emotions can be seen in overstressed midwives. These midwives need support, and a discussion with their supervisor could be helpful here. Some units have staff counsellors in highly stressful areas.

Thus far, the problems and the way midwives communicate have been discussed. To be more effective in communication, our sensitive responsiveness, as defined earlier, needs to be developed. This chapter can only scratch the surface in this respect as communication skills need to be developed experientially as our patterns of communicating are often ingrained from childhood. Having said that, there are things individuals can practise every day which will improve professional practice, particularly listening and empathy. Some pointers will be outlined here but learning these skills needs to take place through experience in order for long-term change in practice to occur.

Listening

Listening skills are essential for a midwife; listening is an active process requiring the full attention of an individual as one needs to listen and fully hear what is actually being communicated, not just what is said. Listening involves the mind, senses and emotions, to pick up what is not said. This is bound up with the development of self-awareness, the awareness of when we fail to listen and attend, which, if addressed, is likely to have a positive effect on future communication. Good communication minimises misunderstanding, poor communication can lead to complaints (Sidgewick 2006).

Part of the process of communication is receiving messages. Obviously, verbal messages are heard but the receiver does need to be actively listening. Passive listening includes encouraging phrases such as 'umm', 'uh huh' as well as non-verbal nodding of the head and eye contact (Balzer-Riley 2012). Passive listening implies understanding but active listening removes the guesswork as it ensures messages are received properly (Balzer-Riley 2012).

Listening skills will differ depending on what we are doing. On some occasions, passive attentive listening will be sufficient. However, if we require more information from clients, or perhaps they are giving an emotional account, then a more active approach is helpful (Kagan et al. 1989). Attending is listening to what is really being said by the speaker, which may also require the skill of appropriate questioning (questioning skills are addressed later). If we focus on our questions then we go back and forth between what is being said and our reply, so we may not really hear what is being said (Rowan 1998). It cannot be emphasised enough that listening is one of the most important communication skills.

Guidelines for listening

- Listen, without interruption as far as possible, and minimise questions.
- Remember what is being said, as if you might be tested on it. Listen to what is not being said, particularly feelings.
- Observe the client's body language as well as your own; are there any clues being given?
- Have an empathic stance; what would it be like if you were in the client's situation?

- Try not to immediately rush in with explanations and answers. The client generally has the answer.
- Look like you have time, or make it clear how much time you have and give your full attention. (Adapted from Jacobs 2000).

Unfortunately, because much of midwifery requires information from the client, we focus on questions and not listening. Questions are so much part of conversation that they seem to have almost replaced the ability to listen or respond in any other way, because we are forming the next question. In order to enable clients to talk and midwives to listen and talk less, it is generally useful to begin with open questions. Open questions usually begin with words such as; would, could, tell me, seem to be, I think, I feel or I wonder. Questions that begin; how, what, where, and particularly *why*, can leave the client feeling they are at the Spanish Inquisition, whereas an open question allows them to explain their experience.

Activity 1.1

One of our jobs is to ask questions which are of a personal nature. Some of us find these easier to ask than others. However, you still need to ask them. So think about asking the following; could they be rephrased into more open questions?

- When was the first day of your last menstrual period?
- Have you had your bowels open?
- When did you last have sex?
- Can I see your sanitary towel?
- How are your breasts?

The following are some of the activities for daily living which may be used on admission forms. How would you phrase the questioning order to gain the information you need? How could you broach the question on issues such as:

- expressing sexuality?
- death?
- safer sex?
- termination of pregnancy?
- use of alcohol?
- domestic violence?
- mental health?

When trying to establish legal responsibility for a child, how will you ask this when the child has a different surname from the mother and the 'next of kin' who is the 'father'?

Further reading: England C, Morgan R (2012) *Communication Skills for Midwives: challenges in everyday practice*. Buckingham: Open University Press.

Listening to what is not being said

In ordinary listening, we are often interested in the content or subject. We generally try to relate this to our own experience (this is sympathy), thinking of interesting replies to carry the conversation on. In contrast, in a therapeutic relationship we are listening to the content but also the message under

16

the message. This may be about the client's emotions and if our own thoughts, experiences and emotions arise, we try to put them aside because it is the client's experience that is the focus (Rowan 1998).

Jacobs (2000) suggests we listen to the 'bass line' in conversations, as if it were a piece of music. Under a melody there is a bass line. This invites us to listen to what is not being openly said but possibly being felt by the client.

Case study 1.1

Tom's Story

'My partner Amy and I arrived early this morning to get things started. Our baby was due last week. It's been awful having people phone constantly asking what is happening. So we really want this induction thing. Amy is scared and disappointed as she wanted a 'natural birth', but I think it's for the best and it's great to know we will have a baby today.

Well, we were kept waiting for an hour before we were seen, then the midwife checked us in, examined Amy, while I had a coffee. But I returned to be told the labour ward is busy and the birth could not be started!

We were sent for breakfast, then lunch. I feel confused and worried as Amy is getting more anxious and nothing is being done. They said the induction was because it's dangerous to go overdue. If that is so then why are we not a priority? The staff all seem rushed and say they will be with us later.'

Tom and his frustrations will be examined below and the interactions with the midwife analysed.

Activity 1.2

A young father-to-be, Tom, is talking about his discontent with his partner's maternity care. Whether or not he is justified in thinking this, what can Tom's bass line tell you? Imagine how you might feel in his position.

What is the bass line saying? He is young, so possibly has less experience of the world, and the transition to parenthood is not without stress, partly due to the unknown. So possibly he is unsure of himself, so any threat might elicit a defensive/attacking response from him. He may be feeling helpless and powerless as he feels he can do little for his new family. He may be concerned for his partner or baby. These are all possibilities, so what are the feelings he could be expressing – anxiety, anger, frustration?

Activity 1.3

A young father-to-be, Tom, is talking about his discontent with his partner's maternity care.

Tom: 'Excuse me, you said you would give my wife some of those tablets to get her started in labour, we have been waiting for hours.'

Think how you would answer. The labour ward has been busy and you were told not to induce her. You also have been frantically trying to discharge clients in order to give beds to the women waiting to clear the delivery ward. The paediatrician has not discharged the babies and the consultant wants to do a round with you.

Midwife: 'I am sorry, we are busy, and have not had time.'
Tom: 'You seem to be making time for everyone else who has babies already.'
Midwife: 'Well, the delivery ward does not have space for you anyway.'
Tom: 'Then why were we dragged in here at 7 am?'
Midwife: 'Well, it's one of those things – we do not know what the workload will be like.'

Now think again about how you could answer differently.

In Activity 1.3, the midwife is polite but defensive, and it sounds like excuses to Tom. The midwife is stressed and is having trouble coping with the workload; her factual response is not demonstrating any understanding or concern for Tom and his wife. Concern and understanding are demonstrated by letting Tom know you have heard him. Giving full attention is difficult in this case; I am sure you have seen this type of conversation occurring while the midwife is on the phone and writing up some notes. Pushing the silent button on the phone, putting the pen down and giving good eye contact may have been the midwife's first reaction, and would go a long way to contributing to Tom's perception that the midwife was listening. Furthermore, reflecting back or summarising what was said might also ensure the midwife understands and Tom would feel heard.

   Here are some possible alternative replies that are more likely to help Tom feel heard and understood.

Tom: 'Excuse me, you said you would give my wife some of those tablets to get her started in labour, we have been waiting for hours.'
Midwife: 'Yes I did, you have been waiting a long time' (reflecting back what he said so he knows you heard him).
Midwife: 'Yes I did, I am sorry you have been waiting so long, it must be very frustrating for you' (empathy).
Midwife: 'You have been waiting a long time, and it's disappointing when you expected the induction to have begun by now' (empathy).

Not only are some of Tom's words being used to help him feel heard, but also the midwife has listened to the 'bass line' and tentatively is reflecting possible feelings. The midwife may be stressed and she might have started the conversation by using factual replies as that is an old habit, but she could recover or repair the communication by demonstrating empathy.

Activity 1.4

Tom: 'Excuse me, you said you would give my wife some of those tablets to get her started in labour, we have been waiting for hours'.
Midwife: 'I am sorry, we are busy, and have not had time.'
Tom: 'You seem to be making time for everyone else who has babies already.'
Midwife: 'You seem concerned that there is no time for you and your wife. You feel anxious because it seems like the induction is never going to happen.'

Empathy

Jacobs (2000) suggests that if you listen to yourself and think how you might feel in a given situation, this might be the first step towards empathy. Empathy involves the capacity to recognise the bodily feelings of another and is related to our imitative capacities. We associate the bodily movements and facial expressions we see in another with the feelings and corresponding movements or expressions in ourselves (Balzer-Riley 2012).

Mothers help babies to regulate their emotions in this way. You may have observed the distressed baby who is cuddled gently by a mother whose facial expression is as pained as that of her infant, her tone of voice and touch mirroring the infant's state, 'Oh dear! There there', gradually soothing into a calmer state with soft voice and holding: 'I know, mummy is here, you can cope' (Gerhardt 2004). Humans also seem to make the same immediate connection between the tone of voice and other vocal expressions and inner emotion. Thus, empathy is a synonym for communicated understanding. It is mentally putting yourself into the shoes of another, so that you can understand how they are feeling without judgement or evaluation, just acceptance (Figure 1.1).

A midwife needs to be empathic and has to understand the woman and provide the care and support needed while watching the process of labour and any deviations from it that might cause concern (Ralston 1998). The midwife who gets this right is truly 'with woman'; by being empathic, she is unlikely to have a different perception from the parents. Midwives also convey compassion, understanding and empathy through touch. Not being touched is related to emotional deprivation; midwives have been observed to touch the fetal heart monitor and not the woman in labour, thus distancing themselves from the intimacy of the relationship (Yearwood-Grazette 1978). Sensitive touch can help relax a person in pain but the midwife also needs to recognise when this becomes intrusive (Ralston 1998), like a mother who is sensitive and does not ignore or overstimulate her baby (RCM 1999).

To be empathic first requires you to listen and identify the emotion. Like the mother–infant relationship, we tune in non-verbally, noticing behaviours. Sometimes we pick up the feeling in our own body, e.g. the stomach is knotted. If these factors are taken into account along with what we imagine it must be like, then we can identify the emotion; however, we also need to communicate this to our client.

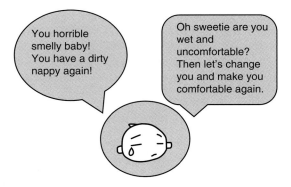

Figure 1.1   Example of empathy.

Midwifery wisdom

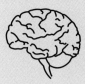 If you find yourself feeling, for example, anxious, maybe because you have a knot in your stomach, consider whether this is your anxiety or the client's? Humans can transfer their feelings and they are picked up by others. If the feeling does not seem to be yours, then say something like 'I notice I am feeling anxious, and I wonder if that is how you are feeling'.

Jacobs (2000) suggests we choose our words carefully when describing other people's emotions; clients may feel you do not understand them if you suggest that they are furious when they are only feeling cross. However, if you truly are sincere and congruent (your words match your own behaviours and emotions), then you will find that people will simply correct you when they respond. Nevertheless, it is important to recognise accurately the shades of emotion which might be present in a particular interaction.

Empathy can be expressed as a phrase, a word or even sensitive touch but first the emotion needs to be identified (Tschudin 1989). For example, a friend tells you she is happy to be pregnant. You already have the information that she is pleased to be pregnant so one emotion you could respond with empathically is 'Happy?' A phrase that might reflect a similar feeling is, 'You look like you're on cloud nine'. Often we congratulate people on their achievements so you could say, 'You must feel delighted with your achievement'. Or you can simply state 'You feel happy because you are pregnant'. Some of these possible responses may not feel right for you but remember, it is how you say them with congruence that shows you are trying to understand. When you respond empathically, the client is aware that you have heard and are trying to understand.

Developing empathic understanding is about staying with the client's experience and not being judgemental or giving advice. One difficulty is that it is easy to be sympathetic and the midwife may identify with her own feelings which arise from the client's message. This transfers the focus from the client to the professional and consequently the listening becomes conversational rather than therapeutic. Here are some classic unhelpful examples which illustrate this:

- 'You think that's bad!'
- 'I'll do that for you.'
- 'Don't worry.'
- 'I remember when I had just the same.'

All of these put the midwife's experience onto the client. Being sympathetic brings out the meaning for the midwife rather than the woman. The difficulty can be putting empathy into practice (Figure 1.2). Tschudin (1989) suggests a formula for an empathic approach. First, it is necessary to identify the emotion in the statement made by the client. Then respond to the words spoken and acknowledge them, by reflecting back that feeling with a rationale for the feeling if possible. For example, 'I don't know what to do' (a mother with twins); the feeling or emotion is confusion or possibly anxiety. The rationale for this feeling is uncertainty about the future. An empathic reply might be 'You feel confused, because you are not sure what to do'. In summary, Tschudin's (1989) 'formula' for empathy is: 'you feel ...because...'.

Sympathy = I know how you
feel, I had just the same. (Let
me cry with you)

Empathy = I understand you feel
awful, let me help you.

Figure 1.2   Empathy and sympathy.

Activity 1.5

Read the examples below and write down your usual response.

- 'Is my blood pressure OK?' (A woman at 32 weeks of pregnancy.)
- 'I'm dying.' (A woman in labour.)
- 'I can't cope.' (A new mother on the postnatal ward.)

Now try to identify what the client is really saying.

As you formulated yours answers, did you notice that the statements used are commonly made by clients to midwives? The client may simply be enquiring about her blood pressure, of course. However, if there is an underlying emotion you will probably hear it in the intonation of the voice. The client may be anxious about her blood pressure, or the growth of her baby. 'I'm dying', sometimes heard in childbirth, is probably an expression of primitive fear. 'I can't cope' is a direct request for help but there may be an underlying feeling of desperation. Appropriate empathic responses might be:

- 'You feel anxious about your blood pressure, because you are worried about your baby?'
- 'You feel terrified because the pain is so bad?'
- 'You feel desperate because of the responsibility?'

You now have a tool for practising empathy when you interact with clients, colleagues and families. The key is to practise, even if you begin by listening to conversations on the bus, in the canteen or on television, and rephrasing the responses in an empathic way in your own mind. For those of us who do not find it natural to be empathic, there is a steep learning curve. Learning to be more empathic can also be scary for the midwife, because their experiences of expressing emotions were not received sensitively, so the fear of hurting another's feelings can overwhelm them. Sadly, when they do not know what to say, they either say nothing or deny the client's emotions in their response. There is nothing wrong with saying 'I don't know what to say'. The fear of getting it wrong is why this needs to be practised experientially. Additionally, the midwife needs to move the conversation to a close sensitively and refer on if needed.

Activity 1.6

Analyse this conversation using the skills discussed so far, i.e. listening, questioning and empathy. Then look at what each student might be feeling at the end of the conversation and how you might continue the conversation.

Two students have just received their results.
Student A: 'What did you get?'
Student B (sadly): 'It's a pass.'
Student A: 'What percentage did you get?'
Student B: '60%.'
Student A: 'Oh, 60%?'
Student B (sounding devastated): 'Yeah.'
Student A: 'Yeah.'

The following activities and comments invite you to exercise the skills described thus far, and illustrate how responses can encourage a conversation through sensitive listening and an empathic stance. They also demonstrate how the responses might draw the conversation to a close.

Note the style of the questions, which are not open. Student A uses an echo statement, repeating Student B's statements, which can be quite useful when you are not sure what to say. I expect Student A also wants to burst out with the news of a '90%' grade, but is sensitive enough not to. Student A did not say she heard the sadness and has not been empathic.

Student A may also be feeling bad that she cannot make it better for student B, but also fears she has opened a can of worms for student B. She could try and make it better, by saying 'that's not a bad grade'. But this denies Student B's emotion and is unhelpful and is not listening. It is like putting a bandage over the 'wound' to cover up the problem. Examine the next part of the conversation in Activity 1.7.

Activity 1.7

Analyse this conversation using the skills discussed so far, i.e. listening, questioning and empathy.

Student A: 'You sound disappointed.'
Student B: 'Yeah, well, I worked really hard on that assignment.'
Student A: 'It's disappointing to only get a 60% grade when you worked so hard?'
Student B (angrily): 'It's just so unfair!'
Student A: 'You feel angry because others do not seem to work so hard but get a better grade?'

Here we observe active listening, open question and empathic responses. Student B has had her emotion heard and is beginning to feel understood. Notice how the empathic response helps clarify the feeling for student B. She can now think more clearly as she can let some of the emotion go. Now analyse the next part of the conversation.

Activity 1.8

Again analyse this conversation using the skills discussed so far, i.e. listening, questioning and empathy. How do you imagine you might feel if you were student A?

Student B: 'Oh, maybe they do work hard, it's just that I am a single parent too, so I have to find time, whereas others don't have responsibility.'
(Student A wants to bring this to a close, so moves the interaction on.)
Student A: 'You do sound stressed. I wonder if you could get more help from someone.'
Student B: 'Um, well, I cannot afford any more childcare.'
Student A: 'That is difficult; I guess you must have to be very organised. Could you ask for more academic help?'
Student B: 'Well, I always seem to just scrape through. But I am concerned I will never finish this course.'
Student A: 'Have you talked to the tutor?'

Student A may be feeling anxious initially that she has opened herself up to being the answer to the problem. Remember, it is not your problem to solve; the other person holds the key. Student A follows with a sensitive answer that demonstrates all the conversation has been heard, and some praise for the difficult place Student B holds. We can imagine that Student B, now having been heard, is likely to ask Student A about her result.

Moving toward more effect communication would improve midwifery care (Kirkham 1993). Observing mothers and babies communicating and facilitating sensitive care are likely to have an impact not only on midwifery but also on society, as responding and communicating effectively with 'small babies make a big difference' (Sinclair 2007), affecting their sociability and thus society as a whole.

It is interesting to note that common errors in general communication are also those found in midwifery. As highlighted in inquiries such as those on Daksha Emerson (Joyce et al. 2003) and Victoria Climbié (Laming 2003), the consequences of poor communication can have devastating effects. The NMC (2009) includes detailed competencies for communication in the skills clusters. These standards of proficiency, that enable the effective delivery of care and support for women in the preconception, antenatal, intrapartum and postnatal periods, embrace the principles outlined in this chapter. Improving listening and empathic skills and the use of open questions in midwifery care as discussed in this chapter would go some way to embracing these standards in practice. It follows that midwives would also help parents to communicate effectively with their infants as they would be modelling these skills in their care.

Conclusion

Effective communication is the cornerstone of good practice and paramount in the provision of good maternity care. This is achieved by intimate and sensitive interaction between midwives and their clients.

This chapter has invited readers to embrace the principles of sensitive responsiveness to enhance their communication skills, and facilitate parent–infant relationships. Midwives need to analyse their own communication and develop more active listening to minimise misunderstanding. Additionally, by developing a more empathic stance, they will be more able to address emotional issues and enhance their care of clients.

Quiz

1. Which is the most empathic response?

   (Sigh) 'I am so tired with this pregnancy.' (35 weeks gestation with a 2 year old)
   a. 'Yes I found my second pregnancy difficult too.'
   b. 'It must be difficult for you coping with pregnancy, work and a little one.'
   c. 'It's normal to feel tired at this stage of pregnancy.'
   d. 'You will feel better soon.'
   e. 'I am sorry to hear that.'

2. Which are the responses of a good listener?

   When I believe I know what someone means but I'm not really sure ...
   a. I let my mind wander until it's my turn to talk.
   b. I give little verbal or non-verbal feedback to the other person.
   c. I ask for clarification or repeat what I believe they have said before I speak.
   d. If I consider the subject boring, I stop paying attention.
   e. I summarise what I believe I heard.

3. Which is the response of an active listener?

   When someone is telling me a story or making a point about something, as soon as I realise what he is thinking, I respond as follows:
   a. 'That's nothing, let me tell you what happened to me.'
   b. I try to give him appropriate advice.
   c. I wait and reflect back his point.
   d. I tell him he is rambling and ask him to get to the point.
   e. If I disagree with the point, I stop listening and begin formulating in my head what I want to say to refute what he has said.

4. Which statements are more likely to leave a client even more angry because she has not been heard?

   A term pregnancy has just been diagnosed as a breech, and the client has been told she must have a caesarean. She says angrily 'I don't want a caesarean!'.
   a. 'I know how you feel.'
   b. 'Try to cheer up. These things happen.'
   c. 'Try to pull yourself together.'
   d. 'You are angry because as your pregnancy is a breech, a caesarean is advised.'
   e. 'I expect you are very disappointed because you wanted a natural birth.'
   f. 'It looks like you'll just have to tough it out.'
   g. 'I'm sorry you feel that way.'

5. A client has been diagnosed with a Down's fetus. Still in shock, the parents look to you for reassurance. Which responses are most helpful?
   a. 'Perhaps this is God's will.'
   b. 'This could have happened to anyone.'
   c. 'It's not your fault, you have looked after yourself and done all the right things.'
   d. 'You will just have to decide if you can cope with a Down's child.'
   e. 'You're a tough person – I'm sure you've been through worse.'

    f. 'This must be a difficult time, and I will be working to help you through this.'

    g. 'I am saddened to hear of your situation, and want to express my condolences.'

    h. 'Remember when we talked about some of the risks that can't be anticipated or prevented? Well, this is one of those instances. But there are several actions that we're going to take to help you, and we'll answer your questions so that you and your family are aware of what we're doing.'

6. On a postnatal visit to a woman who had a caesarean birth, she says she is still traumatised about her birth experience. Which of the following will allow the client to say as much as she needs to share about this experience?

    a. 'Just be happy you have a healthy baby.'

    b. 'Traumatised?'

    c. 'Be grateful; a hundred years ago you both would have died.'

    d. 'You feel traumatised because it was a caesarean birth?'

    e. 'Could you say more about the experience for you?'

References

Balzer-Riley J (2012) *Communications in Nursing*, 7th edn. St Louis, MO: Elsevier Mosby.

Bolton R (1997) *People Skills: how to assert yourself, listen to others and resolve conflicts*. New York: Touchstone.

Bowlby J (1980) *Attachment and Loss. Vol. II: Separation*. London: Random House.

Brazelton TB, Kolski B, Main M (1974) The origins of reciprocity: the early mother–infant interaction. In: Lewis M, Rosenblum L (eds) *The Effect of the Infant on Its Caregiver*. London: John Wiley & Sons.

Commissioning Board Chief Nursing Officer and DH Chief Nursing Adviser (2012) *Compassion in Practice. Nursing, midwifery and care staff, our vision and strategy*. London: Department of Health. Available at: www.dh.gov.uk/ health/2012/12/nursing-vision/ (accessed December 2012).

Department for Education and Skills (DfES) (2006) *Every Child Matters. Change for children, parenting support, guidance for local authorities in England*. London: Department for Education and Skills.

Department of Health (DH) (2004) *The National Service Framework for Children, Young People and Maternity Services*. London: Department of Health.

Department of Health (DH) (2009) *Healthy Child Programme: pregnancy and the first five years of life*. London: Department of Health.

Gerhardt S (2004) *Why Love Matters*. London: Routledge.

Griffin J, Tyrrell I (2004) *Human Givens*. East Sussex, Human Givens Publishing.

Jacobs M (2000) *Swift to Hear. Facilitation skills in listening and responding*. London: SPCK.

John V, Parsons E (2005) Shadow work in midwifery: unseen and unrecognised emotional labour. *British Journal of Midwifery* **14**(5): 266–271.

Joyce L, Hale R, Jones A, Moodley P (2003) *Report of an Independent Inquiry into the Care and Treatment of Daksha Emerson MBBS, MRCPsych, MSc and her Daughter Freya*. London: North East London Strategic Health Authority.

Kagan C, Evans J, Kay B (1989) *A Manual of Interpersonal Skills for Nurses. An experiential approach*. London: Harper and Row.

Kirkham M (1993) Communication in midwifery. In: Roche S, Alexander J (eds) *Midwifery Practice: a research based approach*. London: Macmillan.

Kirkham M, Stapleton H, Thomas G, Curtis P (2002a) Checking not listening: how midwives cope. *British Journal of Midwifery* **10**(7): 447–450.

Kirkham M, Stapleton H, Thomas G, Curtis P (2002b) Stereotyping as a professional defence mechanism. *British Journal of Midwifery* **10**(9): 549–552.

Laming WH (2003) *The Victoria Climbié Inquiry. Report of an Inquiry by Lord Laming*. London: Stationery Office.

Mapp T, Hudson K (2005) Feelings and fears during obstetric emergencies – 1. *British Journal of Midwifery* **13**(1): 30–35.

MacFarlane A (1977) Mother–infant interaction. *Developmental Medicine and Child Neurology* **19**(1): 1–2.

McFarlane K (2012) Love: taking a stance. *Psychotherapist* **52**, 24–25.

Murray L, Andrews L (2010) *The Social Baby*. Surrey. CP Publishing.

Nichols P (2009) *The Lost Art of Listening*. New York: Guilford Press.

Nursing and Midwifery Council (NMC) (2009) *Standards for Pre-Registration Midwifery Education*. London: Nursing and Midwifery Council.

Paavola L (2006) Maternal sensitive responsiveness characteristics and relations to child early communicative and linguistic development. PhD dissertation. Oulu, Finland: Oulu University Press.

Pease A, Pease B (2006) *The Definitive Book of Body Language: how to read others' attitudes by their gestures*. London: Orion.

Pert C (1999) *Molecules of Emotion*. London: Pocket Books.

Ponsford C (2006) The emotional needs of the under 3s and good practice in their care. What About The Children? Annual Conference. Kent: WATch.

Ralston R (1998) Communication: create barriers or develop therapeutic relationships. *British Journal of Midwifery* **6**(1), 8–11.

Rowan J (1998) *The Reality Game: a guide to humanistic counselling and therapy*. London: Routledge.

Royal College of Midwives (RCM) (1999) *Transition to Parenthood*. London: Royal College of Midwives.

Royal College of Midwives (RCM) (2012) *Maternal Emotional Wellbeing and Infant Development: a good practice guide*. London: Royal College of Midwives Trust.

Sidgewick C (2006) Everybody's business: managing midwifery complaints. *British Journal of Midwifery* **14**(2): 70–71.

Sinclair A (2007) *0-5: How Small Children Make a Big Difference*. London: Work Foundation.

Stapleton H, Kirkham M, Thomas G, Curtis P (2002) Language use in antenatal consultations. *British Journal of Midwifery* **10**(5): 273–277.

Steele H (2002) Attachment. *Psychologist* **15**(10): 518–523.

Stern D (1998) *The Interpersonal World of the Infant*. London: Karnac Books.

Tschudin V (1989) *Beginning with Empathy*. London: Elsevier Health Science.

Yearwood-Grazette H (1978) An anatomy of communication. *Nursing Times* **October** 12: 1672–1679.

2

Effective Documentation
Carole Yearley and Celia Wildeman

Aim

The aim of this chapter is to explore and apply the legislative framework of the NMC (NMC 2008, 2009a, 2012a) that relates to the role and responsibilities of the student midwife and midwife in the context of effective documentation and professional practice.

Learning outcomes

It is expected that at the end of this chapter you will be able to:

1. describe the importance of record keeping standards in the context of your professional and legislative framework
2. analyse the implications and consequences of poor or absent record keeping
3. identify strategies to improve standards of record keeping
4. using practical exercises, self-analysis and discussion, enhance your knowledge and skills to enable you to undertake self and peer audit of record keeping
5. demonstrate the necessary knowledge and skills to evaluate your own and others' standard of record keeping
6. identify and address areas for development to enhance the quality of your record keeping

Introduction

This chapter discusses and analyses the legal and professional framework that governs midwifery practice and the accountability of the midwife in relation to the documentation of her records. Activities and practical exercises are included throughout to help you to integrate the theory of the topic area with

The Student's Guide to Becoming a Midwife, Second Edition. Edited by Ian Peate and Cathy Hamilton.
© 2014 John Wiley & Sons, Ltd. Published 2014 by John Wiley & Sons, Ltd.

practice and offer some practical advice and guidance for how you can improve your personal standard of record keeping.

The standards and guidance produced by our regulatory body, the Nursing and Midwifery Council (NMC), concerning the role and responsibilities of the midwife in the context of effective documentation and professional practice (NMC 2008, 2009a, 2012a) will be explored, analysed and applied to practice. It is anticipated that having read this chapter, the reader will be able to describe the various forms of record keeping used in contemporary practice and discuss the rationale for maintaining comprehensive, contemporaneous records in relation to professional accountability. A self and peer audit tool for monitoring the standard of records will be introduced to enable the reader to apply the knowledge and skills in practice, to evaluate and enhance the development of their own record keeping competencies.

The importance of effective documentation

The Nursing and Midwifery Council came into being on 1 April 2002. It succeeded the former professional body, the United Kingdom Central Council for Nursing, Midwifery and Health Visiting (UKCC). With the establishment of the NMC, the new rules for midwives came into effect on 1 January 2013 and the NMC will continue to state the requirements for practice and provide guidance on what standard would reasonably be expected from a midwife's practice.

Rule 6 relates specifically to records (NMC 2012a, p16). The NMC states that:

> Good record keeping is an integral part of nursing and midwifery practice, and is essential to the provision of safe and effective care. It is not an optional extra to be fitted in if circumstances allow.
>
> (NMC 2009a, p3)

The *Midwives' Rules and Standards* make it clear that midwives are accountable for the quality and retention of their documentation (NMC 2012a). 'All records relating to the care of the woman or baby must be kept securely for 25 years' (p18). This ruling applies wherever the midwife carries out her duty, whether in a private, agency, independent or National Health Service (NHS) context.

Effective documentation is part of the midwife's duty of care. Within this, the midwife is expected to use professional judgement to make decisions that will enhance client care through her documentation. The NMC states in the *Guidelines for Records and Record Keeping* that it 'is not a rule book that will provide the answers to every question or issue that could ever arise' (NMC 2005, p5). However, the intention is that it should be used for guidance together with the *Midwives' Rules and Standards* to strive for excellence in record keeping.

The importance of accurate and contemporaneous record keeping cannot be overstated. Indeed, according to Gallagher and Hodge (2012, p18), 'a way of protecting yourself from allegations of incompetence, unprofessional practice or other breach of codes, is records, records and yet more records'.

Good record keeping equates with good care

'Good record keeping helps to protect the welfare of patients and clients' (NMC 2005, p6). Its value has been consistently identified and highlighted in various professional guidelines (NMC 2005, 2006, 2011c, DH 2006).

In summary, good record keeping promotes:

- high standards of clinical care
- continuity of care
- better communication and dissemination of information between members of the interprofessional healthcare team

- an accurate account of treatment, care planning and delivery
- the ability to detect problems, such as changes in the patient's or client's condition, at an early stage
- the professional duty to keep adequate and accurate records
- the ability of the midwife practitioner to meet legal requirements.

The NMC asserts that the quality of your record keeping is also a reflection of the standard of your professional practice (NMC 2009a).

Activity 2.1

Review a client's record that you have written in during the previous 6 months and assess the quality of the content and style of your documentation. Now go to the feedback box below for guidance and suggestions.

Feedback

Your record keeping would be considered to be of a good standard if it includes the following features:

- It is factual, consistent and accurate.
- It is written as soon as possible after the event or an explanation given when written retrospectively, for example why the delay in writing the records became necessary.
- It is clear, concise and legible, written in ink (must be able to be photocopied if necessary) (Dimond 2005).
- It is signed and your name printed (according to the format for the trust or other employer).
- It should be dated and the time included using a 24-hour clock.
- Jargon, abbreviations, irrelevant speculation and offensive subjective statements should not be included.
- Any dialogue with the patient/client should be included in a form that would provide evidence of client participation in their care.
- Any alterations or additions are dated, timed and signed in such a way that the original entry can still be clearly read.
- There is evidence that the client collaborated with the practitioner in the construction of the records; for example, statements from the client are included in language that supports the client's involvement.
- The tone and quality of the communication are such that the client's understanding is ensured.

How did your record keeping compare with the contents of the feedback section? Reflect on this exercise and identify areas for further development.

Record keeping: the extent of the current challenges

The NMC is the statutory body which regulates the practice of nurses, midwives and specialist community public health nurses. The roles and functions of the NMC and how these impact on practitioners are explored in greater detail in Chapter 13 [ED: please check chapter cross-reference]. One of the largest departments at the NMC is the Fitness to Practise Directorate. This manages all complaints of allegations relating to the standards and conduct of practitioners' practice. Each year a Fitness to Practise Report is published which reviews the nature of the complaints that have been reported to the NMC throughout the previous year, how they have been managed and the outcome of the hearings. In the most recent report, 2010–2011 (NMC 2011a), the NMC states that there are almost 670,000 nurses and midwives registered to practise in the UK and there were 4,211 new cases referred to the NMC for investigation during 2010–2011. To put this in context, this accounts for only 0.3% of all practitioners, and midwives make up only a small proportion of this percentage because there are significantly fewer midwives on the register compared to the numbers of nurses. However, the Fitness to Practise Directorate generates the highest expenditure of all the NMC departments as it is a costly exercise to investigate a registrant's conduct and therefore utilises most of the finances from practitioners' annual fees.

When we look further to ascertain the categories of complaints received by the NMC (2011a), record keeping, including failure to maintain adequate records, accounts for approximately 4% of all complaints, coming in at a shared fourth place in a total of 12 categories (dishonesty, including theft or obtaining goods by deception, being the most common complaint). One could argue that dishonesty is to do with conduct, whereas the skill of record keeping is a competency-based activity and if we adopt that view, then record keeping could be included within the second most common category, competency issues. Poor record keeping is a significant practice issue, which could ultimately mean that a midwife could be removed from the register if she fails to reach the required standard.

Included in its other statutory functions, the NMC also has a responsibility under the Nursing and Midwifery Order 2001 (SI 2002 No. 253) to monitor the performance of the local supervising authorities (LSA) to ensure they are meeting the required standards for statutory Supervision of Midwives. Supervision of Midwives is a framework for supporting midwives and safeguarding mothers and their babies and provides a mechanism for every practising midwife in the UK (LSAMO National Forum 2009). It is a unique instrument, in that midwifery is the only profession to enjoy the benefits of Supervision of Midwives (SoM). Chapter 19 [ED: please check chapter cross-reference] explains the function of Supervision of Midwives further. Under the current Midwives' Rules (rule 13) (NMC 2012a), each of the 15 LSA regions must submit an annual report to the NMC, which analyses the contents to ensure the standards for SoM are being met. One of these standards determines the 'Details of how the practice of midwives is supervised' (NMC 2012b, p28). As record keeping is a key aspect of midwifery practice, this will impact on many areas identified in the annual report *Supervision, Support and Safety: NMC quality assurance of the LSAs 2010–2011* (NMC 2012b).

Midwives are working in increasingly demanding clinical environments. Examples include increasing birth rates, increasing numbers of women with diverse cultures and complex physical needs, such as obesity, women with high-risk pregnancies wishing to birth at home and in some areas, midwives working with limited resources and staff shortages. Whilst 'being busy' is by no means a mitigation for poor or absent record keeping, given the pressures some midwives face on a regular basis, one could see how for some, record keeping might not always be the top priority. However, this view would not be shared by the NMC at a Fitness to Practise Conduct and Competence Committee. Of the themes arising from all LSA investigations undertaken in the preceding year, record keeping features as the third most common factor resulting in supervised practice. Substandard record keeping is also mirrored in the Annual Fitness to Practise Report (NMC 2011a) and in the Confidential Enquiry into Maternal Deaths report (Centre for Maternal Child Enquiry 2011). There is no question that poor or absent record keeping is still one of the most common issues in nursing and midwifery, affecting care for babies and mothers. Despite the increasing levels in education for pre-registration programmes and the move towards an all-graduate profession for nurses and direct-entry midwifery (NMC 2009b, 2010), the standards of record keeping remain variable from year to year.

The NMC's Fitness to Practise processes focus on individual practitioners. This is appropriate as every nurse and midwife is accountable for her own practice. This means she/he is professionally accountable to the NMC and furthermore, she/he has a contractual accountability to her employer, in addition to UK law, for her actions. Students are accountable to the approved education institute at which they are registered to undertake their nursing or midwifery training and must also abide by the policies and protocols of the trust where they undertake their clinical practice placements (NMC 2011b). The code explains 'accountability' in terms of taking individual responsibility, stating that, 'As a professional, you are personally accountable for actions and omissions in your practice and must always be able to justify your decisions' (NMC 2008, p1). With regard to record keeping, to put it simply, you are responsible for the content and quality of your records and cannot blame someone else or the circumstances if your record keeping is not up to standard.

Activity 2.2

NMC Annual Fitness to Practise Reports and Statistics

Follow the link below to the list of Fitness to Practice reports:www.nmc-uk.org/About-us/Statistics/Statistics-about-fitness-to-practise-hearings/

Review the content of the most recent report.

- How many new cases were referred to the NMC in the most recent report and what percentage of these were women?
- How many men and women received a striking-off order?
- Who is the most common source of referral of cases to the NMC?

Compare and contrast the contents of the last three published reports. In particular, compare and contrast the tables of statistics of the Conduct and Competence Committee allegations, included towards the back of the reports.

- In relation to standards of record keeping, compare and contrast the percentage of cases of poor record keeping in the reports.
- Consider the factors that could impact on the percentage rates.

Case study 2.1

 A review of a recent case that came to the Fitness to Practise Conduct and Competence Committee hearing illustrates how a midwife's record keeping which did not meet the required standard was her responsibility. However, the organisation where she was employed operated a practice culture which did little to proactively support good standards of record keeping. A series of events combined on a particular day and resulted in a series of life-threatening events for the mother and her baby. Below is a summary of the case. Read it, and then use the activities to reflect by yourself or with your colleagues on the accountability of Midwife B and the other factors which contributed to the events.

Summary of the case

Sophie, a gravida 3, para 2, was admitted to the antenatal ward from home in the late evening, with a full-term pregnancy, having irregular contractions, membranes intact. On admission, it was identified that she was high risk due to a previous caesarean section. On abdominal examination, the presenting part was found to be cephalic and 4/5th palpable abdominally; thus a second risk factor of a 'high head' was identified. On auscultation, the fetal heart was within normal parameters.

The recorded plan of care was for her to be transferred to the delivery suite for a review by the obstetric registrar; this would be likely to include an examination per vaginum and controlled artificial rupture of membranes, depending on the progress of her labour. Sophie was closely observed on the antenatal ward where her contractions became more regular, intense and painful. It was a particularly busy night on the delivery suite with all the rooms being occupied. A bed on the delivery suite eventually became available and she was transferred. Midwife A was allocated to care for Sophie but she was also caring for another woman, who was also in labour. Sophie was coping well with her contractions, using nitrous oxide and oxygen via the Entonox apparatus for pain relief with good effect. Midwife A informed the obstetric registrar that Sophie was high risk and would require an obstetric review, but the obstectrian was in theatre with another case and did not review Sophie. Midwife A updated the labour ward co-ordinator on the situation, who was aware that Midwife A was caring for two women. The delivery suite co-ordinator was also aware that the obstectrian was busy in theatre.

Midwife A's entries in Sophie's notes showed that her admission records to the delivery suite were of an acceptable standard, the risk factors had been identified and a plan of care for an obstetric review was included. However, there were periods when there were gaps in the notes.

The day staff came on duty at 07.30 and Midwife A provided a brief verbal handover to Midwife B, the day-shift midwife. Midwife B surmised from Sophie's behaviour that she was in advanced labour; her contractions were very strong and regular and Sophie said that she wanted to push. Her membranes were intact. Midwife B felt sure that the delivery was imminent; she gathered a trolley and an amnihook and proceeded to undertake a vaginal examination with a view to rupturing the membranes as she thought that the delivery was likely to happen very soon. As soon as Midwife B inserted her fingers into Sophie's vagina, she felt the membranes bulging and was able to 'tip the presenting part'. At that moment, the membranes ruptured spontaneously and a loop of cord prolapsed with a gush of liquor. Midwife B pressed the emergency buzzer for help; she kept her fingers in place to hold the pressure of the presenting part off the cord. Sophie was rapidly transferred to theatre where she underwent an emergency caesarean section as the cervix was not fully dilated.

Outcomes from the case study

Details of the NMC charges against Midwife B included the following:

- She did not check the patient's history.
- She did not assess the patient, including undertaking an abdominal examination.
- She did not refer the patient to the registrar for vaginal examination in view of the baby's head being high.
- She did not maintain contemporaneous record keeping when providing care for the patient.
- She recorded incomplete information in the patient's notes.

Outcomes for Sophie and her baby

Sophie was delivered of a live male by emergency caesarean section, minutes after the cord prolapse, with Apgar scores of 8 at 1 min, 9 at 5 min and 9 at 10 min. Both mother and baby recovered well from their ordeal and were discharged home 3 days later with the baby breastfeeding. However, the events which led to Sophie enduring a frightening experience could have been avoided and although she might still have required a caesarean section for delivery, the urgency of this situation and its associated risks could have been prevented.

NMC panel decision for Midwife B

As part of its review of the evidence, the NMC panel scrutinised the contents of the records. It was noted that there were no entries in Sophie's notes by Midwife B when she took handover from Midwife A. On questioning, it became evident that Midwife B had in fact not made any entries at all until 2 hours after the cord prolapse. When questioned as to why this might be, she explained that she was distracted by what she perceived to be Sophie's imminent birth. Midwife B stated that it would have been her intention to complete the records more fully in retrospect. Asked if this was her normal practice, Midwife B replied that it was common practice for staff to leave gaps in clients' records to complete after events. Midwife B went on to explain that a 'gap' had been left by a colleague for her to complete Sophie's records. However, this space was only five lines and reviewing Midwife B's retrospective entry, it was an incomplete and minimal account of events.

   The panel followed a series of processes during a hearing, the steps of which are detailed on the NMC Fitness to Practise website: www.nmc-uk.org/Hearings/. In this case, the panel concluded that Midwife B's behaviour amounted to misconduct. She had breached the NMC Code (NMC 2012a) which was in force at the time of the events, in particular the following paragraphs (p3):

As a registered nurse, midwife or specialist community public health nurse, you must:

- *Protect and support the health of individual patients and clients, act in such a way that justifies the trust and confidence the public.* [Paragraph 1.2.]
- *You have a duty of care to your patients and clients, who are entitled to receive safe and competent care.* [Paragraph 1.4.]
- *Health care records are a tool of communication within the team. You must ensure that the health care record for the patient or client is an accurate account of treatment, care planning and delivery. It should be consecutive, written with the involvement of the patient or client wherever practicable and completed as soon as possible after an event has occurred. It should provide clear evidence of the care planned, the decisions made, the care delivered and the information shared.* [Paragraph 4.4.]

The panel concluded that Midwife B's fitness to practise remained impaired in the light of the findings; the sanction imposed was a Condition of Practice Order. This requires that Midwife B must comply with set conditions of practice for a period of up to 3 years. This sanction would protect the public and enable her to take rehabilitative steps to address her record keeping and decision-making skills through a structured programme of supervised practice, the specific objectives of which must include record keeping and decision-making skills.

Activity 2.3

In the case of Midwife B, the panel decided that her fitness to practise was impaired and reached a unanimous decision to impose a Condition of Practice Order to protect members of the public. Aside from Midwife B, this case study also highlights issues related to the practice of other staff on duty. Whilst they might not have individually breached any rules, their collective actions might have exacerbated the situation and actions of Midwife B which culminated in the serious incident.

- What is your opinion of Midwife A's standards of record keeping?
- Were there any actions that Midwife A could have taken to ensure that Sophie was reviewed by the obstetric registrar (or consultant) following her admission to the delivery suite?
- Were there any actions that the delivery suite co-ordinator could have taken to help the situation, given the high levels of clinical activity during the shift?
- Discuss or list, in order of priority, the actions that Midwife B should have taken to gain a clearer picture of the situation around the time of Midwife A's handover of care.
- In the light of your reflections/discussion, what recommendations would you make for the trust to develop the overall standard of record keeping for staff?

For more information about NMC hearings and how the process works, follow the link: http://www.nmc-uk.org/Hearings/

Enhancing your record keeping skills

Having reviewed the importance of effective documentation, why we must maintain records, the implications of poor record keeping, the extent of the challenges and the consequences of poor or absent record keeping, it is now be appropriate to explore some strategies that could be used to develop your own record keeping skills.

All NHS foundations and trusts are required to contribute financially to the Clinical Negligence Scheme for Trusts (CNST), an insurance scheme which is responsible for claims against clinical negligence. This scheme provides indemnity insurance for all NHS employers to cover the costs of any negligent acts of employees which occur in the course of their NHS employment (NHSLA 2012). Similar to other insurers' policies, the costs of the scheme are paid for by its members and the annual payment scale for each organisation is dependent on the number of claims; the fewer they are, the lower the annual fee. The CNST Maternity Clinical Risk Management Strategy (NHSLA 2012) reports that maternity services in England account for a significant proportion of all claims reported to the NHSLA each year. The pay-outs are significant as the financial costs required to support a baby damaged through negligence are high and may be ongoing for many years. Aside from the heartache that a family endures as a result of a baby damaged by negligent practice, litigation costs for trusts can be so high that it is in their best financial interests to use their clinical governance frameworks to decrease/minimise risk to reduce the numbers of claims.

Poor standards of record keeping are a feature in many, if not all litigation cases, and initiatives to demonstrate ongoing monitoring and improvement are an important aspect in demonstrating that trusts are proactive in their efforts to improve documentation standards. One measurable benchmark includes the audit of maternal records using a tool to measure record keeping standards; these are assessed within the CNST standards at regular intervals, once every 2–3 years depending on the planned attainment CNST level (NHSLA 2012).

Activity 2.4

Review your trust's policies and guidance on record keeping standards.

Ask a supervisor of midwives or a manager to show you the trust record keeping audit tool.

Use the trust record keeping audit tool to audit a set of notes to which you have contributed some entries.

If you completed Activity 2.4, you will probably have observed that the audit tool itself is detailed and lengthy. This is because NHS and foundation trusts must provide evidence to demonstrate compliance with the standards of record keeping specifically against the CNST criteria. As an employee, the midwife must adhere to the local policies and protocols of the organisation in which she is working. In addition to the NMC rules (NMC 2012a), midwives must also abide by the record keeping standards set out in *The Code* (NMC 2008) and *Record Keeping: guidance for nurses and midwives* (NMC 2009a). This also includes nursing and midwifery students who are required to keep clear and accurate records (NMC 2011b): 'Ensure that you are familiar with and follow our record keeping guidance for nurses and midwives (para 37, p14)' and 'Ensure that you follow local policy on the recording, handling and storage of records (para 38, p14)'.

Auditing standards of record keeping is an important component of the risk management process (NMC 2009a) which enables the assessment of record keeping standards against set criteria, to identity shortfalls and address areas for improvement. This will promote quality patient care, improve healthcare outcomes, reduce client risk and subsequently reduce costs to the organisation. Audit activities should be a normative aspect of care which promotes reflective practice and learning (NMC 2011c). Supervisors of midwives have a key role in supporting midwives in practice through a variety of proactive activities to enhance record keeping skills (Yearley 2003), which may also include regular record keeping audits as part of the supervisory review.

Self-assessment through record keeping audit encourages individuals to accurately assess their learning needs and take accountability for improving their own practice skills. If undertaken in a supportive clinical environment such as in a group or with peers, record keeping audit activities emphasise the value of sharing and learning together and promote a dynamic, proactive clinical learning environment. Gopee (2001) supports this, arguing that peer review is both efficient and effective and democratises a shift in power towards the practitioner. Therefore, self and peer review are thought to improve standards of care, increase awareness of personal professional accountability, help individuals identify personal areas of strength and weaknesses and stimulate professional development that promotes mutual learning.

To sum up, in the context of developing the quality of record keeping, self and peer audit can play a vital part in practice to ensure the highest quality of care is delivered to women.

Record keeping in action

Having discussed the value of record keeping audit in the context of risk management along with some tools and activities to enhance the quality of documentation, we can now introduce a self and peer record keeping tool for everyday use to enhance your record keeping skills (see Table 2.1). The development of this simple tool is based on the *Record keeping Guidance for Nurses and Midwives* and reflects the principles of good record keeping (NMC 2009a, p5). The tool is easy to use and emphasises the content and style which contribute to effective record keeping. The idea is that the more it is used, the more you will become familiar with the identified criteria, so that improvements become an integral part of your daily record keeping practice with each documented entry.

For the purposes of explaining its use, each criterion has been numbered (see Table 2.1). Criteria 1–7 inclusive are self-explanatory. For example, if the handwriting is legible (criterion 2) and this is achieved for every entry in the records, the score would be 100%. If this was mostly the case, the score would be measured at 75% and so on, with the appropriate column being ticked accordingly. Table 2.2 provides further guidance and explanation on the expected standard.

Table 2.1   **Self/peer review of record keeping tool.**
This audit form is designed to facilitate self- or peer review to monitor the quality of record keeping. Each midwife should audit 10 records every year. It is anticipated that this will provide a learning experience for all those involved and extend the sharing of good practice
* If criteria are not applicable, you should write N/A

Criterion	100%	75%	50%	25%	0%
1. Records should be readable when photocopied or scanned					
2. Handwriting should be legible					
3. Entries are dated and timed					
4. Entries are signed					
5. Name and job title should be printed alongside the first entry					
6. Records are factual					
7. Entries are consecutive					
8. Full assessment of client is recorded					
9. There is a plan of care recorded					
10. There is recorded evidence that the plan of care has been delivered					
11. Rationale for decisions is recorded					
12. Client is involved in decision making					
13. Frequency of entries is appropriate to client condition					

Table 2.1   *Continued*

Criterion	100%	75%	50%	25%	0%
14. Entries are jargon free					
15. Entries could be understood by client					
16. There is evidence of appropriate communication with medical staff					
17. Communication with supervisor of midwives documented when appropriate					
18. Amendments made must be dated, timed and signed					

In 10 years' time, would the record give a clear picture to the reader of the health and well-being of mother and baby (born or unborn) and the environment of care?

Comment from peer reviewer:

Having undertaken this self and peer review, what changes do you consider should be made to enhance record keeping?

Comment from self-reviewer:

Name: **Date:**

Activity 2.5

Review a set of your notes in which you recently admitted a woman to the antenatal ward/maternity day unit/delivery suite.
    Summarise the sort of information you recorded.
    Now using the self and peer review of record keeping tool (see Table 2.2), specifically in relation to criterion 8, 'A full assessment of client is recorded', review the same entries that you made and decide whether your records included all the necessary aspects for a full client assessment.
  If there is any additional information that you would have liked to include, make a note of this yourself, do not add it to the records, but ensure that you consider including this in your future documentation.

Table 2.2 Guidance and explanation on the expected standard when using the self and peer review of record keeping tool

Criterion	Guidance and explanation on the expected standard
Records should be readable when photocopied or scanned	Black ink photocopies well. There is no requirement that entries must be made in back ink but some lighter coloured inks do not reproduce well on photocopying or scanning. Remember that records are required as evidence and therefore will be photocopied or scanned and the quality must be of a high standard
Handwriting is legible	If writing is legible it will be easy to understand the care and treatment provided
Entries are dated and timed	Maternity records must be retained for 25 years and correct dates and times are essential in following the care process if complaints are lodged or investigations are required for any maternity episode. Every new page should have the date included
Entries are signed	If entries are not signed or staff designation is not included, it is difficult to identify who was involved in any incident. It is difficult to track staff to request statements; this becomes even more complex if they leave the employment of the trust
Name and job title should be printed alongside the first entry	Every new page should have the name printed, designation and signature, e.g. Jane Wood, RM, followed by the signature
Records are factual	They must be a true account of the events that occurred
Entries are consecutive	The entries must follow in the sequence in which they occurred
Entries are jargon free	Most maternity records will have an explanation of some of the words used in midwifery so that clients are aware what those words mean. Entries should be made in full in the initial text with the shortened version in brackets which then can be used in the rest of the notes, e.g. fetal heart heard (FHH)
Amendments are dated, timed and signed	If mistakes are made during writing, a line should be put through the error and the correction made, but it should be dated and signed either over the top of the text or to the side of the text. If notes are written retrospectively, it should be documented that they were written in retrospect and the reason for this. This entry should also be dated and timed

If you were to peer review a doctor's records, you would find this tends to be achieved at every entry. This may be because midwives are consistent at recording *what is happening* rather than planning *what could happen* in the future. In order to be able to recognise deviations from normality in accordance with rule 6 (NMC 2010) and adjust management options accordingly, it is important that a plan of care is recorded and reviewed at regular planned intervals and adjusted according to the findings. It should include a summary of:

- any relevant antenatal/medical or obstetric risk factors
- the onset and progress of labour to date
- the assessment of maternal and fetal well-being
- all existing plans and any obstetric involvement if applicable
- a new plan of care based on your analysis of the above
- a subsequent time to review the recorded plan.

In relation to criteria 10–18 of the self and peer review of record keeping tool, one would expect that provided the plan of care was being reviewed at regular intervals, the rationale for the decisions made would be recorded. In addition, documented evidence of communication with relevant members of the healthcare team, where appropriate, should also be included. If this is so, then the remaining criteria, 10–18, would also be achieved to the standard of 100%. The tool is intended for use in both low and high-risk cases, hence the inclusion of the statement, 'If criteria are not applicable, you should write N/A (not applicable)'. Thus it encourages practitioners to strive for the same standards in record keeping for women categorised as 'high risk' as well as 'midwife-led care' clients, regardless of the environment of care, be it in an obstetric unit, midwifery-led unit or at home.

Activity 2.6

Using the self and peer review of record keeping tool and referring to the guidance above, undertake a:

- **self-review** of five sets of records in which you have been the prime carer and summarise the key findings
- **peer review** of five sets of records in which your peers have been prime carers, summarise the key findings and give constructive feedback to those peers, identifying the positive aspects and the areas which could be strengthened.

This exercise be shared with your named supervisor of midwives and could go towards meeting your PREP requirements.

Conclusion

This chapter has discussed and analysed the legal and professional framework in relation to midwives' responsibilities for record keeping. The importance of effective documentation has been emphasised and contextualised within the clinical governance framework, which is a mechanism for reducing risk and improving the quality of care and services. The extent of the problem has been explored, common record keeping deficiencies have been identified and a case study has been used to illustrate the implications of poor or absent record keeping for mothers, babies and practitioners. Strategies have been presented and discussed to enable readers to enhance their individual record keeping skills and activities, and exercises and examples have been used throughout the chapter to encourage the practical application of knowledge and skills and the ongoing development of proficiencies that will strengthen the skills of effective documentation.

Student midwives and midwives must remember that record keeping and documentation are an intrinsic part of professional activity and that the onus for improving standards of records lies with individual health professionals. All practitioners should have opportunities provided on a regular basis to review their standards of record keeping and reflect whether their own records are congruent with the guidance provided by the statutory bodies. Implementing strategies to improve record keeping standards will enhance professionals' continuing development, benefit organisations and improve outcomes for mothers and babies.

Quiz

Use the following sources to help you find the answers:

NMC (2007) Ownership and sharing of midwifery records. 02NMC/Circular.

NMC (2009) *Record Keeping: guidance for nurses and midwives*. Available at: www.nmc-uk.org/Documents/NMC-Publications/NMC-Record keeping-Guidance.pdf

NMC (2008) *The Code: standards of conduct, performance and ethics for nurses and midwives*. Available at: www.nmc-uk.org/Documents/Standards/The-code-A4-20100406.pdf

NMC (2012) *Midwives' Rules and Standards*. Available at: www.nmc-uk.org/Documents/NMC-Publications/Midwives%20Rules%20and%20Standards%202012.pdf

1. Give five reasons why it is important to have a good standard of record keeping in midwifery.
2. Define the term 'accountability' in relation to record keeping.
3. Give four statements which apply to the minimum standards of record keeping.
4. Give an example(s) of how records could be used in midwifery legislation.
5. We tend to think of records as handwritten clinical notes. List some examples of different records relating to patient care (i.e. documentation on a woman's drug chart).
6. Who owns clients' records?
7. For how long must records be retained?
8. Describe what you understand by the term 'contemporaneous' record keeping.
9. What would you do if you needed to alter or add to the records after the event?
10. When is it permissible to disclose information about a client in your care?

References

Centre for Maternal and Child Enquiries (2011) *Saving Mothers' Lives: reviewing maternal deaths to make motherhood safer: 2006–08*. The Eighth Report on Confidential Enquiries into Maternal Deaths in the United Kingdom. *British Journal of Obstetrics and Gynaecology* **118**(Suppl. 1): 1–203.

Department of Health (DH) (2006) *Safer Management of Controlled Drugs: changes to record keeping requirements*. London: Department of Health.

Dimond B (2005) Abbreviations: the need for legibility and accuracy in documentation. *British Journal of Midwifery* **14**(12): 665–666.

Gallagher A, Hodge S (eds) (2012) *Ethics, Law and Professional Issues. A practice-based approach for health professionals*. London: Palgrave Macmillan.

Gopee N (2001) The role of peer assessment and peer review in nursing. *British Journal of Nursing* **10**(2): 115–21.

Local Supervising Authority Midwifery Officers Forum UK (2009) *Modern Supervision in Action*. Available at: www.nmc-uk.org/Documents/Midwifery-booklets/NMC-LSAMO-Forum-Modern-supervision-in-action.pdf (accessed May 2013).

NHS Litigation Authority (NHSLA) (2012) *Clinical Negligence Scheme for Trusts. Maternity Clinical Risk Management Standards Version 1 2012/13*. London: NHS Litigation Authority.

Nursing and Midwifery Council (NMC) (2004) *Code of Professional Conduct*. London: Nursing and Midwifery Council.

Nursing and Midwifery Council (NMC) (2005) *Guidelines for Records and Record keeping*. London: Nursing and Midwifery Council.

Nursing and Midwifery Council (NMC) (2006) *Confidentiality*. London: Nursing and Midwifery Council.

Nursing and Midwifery Council (NMC) (2007) Ownership and sharing of midwifery records. 02.NMC/Circular. London: Nursing and Midwifery Council.

Nursing and Midwifery Council (NMC) (2008) *The Code: standards of conduct, performance and ethics for nurses and midwives*. Available at: www.nmc-uk.org/Documents/Standards/The-code-A4-20100406.pdf (accessed May 2013).

Nursing and Midwifery Council (NMC) (2009a) *Record Keeping: guidance for nurses and midwives*. Available at: www.nmc-uk.org/Documents/NMC-Publications/NMC-Record keeping-Guidance.pdf (accessed May 2013).

Nursing and Midwifery Council (NMC) (2009b) *Standards for Pre-Registration Midwifery Education*. Available at: www.nmc-uk.org/Documents/NMC-Publications/nmcStandardsforPre_RegistrationMidwiferyEducation.pdf (accessed May 2013).

Nursing and Midwifery Council (NMC) (2010) *Standards for Pre-registration Nursing Education*. London: Nursing and Midwifery Council.

Nursing and Midwifery Council (NMC) (2011a) *Nursing and Midwifery Council Annual Fitness to Practise Report 2010–2011*. London: Nursing and Midwifery Council.

Nursing and Midwifery Council (NMC) (2011b) *Guidance on Professional Conduct for Nursing and Midwifery Students*, 3rd edn. London: Nursing and Midwifery Council.

Nursing and Midwifery Council (NMC) (2011c) *The Prep Handbook*. Available at: www.nmc-uk.org/Documents/Standards/NMC_Prep-handbook_2011.pdf (accessed May 2013).

Nursing and Midwifery Council (NMC) (2012a) *Midwives' Rules and Standards*. Available at: www.nmc-uk.org/Documents/NMC-Publications/Midwives%20Rules%20and%20Standards%202012.pdf (accessed May 2013).

Nursing and Midwifery Council (NMC) (2012b) *Supervision, Support and Safety: NMC quality assurance of the LSAs 2010–2011*. London: Nursing and Midwifery Council.

Yearley C (2003) Guided reflection as a tool for continuing professional development. *British Journal of Midwifery* **11**(4): 223–226.

3

Confidentiality
Celia Wildeman

Aim

The aim of this chapter is to engage the learner in discussion, exploration, critical analysis and practical activities that will enable professional knowledge and skills to evolve in the context of confidentiality. It also aims to highlight the role and responsibilities of the midwife and how these necessitate her working in a confidential manner when providing care to clients and their families so as to promote their dignity and trust.

Learning outcomes

By the end of this chapter you will be able to:

1. define confidentiality and discuss the significance of exploring confidentiality issues and the impact on professional practice
2. engage in practical activities that will provide experience in a safe and engaging environment
3. critically analyse current communication channels and how these may influence the understanding of the concept of confidentiality from a professional perspective
4. discuss alternative approaches to confidentiality and explore the relevance of the legal framework to midwifery practice
5. discuss an example of a model of confidentiality
6. evaluate the NMC's position regarding confidentiality and critically analyse the ethical issues and develop a personal/professional philosophy that will ensure continuing learning and change.

The Student's Guide to Becoming a Midwife, Second Edition. Edited by Ian Peate and Cathy Hamilton.
© 2014 John Wiley & Sons, Ltd. Published 2014 by John Wiley & Sons, Ltd.

Introduction

The British Medical Association (BMA) asserts that confidentiality is central to trust between doctors and patients. Indeed, it holds the view that without assurances about confidentiality, patients may be reluctant to seek medical attention or to give the key information needed in order to provide good care (BMA 2009a). This is equally true of the midwife and woman relationship. It is a complex issue that requires continuing critical analysis and debate in order to understand ethical and legal principles and professional codes of practice (Gallagher & Hodge 2012).

Patient information is generally held under legal and ethical obligations of confidentiality (DH 2010). From professional, legal and ethical perspectives, information provided to the midwife by her clients in confidence should not be used or disclosed indiscriminately. This particularly applies to disclosure in a form that might reveal the identity of the client who may not have consented to this revelation about her. The Health Professional Council (HPC; now known as the Health Care Professionals Council) tells health professionals that information must be treated as confidential and used only for the purpose for which it has been provided (HPC 2008).

It is prudent to be aware from the first day as a student midwife onwards that the patient is entitled to confidentiality of information about her (Dimond 2006). Historically, midwives have enjoyed an enviable position in their relationship with women and their families. In whatever setting she works, mutual trust and respect for the individual are key requirements for the job of midwife. Her sensitivity and openness are axiomatic to her feelings of worth and enhancement of job satisfaction.

In no other aspect of the role of the midwife are these principles more relevant than in the concept of confidentiality. The midwife's personal and professional philosophy around right and wrong, the position she holds around advocacy and other ethical issues that influence the interaction between client and professional will stand her in good stead. Alternatively, her ethical principles may cause tensions that could inhibit the possibility of a smooth pathway in dealings with clients, their families and the wider community.

Personal belief systems will be brought by the student midwife into her chosen profession. These can be modified and possibly change as she engages in education and training activities and as the highs and lows of professional life are experienced. Deeply entrenched personal beliefs and values are extremely difficult to change as they form the core self of the person. The individual can feel threatened and challenged by the constraints of professional life as these might require her to think, act and even conform in ways that are unfamiliar. Indeed, it is important for practitioners, including midwives, to be aware that their perceptions, ideas and beliefs will determine the way they act towards others. However, the midwife has a duty of care to the woman, her unborn child, the child following birth and for some clients' partners. In order to achieve the professional, ethical, legal and contractual requirements around confidentiality, the midwife will need to be receptive to continuing change. She must be ever consciously aware of the depth of responsibility to clients, her employer, the Nursing and Midwifery Council (NMC) and the community to uphold confidentiality. There are exceptions to absolute confidentiality – for example, the breach of confidentiality in the public interest. Indeed, the BMA states that confidentiality is an important duty but that it is not absolute (BMA 2009b). This and other exceptions will be discussed later in the chapter.

Confidentiality: the professional stance

The NMC (NMC 2008) holds a very firm position around confidentiality. It asserts that 'registrants have a responsibility to deliver safe and effective care based on current evidence, best practice, and where applicable, validated research'. This must be based on the concept of confidentiality to ensure that the midwife/client relationship is strengthened through transparency, trust and mutual respect.

Activity 3.1

How would you define confidentiality?

In your response to Activity 3.1, your definition of confidentiality may have included the following: Confidentiality covers information (private or sensitive) revealed to a chosen other but which is protected from being shared with others (McKeown & Weed 2002). The NMC (2008) also states that you must respect people's right to confidentiality. You must ensure people are informed about how and why information is shared and you must disclose information if you believe someone may be at risk of harm, in line with the law of the country in which you are practising (NMC 2008). The NMC asserts that 'a duty of confidence arises when one person discloses information to another in circumstances where it is reasonable to expect that the information will be held in confidence' (NMC 2012).

It is inevitable and essential that clients will need to trust midwives with personal and confidential information. This is a significant matter and the client has every right to expect that information divulged will be kept in the strictest confidence. This means not sharing the information with a third party unless it was made explicit to the client, prior to them divulging the information, that it was likely to be shared. A rationale for why information may be shared should be given and consent sought.

Confidentiality is the principle of keeping records and information given by or about an individual in the course of a professional relationship secure and secret from others (Dimond 2006). It means that a professional must not disclose anything learned from a person who has consulted her, or whom she has examined or treated without that person's agreement.

The essential nature of confidentiality for professional practice

It requires a huge amount of trust for a client to disclose private information to the midwife. Some women may have not previously shared these personal details about themselves with anyone outside their family and in some cases, possibly not with anyone, including their partner, until they have shared the information with the midwife.

Midwifery wisdom

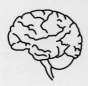

The midwife is in a very privileged position and should understand the sensitive nature of her interaction with the client and must keep this information confidential.

The NMC (NMC 2006, Clause 5) sets strict guidelines that enhance the understanding of the midwife's role and responsibilities regarding confidentiality. The NMC states the following:

- *You must treat information about patients and clients as confidential and use it only for the purposes for which it was given. As it is impractical to obtain consent every time you need to share information with others, you should ensure that patients and clients understand that some information may be made available to other members of the team involved in the delivery of care (for example, if an obstetrician has prescribed a particular treatment and the client refused to consent to the treatment then this information must be divulged to the obstetrician so that appropriate action can be taken). You must guard against breaches of confidentiality by protecting information from improper disclosure at all times. In the example given above, the midwifery practitioner would have complied with the employer's policy and professional guidelines to facilitate proper disclosure of client information.*
- *You should seek patients' and clients' wishes regarding the sharing of information with their family and others. When a patient or client is considered incapable of giving permission, you should consult relevant colleagues, for example a midwifery manager or senior midwife.*
- *If you are required to disclose information outside the team that will have personal consequences for patients or clients, you must obtain their consent. If a patient or client withholds their consent, or if consent cannot be obtained for whatever reason, disclosures may be made only where:*
  1. *they can be justified in the public interest (usually where disclosure is essential to protect the patient or client or someone else from the risk of significant harm)*
  2. *they are required by law or by order of a court*
  3. *disclosure is necessary to prevent or detect a serious crime (Griffiths 2008).*
- *Where there is an issue of child protection, you must act at all times in accordance with national and local standards. These are based on legislative principles which give powers and duties to those involved in protecting children. The central standard being that the child's welfare should be "paramount" in making decisions about her life and property (Kay 2003).*

The NMC is therefore clear about the reasons why the midwife should uphold confidentiality and the way she must act so as to ensure this is achieved.

Activity 3.2

 What does improper disclosure of information mean to you?

In response to Activity 3.2, you might have begun by asking yourself the following questions.

- Who owns the records?
- What is the employer's (work context) policy about disclosure?
- What does my professional body have to say about the issue?
- What is my personal/professional ethical position?
- What might the consequence(s) be if I disclose information?

The above are some of the questions to which you might seek answers to arrive at an understanding of the complex issue of disclosure of sensitive, private information from client to practitioner. It is important that the midwife understands that the duty of confidentiality exits to protect the client.

Activity 3.3

You are a student midwife on duty on the postnatal ward. While you are at the midwifery station, a telephone call arrives from a man claiming to be the partner of Jane. He is enquiring about her and the baby's well-being.

How would you deal with this enquiry?

There are several possible responses to the scenario cited in Activity 3.3. One possible response may be to seek answers to the following questions.

- What questions do I need to ask the enquirer so as to clarify authenticity?
- Who do I need to consult before responding to this request?
- How much information do I need to give?

Additional information is required from the caller – for example, his name, relationship to Jane, how much information he already knows. It is important that Jane is consulted prior to divulging any information in order to confirm her relationship to the caller and in particular what, if any, information she would consent to be divulged about her and the baby. This checking is important because Jane should be the main decision maker in this instance. The student should document the communication between herself, the caller, Jane and any other personnel involved, date and sign the entry.

Whatever decision you have made about what may be considered as improper disclosure of information should be taken in the knowledge that the practitioner should not make a unilateral decision (NMC 2012). You should take into account that, for example, the records of information belong to the organisation where you work; if you work in the NHS, the records belong to the Secretary of State and not the professional staff who construct them (NMC 2007, 2009). The legal right to access information is not automatic. Clients have the right to request access to their records, whether hand held or computer generated. This right to their access is based on the Data Protection Act (1998), the Access Modification (Health) Order (1987), the Access to Health Records Act (1990), the Access to Health Records (North Ireland) Order (1993) and the Data Protection and the Freedom of Information (Scotland) Act (2000).

Procedures for access must be in accordance with the Freedom of Information Act (2000) and the Freedom of Information (Scotland) Act (2002), the Data Protection and Freedom of Information (Scotland) Act (2002) and all other relevant legal frameworks.

All these legal and professional frameworks are in place to ensure that the professional practitioner carries out their duties around client confidentiality in a knowledgeable and confident manner. Indeed, the midwife's responsibility not to disclose confidential information is related to those who are alive and also to those patients and clients who are deceased.

Midwifery wisdom

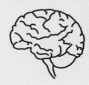

It is important to note that the midwife is personally accountable for any disclosures made.

The midwife is duty bound to keep information which she obtains from or about her clients confidential. The nature of her responsibilities is such that she should be aware that her contract of employment with the employer supports this view. The professional conduct proceedings of the regulatory body, the NMC and her client could all bring an action for alleged negligence if harm was caused as a result of the breach of her duty to maintain confidentiality or an action for an allegation for breach of trust.

To facilitate the midwife's accountability and responsibility, the NMC (2006) in its guidance to midwives supports the view that they should 'respect people's confidentiality' (NMC 2006). The client's right to be informed about how and why information will be shared with the multidisciplinary team is mandatory. Should it become apparent that the midwife needs to divulge private and sensitive information to a third party, it must be made clear to the client, a rationale given and documented in the client's records. In all instances, it is always necessary if possible to gain the client's consent, and such an approach can facilitate and enhance the client/midwife relationship. Awareness of the complex nature of working collaboratively with members of the multidisciplinary team is worthy of note. The dual professional message of respect for client's confidentiality and on the other hand keeping colleagues/team informed will require that the practitioner have a good working knowledge of her responsibilities and accountability. Any diversion from the acceptable standards could result in a breach of confidentiality which is a form of misconduct likely to cause removal from the professional register (NMC 2008).

In today's working environment where technology plays a significant part in the communication channels, the midwife and student of midwifery can inadvertently divulge confidential information. Social networking is one such channel.

Case study 3.1

The midwifery working environment can sometimes be stressful and even overwhelming. You have experienced one such day and, being frustrated, you have decided to communicate your feelings on Facebook to your friends and colleagues. Lots of people (including students) do this. You have disclosed your frustration with a woman who refused to breastfeed her baby as you had a lecture at university that provided credible evidence for exclusive breastfeeding at least for the first 6 months. You believe she is being selfish, particularly because her baby was growth restricted at birth. Your outburst, you believe, did not reveal the identity of the woman.

Thinking about Case study 3.1, what could be the implications of your action? It can be very easy to drift into disclosing information deliberately or accidentally. Social networking has become a huge challenge.

According to Kemp (2010), 'social networking can remove barriers which is both a benefit and a challenge'.

You may think that you kept the woman's identity secure but she, a colleague or a member of her social network may recognise her identity. This could cause untold distress to the woman (Wray 2010). Indeed, the NMC (2012) asserts that 'everything you post on line is public, even with the strictest privacy settings'. It holds the view that 'sharing confidential information on line can be more damaging than sharing it verbally' (NMC 2012).

The issue of professional behaviour is also relevant here (NMC 2012) as there are other readily available sources of support and guidance, for example, your practice mentor, personal tutor or your named supervisor of midwives. The supervisor of midwives provides a confidential 24-hour service and can be accessed at any time of the day or night.

Alternative approaches to confidentiality

Confidentiality is the key element within the midwife/woman relationship as women traditionally appear to have a midwife/client relationship script, one that facilitates complete trust in midwives, which strengthens the ethical obligation to maintain trust between them. Any doubt that the midwife will uphold the confidence of the woman may cause her to be reluctant to give essential information that could positively influence the outcome of her care.

The ethical stance

Haegert (2000) is of the opinion that 'care, together with compassion, forms the foundation of morality'. What does this mean in the context of midwifery practice? This is the essence of being 'with woman' and is a vivid reminder to students of midwifery, and midwives, that our prime purpose is to 'care' for our clients in a sensitive, compassionate manner. This means unconditionally and non-judgementally. This philosophy should be extended to private information and secrets told to midwives by women.

Information, according to constructionists, equates to power (Burr 2003). The midwife needs to be mindful that she occupies a powerful position within the client/midwife relationship. How she acknowledges and executes this power will inevitable depend on, among other things, her ethical perspective. There are various stances she might decide to take depending on her personal belief system, professional and legal directives and guidance.

Utilitarian theory suggests that human nature is such that it will seek pleasure and avoid pain (Singer 2001). If one is swayed by this idea then it would be feasible to assume that one's awareness of one's pleasure and pain preferences would also ensure awareness of those of other people. From a midwifery professional perspective, a practitioner who may consider the disclosure or non-disclosure of sensitive information to be harmful to the client will probably make an ethical decision that would ensure the greater good is achieved.

Gillon (2003) asserted that 'the commonest justification for the duty of medical confidentiality was undoubtedly consequentialist. People's better health, welfare and happiness are more likely to be attained if doctors and other professionals are fully informed by their patients/clients'. This is more likely to occur if they undertake not to disclose their patient's/client's secret.

The deontological view of confidentiality is based on the theory of the absolute and the principle of individual rights – autonomy and privacy (Beauchamp & Childress 2009). *Deon* is the Greek word for duty and deontology considers duty to be central. Deontologists believe that what is good in the world emanates from people doing their duty (Beauchamp & Childress 2009, Hendrick 2004). This principle is uppermost irrespective of the consequences. From a midwifery professional perspective, the concept of 'duty' fits well; the duty of confidentiality may necessitate disclosing or not disclosing information in the interest of the client.

Ethically, it could be argued that the professional's decision whether to disclose information that could be helpful to a third party should be based on the principle of the 'greatest good for the greatest number' (Beauchamp & Childress 2009). The opposing view would support the position that disclosure would lead to erosion and even collapse in the woman/midwife relationship. This utilitarian view is clearly not without problems, with conscience and tension around value systems. It could be argued, though, that in a dominant climate of scarce resources, midwives are faced daily with difficult decision making. This often necessitates a bias towards the majority rather than the minority and possible allegiance to a utilitarian approach. So what determines the position that the professional will take? This may depend on the ethical belief system to which she subscribes and the balance she achieves through exposure to other ethical views, for example deontological.

The ethics of professional practice is not easy to determine. However, professionals make difficult, far-reaching decisions on a daily basis. These choices may affect their clients positively or negatively. Guidance should be sought from the NMC (2008), among other sources of help, including the policy of your employer work and the local supervising authority (LSA 2012). Possibly the key awareness should be the practitioner's commitment to clients and the willingness to be an advocate for the client, who by the very nature of her situation is extremely vulnerable to possible breaches of confidentiality. Continual updating of knowledge and understanding of the professional guidance currently available is the lifeblood of the midwife's practice in this and other areas of care.

The NMC'S (2008) Code of Conduct states that 'people must be able to trust you with their lives and health', and that the professional should 'respect people's confidentiality'. Indeed, it asserts that professionals should 'make the care of people their first concern'. Clearly, from a midwifery professional perspective, the rights of the client enjoy prime position. However, this can create a tension between professional, legal and ethical viewpoints.

Activity 3.4

Tanya informs you that she is having difficulty bonding with her baby. You have been delegated their care for the shift by your midwifery mentor.

How would you deal with this situation?

Activity 3.4 is a realistic scenario that can be faced by a student midwife. Clients frequently confide in students as they feel that they have more time to listen to their concerns. It is important to be aware of the limits to the student midwife's practice. It is helpful to Tanya to be reassuring by being empathic and offering to consult your mentor and/or the midwife in charge.

The confidential nature of the situation is evident. Documentation is crucial. The entry should include details of the conversation, who was consulted, the response of the consultant, what information the client received about what action would be taken and who will be involved in finding a solution that will satisfy the client. All of this interaction should be documented along with a plan of care, designed in partnership with the client and appropriate health professional, for example community public health nurse and/or obstetrician. The date, time, who was involved and the student's signature countersigned by the mentor should also be included in the documentation of the event.

The legal framework of confidentiality

The psychosocial context of midwifery practice and indeed the Clinical Negligence Scheme for Trusts (CNST) statistics (Jones & Jenkins 2004, Nicholson & Saunders 2010) support the view that compared to other caring professionals, the midwife could be considered at particularly high risk of becoming involved in legal situations. Understandably, this occurs because she has potentially three persons for each case in her care: the woman, the unborn child and perhaps the partner (Schott & Henley 2007). The woman's priority will inevitably be her own personal health and safety, that of her child (born and unborn) and that of her partner if this is relevant. Women are today far more informed about pregnancy and child-bearing and their rights through reading, the internet, the NMC's documentation to the public and easy and direct access to the NMC. They are therefore more empowered and alert to any actions or omissions that the midwife makes in her interactions with them. Dimond (2006) also highlights the fact that midwifery clients 'by being comparatively alert and well, will be more willing to seek legal treatments against any healthcare practitioner who may be considered to be the cause of harm to the family unit'.

Jones & Jenkins (2004) remind us of the legal maxim that states: 'the higher the risk, the greater the duty of care'. The midwife makes professional decisions that increase her risk both in 'professional malpractice and in legal liability' (Jones & Jenkins 2004). With the greater risk and the higher duty of care, the midwife must ensure that she weighs up carefully the consequence of the risk in relation to the benefit of undertaking it. The law makes it clear that the practitioner must balance the importance of the object to be achieved against the consequences of taking the risk (Jones & Jenkins 2004). The midwife is reminded that she should be guided at all times by her statutory instruments, including the *Midwives' Rules and Standards* (NMC 2012), Records and Record-keeping (NMC 2004), *Code of Conduct* (NMC 2008) and any other legal and professional guidance, for example, the LSA (2012).

Midwives traditionally have cultivated a sound relationship with women. Informed consent therefore has become the usual way for midwives to go about their work. Indeed, litigation is seldom directed at midwives and other safeguards such as midwifery supervision facilitate midwives in such a way as to enhance their practice and at the same time protect the public (LSA 2012). Midwifery supervision is a statutory provision that ensures quality of client care based on best available evidence and research. Chapter 19[ED: please check chapter cross-reference] in this text discusses the issue of statutory supervision in more detail.

Activity 3.5

Think of a situation when you felt that confidentiality of information you had divulged about yourself to a third party was breached.

How did you feel about the situation?

In your response to Activity 3.5, it may be useful to consider the impact on you and the feelings you might have experienced and the actions you might consider to rectify the situation. This should enable you to think about how a similar situation would probably affect someone else, including the clients in your care. The exploration of your own thoughts, feelings and potential actions should enable you to empathise with, think about and support women in a sensitive way that will prevent them from having cause to take legal action. Women are more likely to consider legal action when communication does not meet the accepted quality standard.

The crux of the matter is that the concept of confidentiality should not be elusive but ever uppermost in the thoughts and deeds of the midwifery practitioner. Confidentiality arises in particular relationships when one party has conveyed (entrusted) information on the understanding that it will not be disclosed without permission.

A duty of confidence arises when one person discloses information to another in circumstances where it is reasonable to expect that the information will be held in confidence (DH 2010). This situation includes the divulging of private information from the client to the midwife.

This legal obligation is derived from case law, is a requirement established in the professional code of conduct (NMC 2008) and must be included within NHS and private employment contracts as a specific requirement linked to disciplinary procedures (Griffiths 2008). Midwives who work independently also have these professional responsibilities.

Women in the care of the midwife entrust the NHS, private and independent sectors to allow them to gather sensitive information relating to their health and other matters. They do so in confidence and they therefore have high expectations that midwives and the multidisciplinary team will respect this trust. Even if the woman is unconscious, the duty to uphold confidentiality does not lapse. 'It is essential, if the legal requirements are to be met and the trust of the women is to be retained, that the NHS provides, and is seen to provide a confidential service' (DH 2010).

Activity 3.6

Revisit Activity 3.4.

Did you include as one of your rationales for thinking, sanctions you would take in pursuit of your legitimate expectation to confidentiality?

Women are known to trust midwives. The relationship of women and midwives is extremely intimate from a physical, social and psychological perspective, and good self-awareness enhances the practitioner's ability to be aware of others' needs and expectations. The realisation that you expected confidentiality to be upheld in your situation should have enabled you to reserve that right to the women in your care.

Civil laws (statutory and case law) enable citizens to claim remedies against other citizens or organisations as a result of a civil wrong (Dimond 2006). A large group of civil wrongs are known as torts, of which negligence is the main one, but the group also includes action for breach of statutory duty, nuisance and defamation (Dimond 2006).

Communication is central to the client/midwife relationship (Schott & Henley 2007). All clients have a right to quality information communicated in a form that can be understood regardless of race, age, culture or any marker of disadvantage (Schott & Henley 2007). The duty of care in the law of negligence may include the duty to give information. Failures in communicating to the client important information relating to treatment and care are considered in relation to the laws on trespass to the person and negligence (Dimond 2006).

There are therefore various legal acts, professional guidance and ethical ways of doing and thinking that ensure women come to no harm. Briefly, it is important that the student midwife is aware of the following in order to understand and execute her role.

The Data Protection Act (1998)

The European Directive on Data Protection, European Commission Schedule 1 and 2 (Dimond 2006) was implemented in the UK by the Data Protection Act (1998). This requires that patients be informed about how their information will be used, who will have access to it and the organisations to which data will be disclosed.

Human Rights Act (1998)

Article 8 of the European Convention on Human Rights, which is given effect in UK law by the Human Rights Act (1998), establishes a right to 'respect for private and family life'. It emphasises the requirement to protect the privacy of individuals and preserve the confidentiality of their health records

Any depth of understanding of the concept of confidentiality and the stance of the midwife must take cognisance of the Data Protection and Human Rights Acts.

Exceptions

The law does provide for exceptions to the duty of confidentiality. Statute requires or permits the disclosure of confidential patient information in certain circumstances, and the court may exercise its right to disclosure (DH 2010).

Public interest

Under common law, staff are permitted to disclose personal information in order to support detection, investigation and punishment of serious crime and/or to prevent abuse or serious harm to others (DH 2010), where they judge that the public good that would be achieved by the disclosure supersedes both the obligation of confidentiality to the individual patient and the broader public interest.

Serious crime and national security

Disclosures to prevent serious harm or abuse also justify breach of confidentiality. Serious crime is difficult to define but includes murder, manslaughter, rape, treason, kidnapping, child abuse or other cases where individuals may suffer serious harm (DH 2010). The student of midwifery may encounter some of these issues, for example, child abuse, particularly in the community midwifery setting. This would probably be a situation for child protection.

In the interest of improving care

It is absolutely essential that patients are informed that information may be disclosed in order to improve the quality of care that they receive (Currie et al. 2004). Some instances when disclosure may be necessary include clinical governance and clinical audits (Currie et al. 2004). These are legitimate reasons for disclosure particularly in the climate of accountability, financial and professional constraints. Disclosure may be requested for research purposes but the client's written consent and the approval of an ethical committee must be sought for this. From the student midwife's and midwife's perspective, in the interest of protection of the client and her infant, information may sometimes be disclosed, either directly or through the midwife mentor, to the supervisor of midwives or the local supervising authority responsible officer. This would be in the interests of health improvement and quality advancement and to safeguard the interest of the client (LSA 2012). The consent of the client is still a primary requirement.

Protecting client information

The Department of Health (2010) guidelines on the protection and use of patient information require that when the disclosure of patient information is justified, only the minimum necessary information should be used. The guidelines also state that this information should be anonymised wherever possible.

To ensure that this ruling was followed, the Caldicott Committee (DH 2010, Griffiths 2008) was established. In relation to the lack of standardisation in the way patient information was handled, the Committee set guidelines and established a network of organisational guardians. Their role is to ensure that information that identifies patients is protected from abuse. Guardians are also responsible for agreeing and reviewing protocols governing the disclosure of patient information across organisational boundaries.

Activity 3.7

 Find out where the Caldicott principles are kept in your maternity unit. Read them and make a written summary. What do they expect from the midwife practitioner?

In whatever sector you are employed, you are required to follow the Caldicott principles as laid down by the NHS Executive. The principles explain the why, how, when and who and the legal framework for professional practice.

Confidentiality model (Figure 3.1)

The Department of Health (2003) has provided guidance to health professionals in the form of a confidentiality model. This model outlines the requirements that must be met in order to realise a confidential service.

The four main requirements of the model are:

- protect
- inform
- provide choice
- improve.

All the four aspects are inter-related and mutually dependent on each other.

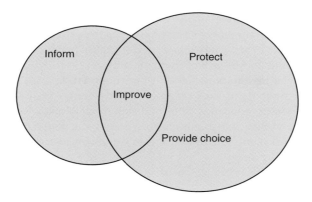

Figure 3.1   Confidentiality model. Adapted from DH (2003).

Protect

Practitioners and student midwives alike must act to protect the client's confidential information. This may include manual, electronic and for some groups of clients professional records, text messages, email communications and telephone interactions. Teenagers often prefer these alternative methods of communication. The Caldicott ruling also includes storage, handling and communication between NHS and non-NHS staff, and the strategies for recording information.

Inform

Clients must be aware of how the information held about them will be utilised. This includes actual and potential uses. Who will have access under what circumstances, what is likely to be divulged and how the sharing of information will influence their care (BMA 2009a, DH 2003).

Provide choice

The informed choice of clients must be part of best professional practice. Women should be empowered to decide whether their information can be disclosed or used in particular ways. Each client is an individual and therefore what would be considered confidential will vary from woman to woman. The DH (2010) therefore advises healthcare practitioners to ask patients for their consent before using their personal information, to respect the patient's decisions to restrict the disclosure or use of information, except where exceptional circumstances apply, and to ensure that clients understand what the implications may be if they choose to agree to or restrict the disclosure of information. The key message is that even if, in the practitioner's judgement, the client's decision will be detrimental to her health and well-being, the client's decision must be respected (Gallagher & Hodge 2012).

Improve

The DH (2003) advised that it is the role of the practitioner to 'always look for better ways to protect, inform and provide choice'. Keeping up to date with legal, ethical and professional changes that affect client confidentiality is an essential part of professional practice. There is also the expectation that breaches or possible breaches of confidentiality will be reported. This is and has always been a difficult and complex issue for healthcare students and none more so than student midwives, particularly when senior practitioners are involved. They may experience dissonance between their education and training needs and the disclosure of possible breach of confidentiality.

The complex nature of whether the practitioner is duty bound to disclose information may generate immense stress for some students as they grapple with the demands of professional practice. The guidance of the practice mentor, education tutor and supervisor of midwives should be sought. They are key people who as part of their role are facilitators, guides and confidants in professional matters. They act in the best interest of clients and this facilitates a mutual alliance with their students.

Conclusion

Midwives are expected to maintain high standards of ethical conduct in a professional context. This must be evidence based which necessitates being motivated to continue to learn and having a mindset for change.

The guiding principles for professional practice are, according to Gallaher & Hodge (2012):

- respect for persons
- respect for autonomy
- justice
- beneficence
- non-maleficence.

In addition to the midwife's duty of care to the client is also the issue of the multidisciplinary team. It is important for her to understand how and when the sharing of confidential client information will be in the best interest of all concerned. In all situations, the over-riding deciding factor is whether or not client consent is sought and received.

There are two further exceptions to this: compulsion of law and the public interest. The NMC states that midwives have a responsibility to protect confidential information about clients (NMC 2008). The reciprocal nature of confidentiality is important to bring to awareness (Johnson 2006) in order to ensure that the best interest of the client is served by the multiprofessional team. Information sharing between practitioner and client is necessary to facilitate assessment, planning delivery and evaluation of care, so understanding the value of reciprocity and how it benefits clients and practitioners is vital.

Quiz

The following quiz is designed to enable the student of midwifery to revisit and reflect on the content of the chapter, to engage in further reading and to facilitate discussion with practice mentors, personal teachers and the supervisor of midwives.

1. How would you define confidentiality?

   a. Information private or sensitive revealed to a chosen other but which is protected from being shared with others.
   b. Information disclosed by one person to another.
   c. Information written about a client/patient by the consultant obstetrician.
   d. Private sensitive information given by a family member about a client/patient.

2. What is the key role of the supervisor of midwives?

   a. To protect women and babies by actively promoting a safe standard of midwifery practice.
   b. To report substandard care to the public.
   c. To monitor the practice of midwives.
   d. To audit midwifery care and services provided to women and babies.

3. Accountability and responsibility issues are essential to the concept of confidentiality to whom?

   a. Yourself as a student midwife/midwife.
   b. The NMC.
   c. The NMC, employer, women and yourself.
   d. The LSA.

4. What are the Caldicott Principles?

   a. Student midwives must at all times report to the senior midwife.
   b. Protect, Inform, Provide choice and Improve.
   c. Obey guidelines and only inform the midwifery team.
   d. Always keep the interest and welfare of the woman uppermost.

5. The BMA's toolkit on confidentiality has how many information cards?

   a. 16
   b. 7
   c. 5
   d. 3

6. Which organisation provides professional directives and advice on confidentiality?

   a. The GMC.
   b. The NMC.
   c. The NHS trust.
   d. The Independent Police Authority.

7. What is the extent of confidentiality?

   a. To the woman.
   b. To the fetus.
   c. To the community.
   d. To the woman's partner.

8. To whom would you report a breach of confidentiality?

   a. The lead obstetrician.
   b. The supervisor of midwives.
   c. The lead midwifery manager.
   d. The trust board.

9. Mary Jones, a woman who has newly given birth, has disclosed her disappointment with the gender of her baby and asked you to say nothing to anyone. What is your course of action?

   a. Uphold confidentiality and say nothing to anyone.
   b. Promise her complete confidentiality.
   c. Discuss the incident with the multiprofessional team.
   d. Inform the lead midwifery practitioner with the consent of the woman, if possible.

10. What are the legally recognised reasons for breaching confidentiality?

    a. In the interest of quality care, to protect the public, to prevent harm to a third person.

    b. To protect the midwifery practitioner.

    c. Required by the NMC.

    d. Required by the NHS trust by whom you are employed.

References

Beauchamp TL, Childress JF (2009) *Principles of Biomedic Ethics*, 6thedn. Oxford: Oxford University Press.

British Medical Association (BMA) (2009a) *Confidentiality and Disclosure of Health Information Tool Kit*. London: British Medical Association.

British Medical Association (BMA) (2009b) *Confidentiality. Guidance for doctors*. London: British Medical Association.

Burr V (2003) *An Introduction to Social Constructionism*. London: Routledge.

Currie L, Morrell C, Scrivener R (2004) Clinical governance: quality at centre of services. *British Journal of Midwifery* **12**(5): 330–334.

Department of Health (DH) (2003) *Confidentiality: NHS code of practice*. London: Department of Health.

Department of Health (DH) (2010) *Patient Interest Disclosures*. London: Department of Health.

Dimond B (2006) *Legal Aspects of Midwifery*, 3rd edn. Edinburgh: Books for Midwives.

Gallagher A, Hodge S (eds) (2012) *Ethics, Law and Professional Issues: a practice based approach for health professionals*. London: Palgrave Macmillan.

Gillon R (2003) *Philosophical Medical Ethics*. Chichester: John Wiley & Sons, Ltd.

Griffiths R (2008) Midwives and confidentiality. *British Medical Journal* **16**(1): 51–53.

Haegert S (2000) An African ethic for nursing. *Nursing Ethics* **7**(6): 492–502.

Health Professional Council (HPC) (2008) *Standards of Conduct, Performance and Ethics*. London: Health Professional Council.

Hendrick J (2004) *Law and Ethics*. Cheltenham: Nelson Thornes.

Johnson G (2006) Confidentiality and standards of care. *Midwives* **9**(12): 486–487.

Jones SR, Jenkins R (2004) *The Law and the Midwife*, 2nd edn. Oxford: Blackwell Publishing Ltd.

Kay J (2003) *Protecting Children*, 2nd edn. London: Continuum.

Kemp J (2010) Social networking offers new opportunities for midwives. *Practising Midwife* **13**(7): 25.

Local Supervising Authority for England (LSA) (2012) *Statutory Supervision of Midwives National Standards for England*. London: Local Supervising Authority National Forum.

McKeown RE, Weed DL (2002) Ethics in epidemiology and community health. *Applied terms. Journal of Epidemiological and Community Health* **56**: 739–741.

Nicholson S, Saunders L (2010) CNST maternity standards and assessments and other NHSLA risk management initiatives. *Practising Midwife* **13**(7): 14–16.

Nursing and Midwifery Council (NMC) (2004) *Records and Record-Keeping*. London: Nursing and Midwifery Council.

Nursing and Midwifery Council (NMC) (2006) *Confidentiality. Advice Sheet C*. London: Nursing and Midwifery Council.

Nursing and Midwifery Council (NMC) (2007) *Record-keeping Access and Ownership*. London: Nursing and Midwifery Council.

Nursing and Midwifery Council (NMC) (2008) *Code of Conduct. Standards for performance, conduct and ethics for nurses and midwives*. London: Nursing and Midwifery Council.

Nursing and Midwifery Council (NMC) (2009) *Guidance on Professional Conduct for Nursing and Midwifery Students*. London: Nursing and Midwifery Council.

Nursing and Midwifery Council (NMC) (2012) *Midwives' Rules and Standards*. London: Nursing and Midwifery Council.

Schott J, Henley A (2007) *Culture, Religion and Childbearing in a Multi-cultural Society*. Gateshead: Butterworth Heinemann.

Singer P (2001) *Writings on an Ethical Life*. London: Fourth Estate.

Wray J (2010) Think before you type. *Practicing Midwife* **13**(7): 28.

4

The Aims of Antenatal Care
Laura Abbott

Aim

To understand the woman's antenatal care needs, including monitoring and assessment of the woman throughout her pregnancy.

Learning outcomes

By the end of this chapter you will be able to:

1. understand the midwife's role in the antenatal period
2. develop a deeper knowledge of the monitoring and assessment required during the antenatal period
3. examine the types of open questions that can be used in the booking appointment
4. demonstrate an understanding of the tests and screening offered during the antenatal period utilising current evidence and guidelines
5. enhance your understanding of the physical, psychological, sociological and economic factors that influence care in the antenatal period.

Introduction

This chapter addresses issues involved in the monitoring and assessment of a woman's health during pregnancy. Different assessment methods are used and central to these are history taking and the significance of the booking appointment, as well as important issues concerning screening and the type of screening tests available. Palpation and its importance are included, as well as various pregnancy milestones.

The Student's Guide to Becoming a Midwife, Second Edition. Edited by Ian Peate and Cathy Hamilton.
© 2014 John Wiley & Sons, Ltd. Published 2014 by John Wiley & Sons, Ltd.

The chapter discusses antenatal care from four key perspectives:

1. *Physiological*: to recognise any deviations from normal, providing management options, treatment and referral as appropriate. To assess mother and fetal well-being.
2. *Psychological*: supporting the transition into pregnancy, providing emotional support and empowerment for women to make their own choices. Giving the women opportunities for fears and anxieties to be expressed. Supporting and assisting with the formulation of a birth plan.
3. *Sociological*: preparation for parenthood to include partners and other children.
4. *Economic*: to inform and educate regarding maternity rights, employer's duties and time off work for antenatal visits. To advise and inform women with regard to benefits and entitlements.

The midwife's role as antenatal caregiver

To support and act as an advocate in partnership with the woman, providing assessment of maternal and fetal well-being and information in order to make informed decisions and emotional support. The student midwives' curriculum has been guided by the Nursing and Midwifery Council (NMC 2012). Essential skills clusters and reference to the clusters will be highlighted below.

Antenatal assessment and monitoring

The NMC (2012) has outlined certain skills that need to be gained by student midwives. During midwifery education, modules and components studied are linked to these skills clusters. An example could be that the skill of 'communication' can be applied to every skill a student midwife undertakes as each skill will require sensitive communication and consent.

The booking visit

Traditionally, the booking visit took place at around 12 weeks. From a dietary and minor disorder of pregnancy point of view, contact with the midwife could be much earlier in the first trimester in order to offer support, care and advice. The National Service Framework (NSF) (DH 2004) standard 11 for maternity services suggests that the midwife should be the first port of call for the woman when she finds out she is pregnant. National Institute for Health and Clinical Excellence (NICE 2008) guidelines alongside those from *Midwifery 2020* (DH 2010) surmise that each pregnant woman should receive the most current evidence available to help her to make fully informed choices regarding her care. In future, women may well see their midwife earlier than the traditional 12 weeks as government proposals stipulate that the midwife, rather than the GP, should be the first contact a woman has when pregnant (DH 2010).

Case study 4.1

 I was really looking forward to my booking appointment with my midwife. I was 12 weeks pregnant and had finally started to tell all my friends and family. I hate hospitals as my mum died last year and view them as places for ill people and death. My partner and I had read about and researched the area of homebirth and had decided that if all remained well in my pregnancy, I would like to give birth at home. I was excited about discussing this with the midwife and had practical questions I wanted to ask her. When I brought this up at my booking appointment, the midwife told me that having a homebirth was out of the question for my first baby. I said that I had done my research and that this was my choice but the midwife was adamant that nobody would support me. I walked out of that appointment feeling disappointed, angry and let down.

After I had calmed down a bit, I decided to have a look online for other women's stories and I came across the AIMS (Association for Improvements into Maternity Services) website. I telephoned the helpline and was reassured that it was entirely my choice where I gave birth and that I should contact a supervisor of midwives at the local trust. I spoke with a wonderful supervisor of midwives who informed me that of course I had the choice of where I gave birth and that the trust were actively encouraging more women to give birth at home. I was so reassured and especially as I was put in touch with a really supportive community midwife from my area who said that she loved doing homebirths! It seems that the midwife I initially had spoken to was misinformed and the supervisor of midwives assured me that they would be helping her in supporting women in all sorts of choices in the future.

I did get my homebirth and gave birth in my living room to a gorgeous baby girl! I did need a few stitches but other than that everything went well and it was so calm and relaxing being in my own home with just my husband, two fantastic midwives and me!

Taking a comprehensive history from a woman relies on the midwife having excellent communication skills in order to elicit important information as well as gaining the woman's trust. For many, especially first-time mothers, this will be the only time that a woman/couple has met a midwife so this visit is an opportunity to explain the role. The booking visit will paint an overall picture of the woman's physical, psychological and social needs. The woman can refer directly to the midwife and does not need to book in with her GP. NICE (2008) antenatal guidelines have endorsed the view that women should have access to antenatal services between 8 and 10 weeks of pregnancy in order to plan care in partnership with the midwife as well as for early consideration of screening options (NICE 2008).

McCourt (2006) undertook a qualitative study examining the antenatal booking interview and interactions between midwives and women using two models of care. It was found that case-loading midwives who look after a group of women, giving continuity of care and being on call for their births, were less hierarchical, offered more choice and information than midwives who were delivering a more conventional model of care, such as having different midwives for different stages of pregnancy and birth. Box 4.1 provides a checklist for the booking visit.

Midwifery wisdom

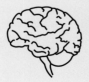

Carry a notebook for prompts to help when you start booking women, ensuring that nothing is written that may breach confidentiality.

> Box 4.1   Booking visit: checklist prompt for midwives
>
> Be attentive
> Personal details (nearest relative, phone numbers)
> Menstrual history, including last menstrual period or date of egg insertion if *in vitro* fertilisation pregnancy
> Medical history, including any mental health illnesses
> Family history
> Known allergies
> Lifestyle, including Body Mass Index, smoking, alcohol and social drug use
> Previous birth history
> Her own mother's birth history
> Physical examination
> Emotional issues, such as relationship difficulties or previous pregnancy losses
> Diet and nutrition, including any eating disorders

Opening questions

The opening questions in the booking visit may be related to this pregnancy. Asking the open question 'How are you feeling?' can elicit a variety of responses and information such as whether the woman is experiencing nausea and vomiting, and if appropriate, information about her employment history and if this pregnancy has been planned. It is important to gain information and document it carefully, but not in such a way that a woman/couple feel that this is a box-ticking exercise. The important things to ask are as follows:

- Has she has had any vaginal bleeding?
- Has she suffered from nausea and vomiting?
- Has she had any recent contact with rubella or any other infectious diseases?
- Does she suffer from varicose veins?
- Does she use any 'social' drugs?
- Is she a smoker or a recent smoker? If yes, what type of tobacco and how much?
- What is her weekly alcohol intake?
- How is her home life with regard to relationships and support?
- How is her work life and does her job impact on her pregnancy?
- Does she have any religious and spiritual beliefs?
- Does she have any specific cultural issues and needs?
- Does she have any pets or live on a farm? If yes, advise on hygiene and avoidance of certain animals such as sheep in lambing season due to the risk of disease.

You may find that as the conversation progresses, you gain more information that you can use to plan the woman's care and in your documentation. Try to build on what she is telling you and listen carefully as this will help in your questioning as the consultation continues. McCourt (2006) found that midwives had different styles of questioning during the booking visit. Some were authoritative, others were professional (information giving) and yet other had a partnership style (offering choice). Midwives who had the partnership style demonstrated most empathy as well as employing a technique of open questioning.

Frye (2004) suggests that midwives observe the woman carefully throughout history taking as well as using senses such as the sense of smell (for example, does she smell of alcohol or tobacco?), which may

---

Box 4.2   Strategies for effective communication

Ask open questions
Make eye contact
Stay at the same level (with chairs the same height)
Have a non-judgemental approach
Observational skills – note any antagonism, bruising, smell of alcohol, for example
Listen
Empathise
Respect choices

give clues to her lifestyle. The woman should be observed to see if there are any scars or bruises and if she displays antagonistic behaviour, in order to try to gain some insight as to why this may be.

It is useful to explore diet when discussing Body Mass Index (BMI). James (2002) notes that eating disorders are within the spectrum of psychiatric disorders. Chizawsky & Newton (2007) uncovered that as many as 15% of women seeking antenatal care may have a history of eating disorders such as anorexia or bulimia. If there is evidence of this, the woman may or may not need a team approach to care, perhaps including a dietician or psychologist experienced in eating disorders. By providing education on nutrition in pregnancy, the midwife may be a useful resource as well as reinforcing positive eating behaviours. *Midwifery 2020* (DH 2010) reinforces the role of the midwife in meeting the public health needs of all women. This includes those women who may suffer from eating disorders or have a high BMI and are therefore classed as 'obese'.

If the woman works, employment issues can be discussed and the woman may want to know her rights with regard to employment or self-employment. It is important that midwives give up-to-date and accurate information. Box 4.2 provides some tips concerning effective communication.

Midwifery wisdom

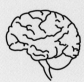

Remember, choice is personal. We all have different preferences, and empathy starts with being non-judgemental.

Emotional well-being

The booking visit can be overwhelming for some women, perhaps because they are receiving a wealth of information. However, it is important to pay attention to their emotional as well as their physical health.

It is useful to explore the labour and birth experiences of the woman's own mother and the mother of her partner as this may have an impact on her hopes and fears and what her influences are with regard to pregnancy and birth. It may encourage further discussion and will also help explore the woman's attitudes to labour and birth. Asking about her family background may also help with exploring feeding issues and attitudes towards breastfeeding as she may come from a family who are very comfortable about breastfeeding or from a family with no close female relatives and who are uncomfortable about it.

A woman may have had a previous difficult or traumatic birth or she may have suffered a pregnancy loss. The booking visit is an opportunity for the woman to talk about a previous experience; she may be coming to the visit with previous birth issues. Holding the booking visit in the woman's home puts the woman in control and is central to her care with you as her guest. With current pressures on our National Health Service, it has been recommended that sometimes bookings take place in a group. Although this may not be ideal, it is important to have an understanding that the booking visit may occur in a variety of places, including hospitals and children's centres as well as in the woman's home. It helps the midwife to assess her social circumstances and affords greater privacy, especially when asking intimate questions. If there are language barriers, it may be useful to have an interpreter, although this may give rise to confidentiality issues.

Case study 4.2

I am an interpreter for the Polish community and I often accompany women to their 'booking visits'. It used to be that we would go to someone's home and meet the midwife there but now I am finding that I attend more group bookings in the local hospital. Recently I accompanied a woman and her partner to one of these group bookings and although it was all very efficient in that all the bloods and scans were done in the same place, I could tell that Ewelina (the woman) felt uncomfortable. She told me she felt a bit out of place not having the same language as all the other women who were chatting amongst themselves. She also wanted to ask about some personal matters to do with finances and her rights as a Polish woman living in the UK. The nature of being an interpreter often means you speak slower and louder and therefore Ewelina did not want to ask the questions in case the other women overheard (we were in a cubicle behind a curtain). I don't think these group bookings are ideal as they take away the individuality for the woman. It is such a special time and I wish the NHS could have a bit more money to invest to get more midwives so they can book all women at home!

Women are entitled to time off work for antenatal visits (Directgov 2012), but this may be difficult if the woman has a job with inflexible hours. She could be self-employed so that time off will affect her business and hence her income. It is important not to pigeonhole women and have an awareness of the great diversity that people have, taking care not to stereotype a woman due to the job that she may do.

Note any hostility. If this is the first time you have met the woman, she may not wish to divulge information straight away. Remember that we are all part of a large multidisciplinary team and liaison with other team members such as health visitors and GPs may be needed if you require further information. It is important not to stigmatise or be judgemental by gaining self-awareness and being sure that the care given is not influenced by personal prejudices. Box 4.3 outlines some of the issues that the midwife may find difficult to raise during the consultation.

Midwifery wisdom

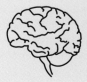

Before asking a difficult question, make sure you know how to respond to a difficult answer.

Box 4.3   Issues that may be hard for the midwife to raise during a consultation

Domestic violence
Previous abuse
Physical and emotional abuse (*Has anyone ever sexually, physically or emotionally abused you?*)
Previous stillbirth/neonatal loss

Medical and family history

The midwife should assess each woman fully, regarding her medical and family history. It may be that there is nothing significant in her history but on the other hand, the woman may remember something previously forgotten, such as a grandmother with a history of pre-eclampsia. It is essential to gain a medical history from a woman in order to plan her care appropriately. For example, if she has a history of thrombosis, she may be at risk of clotting disorders such as deep vein thrombosis or pulmonary embolism during pregnancy and may need to be offered the services of an obstetrician. If she has a history of serious mental illness such as psychotic disorders or a past history of postpartum illness, a team approach may be needed to offer her appropriate care during her pregnancy and support after her baby has been born.

Examples of questions about her medical history include the following:

- Does the woman have any headaches, epilepsy or migraines?
- Does the woman have any high blood pressure, blood clotting disorders, heart disease or thrombosis?
- Does the woman have any respiratory problems such as asthma, tuberculosis or chest infections?
- Does the woman have any digestive disorders, jaundice or anaemia?
- Does the woman have any diabetes mellitus, thyroid disease or hormonal disorders?
- Does the woman have any renal problems, kidney disease or recurrent cystitis?
- Does the woman have any gynaecological disorders, such as pelvic inflammatory disease, sexually transmitted infections, including herpes or thrush, or conception difficulties?
- Is this a planned pregnancy? If it is the result of *in vitro* fertilisation, does the woman know the conception date?
- Does the woman have any known allergies, including hay fever, eczema, foods and drugs?
- Does the woman have any injuries, especially to the back and pelvis?
- Does the woman have any operations or problems with anaesthetics?
- Does the woman have any previous blood transfusions?
- Does the woman have any mental health problems, such as depression, postnatal illness or post-traumatic stress disorder?

Family history

It is important to ask the woman about her family history. You will need to find out whether there is a history of:

- cardiovascular disorders, such as hypertension, heart disease, stroke and blood clots
- epilepsy
- diabetes mellitus or thyroid disease
- congenital abnormalities such as Down's syndrome and spina bifida, or renal and cardiac anomalies, such as tetralogy of Fallot
- multiple pregnancies.

You also need to ask about her partner's health and family history.

Blood tests, urine tests and scans offered at the booking visit will include:

- blood specimens for: blood group, rhesus status, haemoglobin, hepatitis B, HIV, rubella susceptibility, syphilis, asymptomatic bacteriuria (urine test)
- ultrasound scan
- urinalysis.

Midwifery wisdom

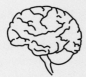

These tests are not compulsory! Never assume consent . . .

Subsequent visits

Antenatal guidelines from NICE (2008) recommend 10 visits for nulliparous (no children) women and seven visits for multiparous (one or more births/children) women in the antenatal period. *Midwifery 2020* (DH 2010) states that within antenatal care, the woman and her partner must be the focus of care. Care should be flexible and focused upon the individual needs of the woman. NICE (2008) recommends that antenatal visits should be structured and purposeful but that this should not detract from giving holistic antenatal care, tailoring it to each woman's individual needs. Although women may receive fewer midwifery visits, more quality time should be spent at each visit (NICE 2008). It is vital that visits are individualised, appropriate and tailored to the individual's needs. The midwife needs to exercise her autonomy and schedule extra visits should the woman's needs dictate this.

In discussing the frequency of antenatal visits, Frye (2004) suggests that reducing the number of visits a woman receives because she is healthy is illogical as midwifery should be about promoting normality. Therefore, if a woman is well and healthy, she still requires her midwife to visit.

Record keeping

The NMC (2010) standards on record keeping and information sharing (including confidentiality) point out that the midwife will be judged (amongst other things) on the standards of her record keeping. The midwife should keep contemporaneous records at all times. *Saving Mothers' Lives* (CMACE 2011) and the NMC (2012) both cite poor standards of record keeping in many cases that have been investigated. The NMC's 2003 annual report noted that the second highest category for removal from the professional register was failure to keep accurate records and the Health Service Ombudsman (DH 1999) equates poor record keeping with poor standards of care. (Chapter 2 discusses the important issue of effective documentation further and Chapter 3 explores confidentiality.)

Tests offered at subsequent visits

A 'dating scan' is offered to women at between 10 and 13 weeks to elicit an accurate 'due date' and to measure gestational age (NICE 2008). Nuchal scan screening is also offered between 11 and 13 weeks

(NICE 2008) and can be combined with a dating scan. This used to be offered in only a few trusts but is now offered free of charge in most NHS trusts in the UK. An anomaly scan is offered between 18 and 20 weeks. No further scanning is recommended. However, if the placenta is low lying at 20 weeks, another scan can be offered at 36 weeks.

Haemoglobin (Hb) is assessed at 16 weeks if there is a low Hb (less than 11 g/dL) at booking (NICE 2008).

- At 28 weeks, Hb is checked again and anti-D is offered to rhesus-negative women.
- At 34 weeks, a second dose of anti-D is offered to rhesus-negative women.
- Women deemed to be at risk of sickle cell disease or thalassaemia should be offered routine testing at around 10 weeks' gestation (NICE 2008).

At each visit the midwife should undertake a variety of physical checks of the health of the woman and her growing baby, including physical examinations, for example, abdominal palpation, observation of vital signs and the general physical condition of the woman. This care should be tailored for each woman. Cronk (2005) recommends that a woman who has had a previous caesarean section should have her pulse rate checked regularly in order for the midwife to determine the woman's healthy heart rate and to establish a consistent baseline that can used when the woman is in labour. If a woman has a high BMI, a larger blood pressure cuff should be used because this gives greater accuracy. Urinalysis at each visit should be provided by the production of a midstream urine sample in order to avoid contamination and thus an incorrect result.

At each visit the midwife should be alert to conditions such as pre-eclampsia when assessing blood pressure and testing urine for the presence of protein, diabetes mellitus when testing urine for the presence of glucose, as well as domestic violence using observational skills and questioning. Blood pressure (BP) and urinalysis should be taken and documented at each visit. Information should be gained about nutrition, attendance at antenatal classes, preferred place of birth and breastfeeding.

The National Institute of Health and Clinical Excellence (2008) stipulates that women should be offered lifestyle advice by their midwives. This should include the latest nutritional recommendation that women should increase their levels of vitamin D intake during pregnancy, particularly if they are in a high-risk group for a lower vitamin D uptake (women who have a high BMI, those who are housebound or have very little sunlight, South Asian, African, Middle Eastern and Caribbean women). The dose recommended by NICE (2008) is an added 10 µg of vitamin D per day to ensure that the levels are adequate to maintain well-being for women and their babies.

Opportunities should be given to the woman to ask questions. NICE (2008) states that there should be continuity of care throughout the antenatal period. This will help the midwife and woman form a trusting partnership.

Assessments at each visit

Palpation

Palpation determines the size, position and growth of the baby by feeling the abdomen with both hands. This should begin at the booking appointment and continue through the woman's pregnancy. The uterus begins to grow and show during the first 20 weeks of pregnancy. As the fetus grows and the pregnancy develops, palpation is essential in assessing the position and movement of the baby, how it is growing and its approximate size.

The midwife must use all of her senses in order to gain skills in palpation.

- Are there stretch marks (striae gravidarum)?
- Is there a linea nigra (dark line of pigmentation extending from the bikini line to above the navel)?

- Are there any rashes?
- Is there evidence of scarring from previous surgery, or bruising?
- Contour: what is the shape of the uterus – for example, oval or slightly displaced to one side? What is the size and shape of the abdomen? This may give clues as to whether the baby is in a posterior position or presenting in the breech position.

It is vital to gain permission prior to touching the woman. Before palpating the abdomen, the midwife's hands must be clean with short fingernails. She should ensure privacy and dignity, make sure the woman has an empty bladder and that she is not flat on her back in order to avoid aortocaval occlusion. NICE (2003) recommends that symphysis–fundal height is plotted on a graph by measuring the uterus from the pubic bone to the height of the fundus.

Abdominal palpation and assessment of the fetal heart

Guidance from NICE (2008) suggests that it is not necessary to auscultate the fetal heart at antenatal visits because it offers no predictive value. However, some women find it reassuring (NICE 2008). Knowledge of movements, the lie of the baby and if the baby is in an optimal position empowers the woman by explaining ways in which she can help to encourage the baby into the ideal position for birth.

Get used to using your Pinard (see Figure 4.1). Wickham (2002) suggests that midwives can learn to hear variability with a Pinard by adding up the number of heartbeats auscultated in 5-min intervals (see

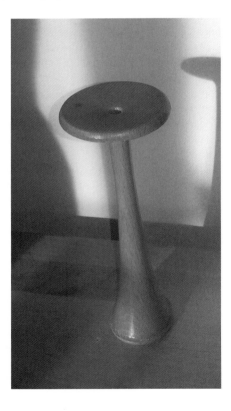

Figure 4.1   Pinard.

Box 4.4   Using your Pinard

Why use a Pinard?
Some women decline electronic monitoring and it is vital that you have this skill.
The batteries in your Sonicaid may run out.
Auscultation with the Pinard gives you more clues as to the position of the baby. This is especially useful if you suspect the baby is in the breech position.
You can hear the fetal heart (FH) from approximately 28 weeks through the fetal shoulder.

How to use a Pinard: five steps to Pinard success

1. Palpate to ascertain the baby's position. Ask the woman where she thinks the baby is. Generally, you are aiming to hear the FH through the fetal back (remember that the baby's lungs are not inflated).
2. Use your knowledge and experience to see where the FH might be for the different positions the baby might be in, and choose your target point.
3. Place the Pinard on your chosen spot, put your ear to the earpiece, take your hand away from the Pinard, listen and keep listening.
4. Feel the maternal pulse at the same time. If it coincides, you have the uterine vessels.
5. If after careful listening you really can't hear anything, repeat the palpation and try the Pinard in another spot.

Source: Wickham (2002).

Midwifery wisdom

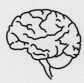

The tall woman may feel small for dates. The short woman may feel large for dates. Use your senses – your eyes to see, your hands to feel, but sometimes the most useful sense of all is your common sense!

Box 4.4). If the number of beats added up in 5-min intervals differs, variability can be confirmed. Wickham (2002) explains that if the number of beats is the same, the baby may be asleep. If so, the midwife should try again in 10 min.

Screening

Midwives need to be able to impart information about screening options with clarity and sensitivity and in a way that clients can understand. How information is given and the language used can ease anxiety for clients. Women are faced with having to make decisions about screening for abnormalities as developments in antenatal care mean that there are ever-increasing ways to screen and detect abnormalities in the fetus. The majority of pregnancies will be normal but for a minority, some test results may come back positive, which means that parents face further decision making about proceeding with more tests.

Referral to other healthcare professionals is needed if the tests detect an abnormality. Ultimately, the question of whether to continue with the pregnancy may have to be faced. Many trusts employ a midwife who specialises in screening and abnormalities, supporting parents through their decision making. Some women may choose to have private scans via a consultant obstetrician. Consultants usually work for the NHS as well but a woman may choose to have care delivered to her privately, giving her greater choice and flexibility over appointment times and more time with a specialist to ask questions. If the woman is being cared for by an independent midwife, she is still entitled to all the screening options provided by the NHS should she choose to have them. If abnormalities are found, the same options will be discussed and offered.

Screening tests

The following tests are offered to all women:

- Nuchal transclucency at 10–13.6 weeks to measure the thickness of the back of the fetus's head in order to calculate a risk factor.
- Serum screening at 14–20 weeks for Down's syndrome, giving a risk factor or probability of Down's syndrome. For example, a 1:2800 risk would mean that if the woman was pregnant with the same baby 2800 times, there would be a risk of Down's syndrome occurring once
- Anomaly scan at 18–20 weeks (checking for abnormalities); for example, looking at the four chambers of the heart, kidneys, brain, face and limbs.

These are only offered to women who may be at increased risk:

- Chorionic villus sampling at 10–14 weeks. A fine-bore needle is inserted into the uterus via the cervix and a small piece of developing placenta is taken for analysis. The chromosomes in the cells are studied to test for abnormalities and inherited disorders.
- Amniocentesis at 16–20 weeks. A small sample of amniotic fluid is obtained by inserting a fine-bore needle through the abdomen into the amniotic sac via ultrasound guidance, looking for chromosomal abnormalities.
- The risk of gestational diabetes should be determined at booking (NICE 2008) (e.g. women who have had a previous macrosomic baby or women with a high BMI) and these women should be offered testing on a regular basis. One way of assessing for gestational diabetes is by undertaking urinalysis for sugar in the urine at each antenatal visit.

Case study 4.3

Deborah, aged 32, was pregnant with her second child. Her daughter was a healthy 7 year old and this was a much-wanted pregnancy with a new partner, Amir. Deborah decided to have the triple test at 16 weeks and thought of it as just another blood test. The results came back as positive.

Deborah was told this by phone on the Friday of a Bank Holiday weekend. Deborah and Amir had no idea what this meant for her or her baby and they spent 3 days desperately worried and frantically searching the internet for clues. Deborah made an appointment on the Tuesday to see her community midwife who informed her that although the test was positive, it did not mean that her baby had an abnormality. The test result of 1:100 meant that there was a higher probability that the baby had an abnormality, but this could only be confirmed by amniocentesis.

Deborah and Amir were faced with a difficult decision as they knew there was a small chance that she could miscarry a healthy baby following an amniocentesis. Deborah felt philosophical and had a 'what will be will be' approach. She would want the baby regardless. Amir, on the other hand, believed that there was no way he could be a father to a child with an abnormality. This resulted in great conflict and arguments. Eventually they decided to go for the amniocentesis. It was stressful for Deborah as she was still uneasy about this choice, but felt she should do it for her partner. The results came back clear – there were no chromosomal abnormalities. Deborah was relieved but also felt angry that she had been through this trauma. She was upset with Amir for persuading her to have such an invasive test that had put their baby at risk. Deborah decided that if she ever became pregnant again she would refuse any screening tests.

Deborah progressed through her pregnancy but still felt anxious about her baby throughout. Deborah and Amir continued to have arguments which always seemed to go back to the same theme of her feeling controlled and bullied by Amir for pushing her into having a test she did not want. Deborah confided in her midwife who helped her decide to go and see her GP. Deborah was diagnosed with antenatal depression and the couple were referred to a counsellor. Amir felt relieved that the depression may have been the cause of Deborah's outbursts and aggression towards him but also concerned about how she would cope with a new baby when she was already so down.

Deborah went on to have a healthy baby boy, but she subsequently developed postnatal depression (PND). With the support of her midwife, GP and health visitor, Deborah attended group counselling with other women who had PND and was prescribed antidepressants. The strategies put in place and the team work helped Deborah overcome her depression, but she always maintained that the unnecessary (in her eyes) screening was the trigger for her developing a mental illness.

Midwifery wisdom

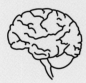

Ask about the baby's movements whilst you are palpating; it will help you in defining the position.

Antenatal Results and Choices, a national charity, provides non-directive support and information to parents throughout the antenatal testing process. Visit the website: www.arc-uk.org.

Box 4.5 outlines key points that should be taken into account when assessing women at each visit.

Case study 4.4

I saw my midwife when I booked at the clinic when I was 12 weeks pregnant and saw another midwife when I was 16 weeks. I had my 20-week scan yesterday and the sonographer said I had a low-lying placenta. My next visit with the midwife is not for 8 weeks! Eight weeks! I was told by the receptionist that because this is my second pregnancy, I am entitled to fewer visits than the first time around. How am I supposed to wait until I am 28 weeks pregnant? I have been on the internet to look at low-lying placentas and am now pretty scared. My friend had a placental abruption last year and her baby died. I just wish I could have a midwife to talk to.

Well, I went for my 28-week midwife meeting and just burst into tears. My midwife was so lovely and asked why I hadn't called her sooner! I didn't know that I could have spoken to a midwife about my worries even though I did not have a meeting scheduled. My midwife gave me her work number and said that I could call and make an appointment if I was ever feeling anxious again.

I have a baby boy! He is now a week old and the rest of my pregnancy went so well that I didn't need to call the midwife and she had put my mind completely at rest. I felt that just by knowing I could contact her at any time that was reassurance enough. It all feels like a distant memory to me now as I hold my son. I had a normal birth as well and no stitches this time!

Box 4.5   Key points to be taken into account when assessing at each visit

At each appointment you should:
observe the woman's appearance: is she tired? Pale? Flushed?
assess the BP (a large woman may need a larger cuff)
undertake a urinalysis
observe for signs of oedema in the ankles, legs and hands
ask about (assess) gestation.

Perform palpation, noting:
abdominal appearance: striae gravidarum? Linea nigra? Bruising?
fundal height: is this equal to dates? Give gestation
lie: is the baby lying oblique, longitudinal or transverse?
presentation: is the baby cephalic? breech?
deep palpation: is the presenting part free? How many fifths palpable?

Assess:
fetal heart: what is the range? For example, 135–148 beats/min
fetal movements. Where? What do they feel like?

Do not forget
Date
Time
Signature
Print your name by your signature

Conclusion

The midwife providing antenatal care needs to understand the physical, psychological, sociological and economic factors that may impact on the woman's care. The needs of the woman from booking throughout pregnancy should be carefully assessed and planned for holistically, using a team approach where appropriate. An in-depth understanding of the physical symptoms of pregnancy at different stages is required in order to be able to educate, inform and reassure the pregnant woman.

Excellent and effective communication skills are vital and the midwife must develop self-awareness in order to be able to provide non-judgemental and unbiased care. Having respect for the choices that women make and valuing the woman as an individual help in the provision of personalised care. The balance between keeping up to date with the latest guidance and recommendations and developing the midwife's personal art of midwifery leads to providing excellence for the pregnant woman and her family.

Quiz

Attempt to answer the following 10 true or false questions pertaining to antenatal care to test your knowledge.

1. A woman can bypass her GP and book directly with her midwife.
2. The booking visit usually takes place at around 14 weeks.
3. All women need to be tested for gestational diabetes.
4. All women must have screening for fetal abnormalities.
5. NICE (2008) recommends that nulliparous women are offered 10 antenatal visits.
6. NICE (2008) recommend seven visits for multiparous women.
7. Women should be offered lifestyle advice to include increasing their levels of vitamin D.
8. It is important that a woman has a full bladder prior to abdominal palpation.
9. Nuchal translucency screening is undertaken at between 11 and 14 weeks. gestation.
10. Women should be offered routine HIV testing at booking.

References

Centre for Maternal and Child Enquiries (CMACE) (2011) *Saving Mothers' Lives: reviewing maternal deaths to make motherhood safer, 2006–08*. Eighth Report of the Confidential Enquiries into Maternal Deaths in the United Kingdom. *British Journal of Obstetrics and Gynaecology* **118**(Suppl. 1): 1–203.

Cronk M (2005) Mary Cronk's MBE thoughts on early detection of scar problems during VBAC. Available at: www.caesarean.org.uk/articles/VBACScarMonitoring.html (accessed May 2013).

Chizawsky L, Newton M (2007) Eating disorders, identification and treatment in obstetrical patients. *AWHONN Lifelines* **10**(6), 482–488,

Department of Health (DH) (1999) *For the Record: managing records in NHS trusts and health authorities*. Health Service Circular HSC 1999/053. London: Department of Health.

Department of Health (DH) (2004) *National Service Framework for Children and Young People*. London: Department of Health.

Department of Health (DH) (2010) *Midwifery 2020: delivering expectation*. London: Department of Health.

Directgov (2012) Available at: www.direct.gov.uk/en/Parents/Moneyandworkentitlements/WorkAndFamilies/Pregnancyandmaternityrights/DG_10026556 (accessed May 2013).

Frye A (2004) *Holistic Midwifery: a comprehensive textbook for midwives in homebirth practice. Vol. 1: care during pregnancy*, 2nd edn. Portland, OR: Labrys Press.

James DC (2002) Eating disorders, fertility, and pregnancy: relationships and complications. *MIDIRS Midwifery Digest* **12**(1): 44–50.

McCourt C (2006) Supporting choice and control? Communication and interaction between midwives and women at the antenatal booking visit. *MIDIRS Midwifery Digest* **16**(3): 318–326.

National Institute for Health and Clinical Excellence (NICE) (2008) *Antenatal Care: routine care for the healthy pregnant woman. Clinical guidelines*. London: National Institute for Health and Clinical Excellence.

Nursing and Midwifery Council (NMC) (2010) *Guidelines for Records and Record Keeping*. London: Nursing and Midwifery Council.

Nursing and Midwifery Council (NMC) (2012) *Midwives' Rules and Standards*. London: Nursing and Midwifery Council.

Wickham S (2002) Pinard wisdom – part 1. *Practising Midwife* **5**(9): 21.

5

Programmes of Care During Childbirth

Laura Abbott

Aim

The aim of this chapter is to explain the different choices that women have in the types of midwifery care they can access and places where they can give birth.

Learning outcomes

By the end of this chapter you will be able to:

1. demonstrate a greater understanding of the different models of care that women may access
2. express a greater awareness of the choices women can be offered in where they can give birth
3. access some of the latest evidence supporting place of birth
4. develop a deeper understanding of the choices women make including supporting their plans in making an informed choice for their birth.
5. demonstrate an awareness of the parenthood education classes that may be offered to women/ couples
6. enhance your own midwifery wisdom in supporting women to make an informed decision about the care they choose for themselves and their families.

Introduction

This chapter covers a variety of topics exploring programmes of care during childbirth, with choice as its central theme. The government's aspirations for women to have choice regarding their place of birth are a central theme for governmental policy (DH 2010) and this is therefore an important

The Student's Guide to Becoming a Midwife, Second Edition. Edited by Ian Peate and Cathy Hamilton.
© 2014 John Wiley & Sons, Ltd. Published 2014 by John Wiley & Sons, Ltd.

element to consider within this chapter. Place of birth is discussed – hospital, homebirth and birth centre. Choices for women are discussed and include the importance of information giving to ensure that choices of care are fully informed. The Department of Health (DH 2010) outlines how equity and excellence can empower and liberate both women and their clinicians. Models of care are discussed, including the different types of midwifery care provision available to women. Childbirth preparation classes are explored, looking at programmes of education that parents are offered and planning for childbirth.

Midwifery wisdom

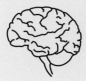

How we arrive at our choices may be deep-rooted. Sometimes we don't even know how we get there. It is not our role to judge a woman who makes decisions very different from the ones we would choose for our families or ourselves.

A woman can choose from a variety of models when planning her care during pregnancy and childbirth. A midwife is skilled and qualified to care for the woman from conception through to birth and the postnatal period. However, in the UK most women see their GP as the first point of contact. GPs may not be expert in the different options for maternity care. The House of Commons Health Committee (2003) describes how some women were frequently referred by their GPs to consultant-led care, thereby limiting choice for women who may be experiencing a normal pregnancy. It was also discovered that women often found it difficult to access maternity care without a referral from their GP. A study undertaken by the National Childbirth Trust (NCT) in 2009 discovered that around 40% women felt that they did not have a choice as to where they gave birth (Dodwell & Gibson 2009).

The National Service Framework (NSF; DH 2004) standard for maternity services states that the midwife should be the first port of call for women when they discover they are pregnant. The House of Commons Health Committee (2003) cites several interesting comments regarding consumer organisations and their opinions concerning choice in maternity services – according to Beech (House of Commons Health Committee 2003), 'Choice is an illusion. The majority of women are conned into thinking they have a choice', while Phipps (House of Commons Health Committee 2003) talks of 'informed compliance rather than informed choice'.

It is essential that the midwife is aware of the choices that the woman can make and provides her with up-to-date information so that she can make informed decisions in partnership with the midwife. The Birthplace Plus Study (Birthplace in England Collaborative Group 2011) has validated the latest policy of ensuring that low-risk women are offered a range of birthplace choices. The study found that birth in midwifery-led units and midwifery-led care are safe for the mother and baby and that these are the best places for low-risk women to give birth. Interestingly, the study discovered that low-risk women planning to give birth in consultant-led units were three times more likely to have an emergency caesarean section, twice as likely to have an instrumental delivery, need a blood transfusion, need intensive care and suffer severe perineal trauma compared to low-risk women choosing to give birth at home or in a midwifery-led unit. These are important findings to share with women when helping them make an informed decision as to where to give birth.

The different places where a woman can choose to give birth will now be explored.

Place of birth

A woman has a number of options when thinking about the place in which she wishes to give birth. For most women, pregnancy and birth is a healthy, exciting and special episode. It is important that the woman makes the choice that is right for her and her family. Options need to be woman centred and focused on meeting the needs of the individual rather than the service. The DH (2010) outlines how personalised care and increased choice can strengthen women's voices, empowering them to make informed decisions. The Birthplace Plus Study (Birthplace in England Collaborative Group 2011) can provide midwives with facts about the health outcomes that birthing in different areas may produce. This is an important and robust study into health outcomes and should be included in discussions with women and couples when they are choosing their place of birth.

Hospital with a central delivery suite

A woman may choose to give birth in a hospital and indeed this is where the majority of babies in the UK are born (Birth Choice UK 2007). Women who have complicated or high-risk pregnancies are offered consultant-led care and the consultant obstetrician will be the lead carer. Examples of pregnancies deemed to be high risk are in women who develop high blood pressure and pre-eclampsia; women with pre-existing medical conditions; and women who are carrying more than one baby. However, for women who do develop complications, there needs to be a team approach, bringing together the skills of midwives, obstetricians, paediatricians and anaesthetists to ensure seamless care for the woman. The Department of Health's (2011) 8th Confidential Enquiry into Maternal Deaths (2006–2008) makes reference to the importance of teamwork in many areas where substandard care has been uncovered.

Healthy women who choose to give birth in hospital do so for a variety of reasons. The woman may feel safer there or wants the reassurance of knowing that an anaesthetist is on hand if she chooses to have an epidural. However, some women may be unaware that they have other options than to go to hospital. In a study about women's choices undertaken by Lavender (2003), it was highlighted that women were reassured by the medical facilities a large consultant unit offered, especially in the event of an emergency. Lavender (2003) attributed this to women's lack of knowledge of the choices available to them and the fact that a medically oriented approach was perceived to be safer than midwifery-led care. Women should be given the opportunity to familiarise themselves with the delivery suite by having a guided tour with the midwives and midwifery assistants who work there. Where it is known that a woman's baby is likely to spend time in a special care baby unit, she should be offered the chance to visit it and meet members of the team.

Case study 5.1

My local hospital has a birth centre attached to it. Most of my friends have had their babies there. I must admit that I am petrified of the pain and want to have an epidural as soon as I go into labour! The midwife has said that I should try the birth centre as it is very homely and has two birthing pools. I don't care about the wallpaper, I just care that there is an anaesthetist on standby as soon as I have the first contraction. I want every drug going.

I am one of the last of my friends to have a baby and have heard so many horror stories of tearing, hours of agony and losing lots of blood and I really don't want to feel anything. If I could have a planned C section, I would but the midwives have told me this is not possible. If I had the money, I would pay for this privately.

Postscript: I am writing this holding my baby boy! When I arrived at the midwifery-led unit I was already 8 cm dilated!! I really wanted them to take me downstairs to the main unit to have an epidural but the midwife who was looking after me was so kind and lovely that she was able to calm me and reassure me. I was even persuaded to get into a birth pool! I gave birth using a bit of gas and air and did not even tear. Looking back, I am so pleased I gave birth normally as I was up and about so quickly. I am now a bit evangelical about childbirth. My friends cannot believe my change in attitude.

Birth centres

Birth centres are also known as stand-alone birth centres, free-standing birth centres or midwifery-led units. They are facilitated and managed by midwives and often have consumer involvement from women who have used the birth centre previously and members of Maternity Services Liaison Committees (MSLCs) and the National Childbirth Trust (NCT). Staffing usually includes midwives, midwifery assistants and housekeepers. Birth centres often provide antenatal care and postnatal support, as well as facilitating parenthood education.

Being midwifery led, birth centres take the focus away from the medical model and concentrate on the social model of care. With regard to medical facilities, birth centres are the same as what is expected from a homebirth – should intervention be required, the woman would be transferred to a hospital just as if she were transferring from home. Birth centres have a wealth of benefits and these have been outlined by Walsh & Downe (2004) and more recently the Birthplace Plus Study (Birthplace in England Collaborative Group 2011):

- Increased normal birth rates
- Fewer assisted births using instruments such as forceps and ventouse
- Reduced caesarean section rate
- Fewer women using strong pain-relieving drugs, such as pethidine and diamorphine
- Fewer women using epidurals
- Reduced rates of induction of labour
- Fewer women needing episiotomies
- Fewer vaginal examinations
- Shorter labours
- Reduced incidence of shoulder dystocia (when the baby's shoulder becomes impacted behind the woman's pubic bone)
- More intermittent fetal monitoring and less use of continuous electronic monitoring
- Higher maternal satisfaction
- Increased midwifery job satisfaction
- Increased breastfeeding success
- Cost-effective

Walsh (2005) defines a birth centre as a place that provides midwifery care in childbirth, with importance placed on relationships and the environment rather than on machinery and drama. Many birth centres offer birthing pools or large baths as pain relief and may have options for low lighting, birth balls, birth stools and music. The environment in a birth centre usually facilitates normality. The birth environment is important to women and has been highlighted in the NSF (DH 2004) and by the NCT (Dodwell & Gibson 2009). The NCT issues awards for midwifery-led units that facilitate the best birthing environments for women with the aim of celebrating innovations in practice that enhance women's experience of labour and birth. Lavender (2003) found that many women believed that a midwifery-led unit on the same site as a consultant unit offered safety but with a more homely environment, and 51% of women said that it was important to them to have a midwife help them to give birth naturally without medical intervention.

Case study 5.2

I was the 100th mum to give birth in the Hemmingway birth centre. It is such a great environment to give birth. The midwives and staff are so calm and professional and just let you get on with the business of labour. I spent my early labour in the 'sensory room' where it was dark and relaxing with gentle music and aromatherapy oil burning. I had bean bags to lean on and a birth ball to sit on. When I got to 8 cm dilated (with no drugs) I transferred into the dolphin room (aptly named because of the deep pool). The warm water was just what I needed as I was really howling the place down by then! It wasn't long before my baby boy was born into the water and into my and Lynda's (the midwife) hands. He looked into my eyes and I fell in love instantly and all the pain of labour just melted away. I was on cloud nine. I did it.

Midwifery wisdom

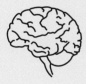

At a homebirth, you are the guest. This puts the woman in control. Homebirth truly empowers the woman and enables the midwife to be 'with woman' without interruption.

Midwifery caseloading

Caseloading teams of midwives provide total care for women and their babies throughout pregnancy until 6 weeks post delivery. Midwifery caseloading teams offer hospital, community maternity unit and homebirths. Although this is predominantly primary maternity care, midwives will usually continue caring for women whose pregnancies become complicated but in conjunction with the hospital obstetrician. Caseloading midwives will often work in small teams and spend time getting to know a group of women, focusing on their individual needs and working in partnership with the women. Within NHS trusts this can often be as many as 30 women a year, depending on whether the midwife works full or part time. In one area of the UK, caseloading exists in contract between a group of self-employed midwives and an acute trust. Walsh (1999) explored caseloading midwifery using an ethnographic approach and described the caseload midwife as a 'professional friend' to the woman. *Midwifery 2020* (DH 2010) discusses caseloading midwifery as a model that demonstrates positive benefits for women and for their midwives.

One practice in South London (the Albany Practice) was evaluated by Sandall et al. (2001). They describe how the normal birth rate, the homebirth rate and breastfeeding rates all increased for women being caseloaded by the midwives at that practice. Rawnson et al. (2009) explored the benefits of student midwives undertaking caseload midwifery as part of their education and found that the experience was extremely valuable for both the student midwife and the woman and her family. *Midwifery 2020* (DH 2010) recommends that women receive continuity of care and suggests that the midwife is the co-ordinator of care with the support of the multidisciplinary team where appropriate.

Homebirth

There is a large body of evidence that suggests that homebirth is at least as safe as hospital birth for healthy pregnant women. The Birthplace Plus Study (Birthplace in England Collaborative Group 2011) describes how morbidity is higher among women who have babies in an institutionalised setting such as large consultant-led units, and a large majority of women who experienced both hospital and home delivery preferred the homebirth. More recently, the Birthplace Plus Study has shown that low-risk women who choose to give birth in consultant-led units are three times more likely to end up having an emergency caesarean section and twice as likely to need an instrumental delivery (Birthplace in England Collaborative Group 2011). A Cochrane review by Olsen & Jewell (2005) found no compelling evidence to suggest that hospital birth was safer than homebirth for low-risk women.

Case study 5.3

 I was pregnant with my first baby and really keen to plan a homebirth. However, when I went to see the midwife, she told me that I couldn't have a homebirth with my first child as I had an 'untried pelvis'. She was quite adamant about this. I had really wanted my midwife's support. My partner was nervous about the idea of homebirth and I was hoping that the midwife would put his mind at rest. After the midwife implied it was dangerous, my partner said there was no way he would let me have the baby at home. I ended up in hospital with a ventouse and a third-degree tear. I wish I had stayed at home. I wish my midwife had supported my choice. Instead, I felt cajoled into doing something I didn't want to do. I must admit, I felt a bit powerless; I am sure my postnatal depression has something to do with feeling as though I had no control over my decisions.

This all had a big impact on my relationship with my partner and caused us to drift apart. I am not sure whether my postnatal depression was the cause or whether it was just the fact that I felt so disempowered by the whole birthing process. I wish midwives and doctors understood sometimes that yes, it is essential that a healthy baby is the outcome of the birth experience but also a woman's mental health is vital too.

Having a homebirth usually results in fewer unnecessary interventions such as episiotomy or assisted birth, and being in familiar surroundings the woman is more likely to feel relaxed, enabling labour to progress effectively. The National Service Framework (DH 2004) standard 11 states that women should be able to choose their place of birth and that normal childbirth should be facilitated wherever possible. This includes being offered the choice of homebirth. The National Institute for Health and Clinical Excellence (NICE) states: 'During their discussions about options for birth, healthy pregnant women should be informed that delivering at home reduces the likelihood for caesarean section' (NICE 2008).

The Nursing and Midwifery Council (NMC 2012) stipulates that midwives have a duty to respect women's choices when choosing homebirth. If there is a perceived conflict between risk and a woman's choice, midwives should seek guidance from a supervisor of midwives whose role is to empower midwives in acquiring and maintaining skills in facilitating normality. The role and function of supervisor of midwives are discussed in more detail in Chapter 19.

Women having their babies in a birth centre or at home may choose to labour and/or give birth in water. The Royal College of Midwives (RCOG/RCM 2006) states that 'women experiencing normal pregnancy, who choose to labour or deliver in water should be given every opportunity and assistance to do so'. Birth in water is considered a normal birth and just like homebirth, it gives midwives a chance to practise autonomously, using their 'with woman' skills. Women have said that water birth has given a greater sense of control and movement as well as providing good pain relief and immersion in water during labour has many benefits for the woman and has high levels of safety (Cluett et al. 2004). More recently, NICE (2007) guidelines say that water birth should be offered as an option for pain relief, especially for those women who have a low-risk pregnancy.

Midwives have a responsibility to ensure they are competent and accountable for their actions and omissions, and all units should develop guidelines for water birth. Midwives have a responsibility to reflect on rules and ensure accountability for their own practice. One of the roles of the supervisor of midwives should be to help other midwives acquire and sustain their skills in water birth.

Midwifery wisdom

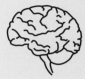

Remember, it is the woman's choice to make. Count to ten before you ever hear yourself saying to her 'you can't' or 'you're not allowed'.

Box 5.1 provides a list for parents to enable them to prepare for a homebirth. Box 5.2 describes the contents of a hospital bag.

Box 5.1   Homebirths and equipment

Equipment for parents to provide
- Something waterproof (e.g. waterproof tablecloth, shower curtain) to protect carpet/sofa/bed or wherever you end up. (NB. Not all shower curtains are waterproof. Plastic sheets available from garden centres are.)
- Old sheets or linen
- Bin bags
- Torch with spare batteries
- Nourishing, easily digestible food and drink, e.g. bananas, honey, sugary sweets, chocolate, yoghurts, glucose tablets, Lucozade, Ribena and fruit juices
- Bendy straws to drink from
- Comfortable clothes, e.g. large, baggy T-shirt
- A large soft towel to cover mum and baby together after the birth
- Towels for the baby
- Sanitary pads (large maternity type)
- Two or three new face cloths
- Hot water bottle (to put on back for labour or tummy for after-pains)
- Snacks for your midwife to eat whilst you are in labour!

Optional
- Mirror so that you can see the birth
- Camera/video to record the birth and to take the first pictures of your baby
- Lavender oil, homeopathy, alternative therapies

Equipment provided by the midwife
- Large absorbent pads
- Sphygmomanometer (for reading blood pressure) and a stethoscope
- Thermometer
- Mobile phone in case of emergency
- Pinards and underwater Sonicaid to listen to the baby's heartbeat
- Baby resuscitation equipment, including oxygen, a bag and mask
- An adult bag and mask should oxygen be required
- Entonox (three cylinders) and mouthpieces
- IV fluids, cannulae and giving set
- Syntometrine, Syntocinon and ergometrine (drugs used to prevent heavy bleeding)
- Baby weighing scales
- Sterile cord scissors and clamps, episiotomy scissors
- Suturing materials, including local anaesthetics
- Warm electric pad

The majority of equipment provided by the midwife is there as a precaution and is rarely used.

Box 5.2   Suggested contents of a hospital bag

It is essential to have a hospital bag ready. If you do need to transfer to hospital there will be no time to wait for someone to pack!

- Two or three nightdresses or large T-shirts, dressing gown and slippers
- One pack of night-time or maternity sanitary pads
- Toilet bag with soap, toothbrush, toothpaste, etc., tissues
- Change for the public pay phone, list of telephone numbers
- Clothes and shoes to come home in
- Lavender oil, homeopathy
- Large paper pants or old knickers
- Two face cloths
- Charged mobile phone and camera battery

For the baby
- Towel
- Nappies
- Cotton wool
- Baby clothes (vest, Babygro) and blanket (include warmer clothing for coming home in)

Case study 5.4

Giving birth to my third child at home was an amazing experience for all of us. My older children were there to witness their little sister being born and my midwife was fantastic and so supportive. However, the best part was having a relaxing bath afterwards in my own bath and then snuggling down into my own bed with my gorgeous new daughter!

I am 41 years old so at first when talking to my midwife about homebirths, she needed to let me know the risks of having a homebirth as an 'older' mother. However, I know my own body and was able to let the midwives know that I would take full responsibility for my decision. I am a healthy 'older mother' and really did want a normal birth experience at home. The midwives were really supportive but had to let me know all the pros and cons so that I was aware and could make that important choice being in full possession of all the facts. It was lovely to have such a great team of midwives around, supporting my choice. Having my children around during the labour made the birth of their baby sister such a family experience. I did have my Mum and a neighbour 'on stand by' to look after the children if I had needed to go to hospital. Luckily I didn't need to and they were there to meet their little sister as she gently entered the world!

Midwifery Wisdom

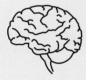

Remember to pack some food or drink. The midwife needs to be cared for too!

Independent midwives

Independent midwives (IMs) are self-employed and work outside the NHS in order to be able to offer continuity of care for a caseload of women throughout pregnancy, birth and for 6 weeks postnatally (ensuring the woman has ongoing care and that issues such as mental health problems, support when the partner goes back to work and certain physical problems such as mastitis are identified and the woman has support), providing women with the care that they choose. This usually involves homebirth. Women choose independent midwives for a variety of reasons. One is to ensure continuity of care and knowing who will be supporting them at the birth. IMs usually support women wanting a homebirth, but may also support them in hospital if needed.

Any midwife can choose to work in this way whether she has just qualified or has 20 years' experience. IMs work using the *Midwives' Rules and Standards* (NMC 2012) as their guide and the latest midwifery evidence to support their practice. IMs, like NHS, agency and bank midwives, have a named supervisor of midwives chosen from the local supervisory area in which they work.

Case study 5.5

I had complications in my first birth, which left me feeling quite distressed. I ended up suffering from post-traumatic stress disorder and it took me some years to decide to get pregnant again. I wanted to know my midwife in my next pregnancy and so we took out a small loan in order to employ an independent midwife to look after us. The visits all took place at our house and lasted at least an hour. I really felt that my midwife spent a lot of time listening to me and respecting my choices. She did all the physical checks, such as assessing the growth of the baby, taking my blood pressure and testing my urine. She also took my blood to test my iron levels and screening tests.

I had not decided where I wanted to give birth but by the time I was 40 weeks chose to have a homebirth. My midwife respected my choice and had always said that it was up to us and she would support me wherever we chose to have our baby.

My labour with my daughter was quite long and tough, but my midwife was by my side the whole time supporting me. The birth of my daughter was so much better than with my first child. I felt that having a trusting and continual relationship with my midwife made all the difference. My midwife visited us for 6 weeks following birth and was really helpful with assisting me to establish breastfeeding (something I had not managed to do before). She was also able to reassure any concerns I had and check that we were coping psychologically as well as physically.

By the time I was discharged from my midwife's care I felt I had laid to rest the ghost of my first birth and could get on with family life. It was the best money I had ever spent.

Independent Midwives United Kingdom (IMUK) has set up an audit of independent midwifery practice in the form of a database project registering clients at the time of initial contact to give the study credibility. The ongoing study has consistently shown that IMs have a high rate of normal births even amongst women who have risk factors (Milan 2005). The IMs also have a 14% caesarean rate compared with a national average of 22% (Birth Choice UK 2007). This is with over 70% of the clients that they book with one or more risk factors (Milan 2005). IMs give informed choice and often support women who have made difficult decisions.

The IMUK is respected politically and has members who provide advice and guidance to the Department of Health on issues pertaining to maternity care. Currently, the IMUK is proposing that the NHS Community Midwifery Model (NHSCMM) is implemented (van der Kooy 2005). The NHSCMM proposes that when a woman becomes pregnant, she is given direct access to a list of midwives in her area. The woman then contacts them and chooses the one she feels most comfortable with. That midwife then enters into a standard contract with the NHS who pays on a set fee per case basis. The NHSCMM would be available to those women who want it, no matter where they live or what socio-economic background they come from.

There is much behind-the-scenes work that IMs do. Boxes 5.3 and 5.4 are examples of the kind of letters that IMs send to various people/organisations.

One of the current challenges IMs face is the fact that they are unable to obtain professional indemnity insurance (PII). The NMC (2012) has stipulated that all midwives must ensure that if they are working without indemnity insurance, the woman and her partner must be informed of this. IMUK have been campaigning to ensure that independent midwifery remains a choice for women. At present IMs are able to practise but the results of a consultation and bid for insurance are not yet available.

Box 5.3 Examples of letters to child health records requesting a NHS number and a request for Guthrie results

Dear Child Health Records,
I am enclosing the birth notification for the baby of Mrs B. Please could you send me the baby's NHS number ASAP in the stamped addressed envelope enclosed in case of admission to hospital and/or for neonatal screening.

Please do contact me if you have any queries.

Yours faithfully,
Independent Midwife

Dear Sir/Madam,
Please could you provide me with a photocopy of the Guthrie results for my records. I have provided a stamped addressed envelope for your convenience.
With many thanks,

Box 5.4 Examples of letters to the supervisor of midwives and the general practitioner

Dear Supervisor of Midwives,
I am writing to inform you that I have been requested to provide midwifery care for:

NAME: Mrs M
ADDRESS:
EDB: 01.01.2012 24.11.2012

I have been asked to attend the homebirth of the above named client as well as provide all antenatal and postnatal care.
    In the event of emergency transfer to your hospital I would be grateful if you could provide the direct line numbers for:

Delivery Suite
SCBU
Ambulance Control

I would appreciate it if you could send us some Guthrie cards and an address to which the completed card needs to be sent. Could I also have the address for the Child Health Department in order to send the birth notification after the baby has been born?
    I have completed Intention to Practice notifications which include working in your area.
    Please do not hesitate to contact me if you have any queries.

Thank you.
Yours sincerely,
Regarding: *Mrs B*

ADDRESS:
EDB: 01.01.2012 24.11.2012

Dear Dr.
I have been requested by Mrs B to provide midwifery care and to attend her homebirth. Should a problem arise as a direct result of Mrs B's pregnancy, I will be referring directly to an obstetrician. However, if a non-pregnancy health-related issue should occur, I hope to refer directly to you. If there are any health issues that you feel would be useful for me to be aware of please do get in touch. Please do not hesitate to contact me if you have any queries.

Thank you.
Yours sincerely,

Sure Start programmes of care

The NSF (DH 2004) recognised that midwives have an essential role to play in caring for vulnerable women, including those with mental health problems, suffering domestic violence, non-prescription drug users, disadvantaged minority groups and pregnant teenagers. The aim of Sure Start is to provide a better start in life for children under 4 years who live in disadvantaged areas so that they may have greater opportunities when they start school and also better health. Sure Start programmes have developed and children's centres are now opening in many disadvantaged areas where more midwives will be situated.

In an article about Sure Start midwifery, Rosser (2003) outlines an essential area for consideration – the fact that young, vulnerable women living in poverty have urgent needs that can be provided for by the clinical midwife. The problems faced by women offered Sure Start midwifery may be multifaceted. The women and families requiring Sure Start programmes are often disadvantaged. The government has plans to tackle inequalities in healthcare to ensure a reduction in the mortality rate of babies under 1 year. Policies such as the NSF (DH 2004) and *Tackling Health Inequalities* (DH 2003) have set targets to improve the health of those most vulnerable. Rosser (2003) poignantly writes of a young woman whom she has helped with some aspects of her life, such as stopping smoking, accessing and using counselling, and help with form filling. *The Strategic Review of Health Inequalities in England – Post 2010* (Marmot Review 2010) built upon previous government policies to tackle social inequalities and strengthen fairness and social injustice in England. This has an impact on midwifery care, ensuring that all members of society have access to excellent care, reducing inequalities in health.

There is no doubt of the support that Sure Start midwifery can potentially offer to vulnerable families. However, a recent national survey commissioned by the Daycare Trust (2011) has found that the majority of Sure Start centres have a reduced budget and reduced staffing levels, and that 7% of centres are set to close in the next few years (Daycare Trust 2011).

Midwifery wisdom

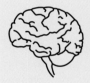 We cannot fix everyone, but the small gestures that go beyond the call of duty may make a difference to the woman who is vulnerable.

Families can apply to pay off debts and apply for benefits to buy food and a cooker. Sure Start is an area where the public health role of the midwife and clinical midwifery really combine and *The Strategic Review of Health Inequalities in England – Post 2010* (Marmot Review 2010) ensures that midwives play a key strategic role in promoting health and reducing inequalities for women.

See Boxes 5.5 and 5.6 for the seven Sure Start principles of care and the Sure Start targets.

Parenthood education programmes

There is a variety of ways in which parents can access childbirth education. This section outlines the options available. Parenthood education classes are also discussed. Parenthood education is a helpful way for prospective parents to meet others and build up a support network for the latter stages of pregnancy and after the baby is born. Parents can access parenthood education and attend childbirth classes in a number of ways and it is important that the midwife offers different choices to the woman and her partner.

Box 5.5   The seven Sure Start principles of care

1. Working with parents and children
2. Services for everyone
3. Flexible at the point of delivery
4. Starting very early
5. Respectful and transparent
6. Community driven and professionally co-ordinated
7. Outcome driven

Source: DfES (2002)

Box 5.6   Sure Start targets

- Ten percent reduction in children admitted to hospital with gastroenteritis, severe injury or respiratory infection
- Support and guidance on breastfeeding
- Identifying and supporting women with postnatal depression
- One hundred percent contact of all families within 2 months of birth
- Smoking reduction of at least 6%
- Antenatal information and support for parents
- Increased incidence of children having normal levels of language, communication, speech and literacy
- A 12% reduction in children who live in households in which neither parent works

NHS classes

These classes are facilitated by midwives and occasionally have input from other healthcare providers, such as health visitors and physiotherapists. The classes are often held at the local hospital, birth centre or GP surgery; they are free and available in the evenings when both parents can attend. Midwives may also run parenthood education for different groups of women, such as teenage mothers, lone mothers, couples or parents wanting to achieve a vaginal birth after a caesarean section.

Active birth classes

Active birth classes are fee based and are run by antenatal teachers who have been trained by the Active Birth Centre. Yoga is usually included, with an emphasis on relaxation, breathing and self-help methods for coping with labour. Many of the exercise and yoga classes are for women, incorporating the couple in the childbirth preparation and education classes.

National Childbirth Trust classes

Classes are provided by antenatal teachers trained by the NCT. They are kept to a maximum of around six couples and are held in community centres or at the teacher's home. The fee may be negotiated if a woman is on a low income. The focus is on informed choice and decision making, and issues such as pain relief, positions for labour and life with a new baby are addressed. There is also discussion around the medicalisation of birth and how to avoid a cascade of intervention and plan for a natural birth.

Parenthood education classes provide an opportunity to ask questions and explore areas of concern. As the classes usually involve couples, it is a way of including the partner in the pregnancy and birth, as well as providing information associated with support for the woman.

Birth plans

A birth plan is a means by which a woman can communicate her wishes to her midwives and hospital doctors. It may include choices such as wanting to use water for birth, avoiding the use of pethidine and wanting skin-to-skin contact with the baby immediately after birth (DH 2010, NICE 2007). The midwife can help the woman write her birth plan. Midwives need to ensure that they are the woman's advocate and that the woman is given balanced, non-judgemental and appropriate information at every stage so that she is able to make informed choices.

Midwifery records should reflect discussions and plans of how choices can be implemented. The latest NMC guidance determines that it is the midwife's duty to support and respect the woman's choice. The supervisor of midwives' integral role is supporting the midwife in facilitating the woman's choice (NMC 2006). The NMC (2006) notes that withdrawing a woman's choice of a homebirth is similar to an NHS trust withdrawing hospital services. Midwives need to have the courage to be advocates for the women they are supporting.

Midwifery wisdom

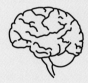

Birth wishes may not always go to plan for a couple, but always respect the woman's birth plan if possible. She has thought long and hard about what she wants and has taken the time to write it down. That in itself deserves your attention and respect.

When to call the midwife

When discussing choices and birth plans, it is useful for the woman to have information about when to call her midwife. She should be given information on how to make contact with her midwife and when to call, particularly when symptoms such as severe headache or reduced fetal movements may indicate that there could be a problem (see Box 5.7). It is useful for women and couples to know what is normal and when to call the midwife if they think labour has started.

Midwifery wisdom

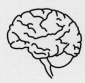

When a woman or her partner calls to say they think that labour may be beginning, they may have thought long and hard before picking up the phone so ensure you listen carefully to what is being said.

Box 5.7   Advice for women on when to call the midwife

- Baby's movements reduced
- Severe headache
- Severe itching
- Visual disturbances
- Epigastric (upper abdominal) pain
- Bleeding
- Abnormal discharge
- Spontaneous rupture of the membranes
- Contractions have started
- Needing reassurance

Conclusion

Choice for pregnant women is a key issue which the current government is keen to promote (Birthplace in England Collaborative Group 2011). The midwife has a responsibility to inform women of their choices. The DH (2010) endorses the importance of choice for all women where the midwife is the main co-ordinator of care. The different options available are particularly important for the midwife to explore with the woman when it comes to place of birth. Women may not know that they have the option of a birth centre or a homebirth, and these options should be given from the first booking appointment. Once the place of birth has been decided, the woman needs to know she can change her mind should she wish. A woman should be encouraged to write down or communicate her plans for birth. This can help her in exploring the options available and outline her wishes in respect of labour and the birth of her baby.

Parenting education is an important way of giving information to couples to help them arrive at their choices. There are many ways in which a woman can access classes and the midwife can inform her of what is available in her area. Models of care also vary in each area. There are different ways in which midwives can practise midwifery, from working within a hospital or birth centre to working outside the NHS as an independent midwife or caseloading for a group of women.

Models of care may vary but all women require information and respect and to be given the opportunity to make choices that meet their individual needs.

Quiz

Attempt the following 10 true or false questions related to programmes of care during childbirth to test your knowledge.

1. Giving birth in a consultant-led unit is more likely to lead to a normal birth.
2. Independent midwives are employed by the NHS.
3. Birth centres are managed and facilitated by midwives.
4. Birth centres for low-risk women have a variety of benefits including an increased normal birth rate and shorter labours.
5. Women who give birth in birth centres are less likely to breastfeed.
6. The safest place for a low-risk woman to give birth is in a consultant-led unit.
7. Sure Start programmes of care have been developed to support vulnerable women and families.
8. Parenthood education classes are facilitated by GPs.
9. Birth plans are written by the midwife for the woman to follow.
10. National Childbirth Trust classes are free.

References

Birth Choice UK (2007) Available at: www.birthchoiceuk.com/ (accessed May 2013).

Birthplace in England Collaborative Group (2011) Perinatal and maternal outcomes by planned place of birth for healthy women with low risk pregnancies: the Birthplace in England national prospective cohort study. *British Medical Journal* **343**: d7400.

Cluett ER, Pickering RM, Getliffe K, St George Saunders NJ (2004) Randomised controlled trial of labouring in water compared with standard management of dystocia in first stage of labour. *British Medical Journal* **328**: 314.

Daycare Trust (2011) Available at: www.daycaretrust.org.uk/pages/250-sure-start-childrens-centres-face-closure-within-a-year.html

Department for Education and Skills (DfES) (2002) *About Sure Start. Sure Start Unit.* Available at: www.education.gov.uk/childrenandyoungpeople/earlylearningandchildcare/delivery/surestart/a0076712/sure-start-children's-centres (accessed May 2013).

Department of Health (DH) (2003) *Tackling Health Inequalities: a programme for action.* London: Department of Health.

Department of Health (DH) (2004) *National Service Framework for Children and Young People.* London: Department of Health.

Department of Health (DH) *Midwifery* 2020: *delivering expectations.* London: Department of Health.

Department of Health (DH) (2011) *Saving Women's Lives: 2006–2008. Report of the Confidential Enquiry into Maternal Deaths.* London: Royal College of Obstetricians and Gynaecologists.

Dodwell M, Gibson R (2009) *An Investigation into Choice of Place of Birth.* London: National Childbirth Trust.

House of Commons Health Committee (2003) *Choice in Maternity Services.* Ninth Report of Session 2002–2003, Vol. 1. London: Stationery Office.

Lavender T (2003) *Report to the Department of Health Children's Taskforce from the Maternity and Neonatal Workforce Group.* London: Department of Health.

Marmot Review (2010) Available at: www.instituteofhealthequity.org/projects/fair-society-healthy-lives-the-marmot-review (accessed May 2013).

Milan M (2005) Independent midwifery compared with other caseload practice. *MIDIRS Midwifery Digest* **15**(4): 548–554.

National Institute for Health and Clinical Excellence (NICE) (2007) *Intrapartum Care Guidelines.* London: National Institute for Health and Clinical Excellence.

National Institute for Health and Clinical Excellence (NICE) (2008) *Routine Antenatal Care for Healthy Pregnant Women.* London: National Institute for Health and Clinical Excellence.

Nursing and Midwifery Council (NMC) (2006) *Midwives and Homebirths Circular.* Available at: www.nmc-uk.org/Documents/Circulars/2006circulars/NMC%20circular%2008_2006.pdf (accessed May 20013).

Nursing and Midwifery Council (NMC) (2012) *Midwives' Rules and Standards.* London: Nursing and Midwifery Council.

Olsen O, Jewell MD (2005) Home versus hospital birth. *Cochrane Database of Systematic Reviews* **3**: CD000352.

Rawnson S, Brown S, Wilkins J, Leamon J (2009) Student midwives' views of caseloading: the BUMP study. *British Journal of Midwifery* **17**(8): 484–489.

Rosser J (2003) How do the Albany midwives do it? Evaluation of the Albany Midwifery Practice. *MIDIRS Midwifery Digest* **13**(2): 251–257.

Royal College of Obstetricians and Gynaecologists (RCOG)/Royal College of Midwives (RCM) (2006) *Royal College of Obstetricians and Gynaecologists/Royal College of Midwives Joint Statement No.1. Immersion in water during labour and birth.* London: Royal College of Midwives.

Sandall J, Davies J, Warwick C (2001) *Evaluation of the Albany Midwifery Practice. Final Report.* London: King's College.

Van der Kooy B (2005) *The NHS Community Midwifery Model (NHS CMM).* London: Independent Midwives Association. Available at: www.independentmidwives.org.uk (accessed May 2013).

Walsh D (1999) An ethnographic study of women's experience of partnership caseload midwifery practice: the professional as a friend. *Midwifery* **15**: 165–176.

Walsh D (2005) Birth centre care: a review of the literature. *Birth Issues* **13**(4): 129–134.

Walsh D, Downe S (2004) Outcomes of free-standing, midwifery-led birth centres: a structured review of the evidence. *Birth* **31**(3): 222–229.

6

Interprofessional Working: Seamless Working within Maternity Care

Jenny Lorimer

Aim

The aim of this chapter is to help you to identify the people who you need to collaborate with and recognising some ideas and strategies to support you in working with them successfully. Achieving this success will be crucial to you in maintaining the standard of the care you provide throughout your professional working life.

Learning outcomes

By the end of this chapter you will be able to:

1. consider the professional standards of midwifery and other professions and how they impact on the people being cared for
2. examine the interprofessional aspects of a care pathway
3. consider the opportunities for and barriers to collaborative working
4. discuss theories and concepts behind successful team working
5. consider how knowledge of complexity theory can support work in the clinical environment.

The Student's Guide to Becoming a Midwife, Second Edition. Edited by Ian Peate and Cathy Hamilton.
© 2014 John Wiley & Sons, Ltd. Published 2014 by John Wiley & Sons, Ltd.

Introduction

Any student new to midwifery will very quickly become familiar with the Nursing and Midwifery Council (NMC) standards of conduct, performance and ethics. Students registered on any midwifery programme will remain familiar with these important standards throughout their programmes and then through their working lives.

The focus of this chapter is to integrate the following statement from these standards: 'the people in your care must be able to trust you with their health and well-being' (NMC 2008, p2) within the concept of inter-professional working. If we explore what is involved in how this trust is achieved, it inevitably leads us to our working relationships with other professionals as much as our relationships with the people in our care. Building on this, Midwifery 2020 (DH 2010) is more explicit in explaining the role of the midwife within multidisciplinary or multiagency teams. The vision described in this paper places the midwife firmly as the 'key co-ordinator within the multidisciplinary team' (DH 2010) for women with complex pregnancies. With direct reference to midwifery education, it states that there will be an 'increased emphasis on the principles of autonomy and accountability within multidisciplinary and multiagency teams' (DH 2010).

Other healthcare undergraduates such as nursing, physiotherapy and pharmacy have similar needs through their education and working practice. To help the undergraduate on a healthcare programme prepare for these responsibilities, higher education institutions have incorporated interprofessional education (IPE) within their healthcare programmes.

There has been a national mandate for interprofessional collaborative working within health and social care for many years. Initially, the need was identified and explored by the World Health Organization during the 1970s. This was followed in the UK by an acceleration of development because of the influence of government policy during the 1980s and 1990s. Continued well-publicised failures in the care of patients/service users/clients have meant that currently many healthcare regulatory bodies include the necessity of interprofessional collaborative working within their standards (GMC 2009, HCPC 2009, NMC 2008). Such is the fundamental importance of successful interprofessional working that healthcare programmes will usually incorporate elements of interprofessional education. The over-riding goal of interprofessional education must be to ensure that graduates are equipped with the knowledge, skills and attitudes to ensure they are able to work collaboratively for the benefit of their patients/service users/clients throughout their working lives.

Activity 6.1

Look up the reports of one of the following cases and read the summary.

- The Protection of Children in England: A Progress Report: www.education.gov.uk/publications/eOrderingDownload/HC-330.pdf (accessed May 2013)
- The Victoria Climbié Inquiry: Report of an Inquiry by Lord Laming: www.publications.parliament.uk/pa/cm200203/cmselect/cmhealth/570/570.pdf (accessed May 2013)
- The Inquiry into the Management of Care of Children receiving Complex Heart Surgery at the Bristol Royal Infirmary: webarchive.nationalarchives.gov.uk/20090811143745/http://www.bristol-inquiry.org.uk/final_report/rpt_print.htm (accessed May 2013)
- Final Report of the Independent Inquiry into Care Provided by Mid Staffordshire NHS Foundation Trust (The Francis Report): www.midstaffsinquiry.com/pressrelease.html (accessed May 2013)

Activity 6.2

Make a list of the points that are relevant to you in your professional practice as a midwife.

Central to the goal of IPE is a usable definition. It is most commonly described as 'when two or more professions learn with, from and about each other to improve collaboration and the quality of care' (CAIPE 2002).

We need to explore the meaning of interprofessional collaborative working in the context of midwifery. Services that are involved in providing maternity care for women may be from the NHS, social care, the voluntary sector or other organisations such as government agencies. Some women will have their care provided in the community, others in the hospital setting. Care will often be provided by midwives and obstetricians. However, the situation is not always as conveniently straightforward. There are women who will have more complex needs, some of which may be social needs. Maternity care may then involve organisations such as children's services, learning disability and mental health teams, domestic abuse teams and drug and alcohol teams. Using this more complicated example, the situation can be more obviously seen to require interprofessional, interagency and cross-organisation collaboration in order to achieve seamless maternity care. The aim of the care would be for all the professionals in all the agencies to be communicating and collaborating effectively. Thinking of the most complex maternity care scenarios illustrates how important, and yet challenging, true collaborative working can be.

Working with other professionals

When you look at the codes of conduct of different professions, you will find many similarities between them. There are some general principles that apply to all healthcare professions. Some examples include always trying to do the best for the people in our care and co-operating with colleagues. Can you think of some others?

To help you learn more, look at the Nursing and Midwifery Council (NMC) code of conduct, performance and ethics and write a list of the qualities you need to consistently demonstrate throughout your professional life. Now think of a colleague from a different profession with whom you work regularly in the clinical environment. This could be a medical practitioner, paediatric nurse, radiographer or any other you think is particularly relevant to you. Look up their professional body's code of conduct, performance and ethics and write a list of the qualities that they need to demonstrate. Place the two lists side by side and highlight all the similarities. Are there any significant differences? What are the consequences of the similarities and differences in the two sets of qualities for the people in our care?

To help you in this task, Box 6.1 gives a list for the profession of diagnostic radiography.

Now we are going to consider an episode of care where the interprofessional working was less than ideal. Use the example below to help you think of an episode that you were either involved in or know about. Start by writing a brief description of an event. Where were the challenges in achieving

Box 6.1   Standards of conduct, performance and ethics (HCPC 2012)

The registrant must...

Act in the best interests of service users.
Respect the confidentiality of service users.
Keep high standards of personal conduct.
Provide (to us and any other relevant regulators) any important information about your conduct and
     competence.
Keep your professional knowledge and skills up to date.
Act within the limits of your knowledge, skills and experience and, if necessary, refer the matter to
     another practitioner.
Communicate properly and effectively with service users and other practitioners.
Effectively supervise tasks that you have asked other people to carry out.
Get informed consent to provide care or services (so far as possible).
Keep accurate records.
Deal fairly and safely with the risks of infection.
Limit your work or stop practising if your performance or judgement is affected by your health.
Behave with honesty and integrity and make sure that your behaviour does not damage the public's
     confidence in you or your profession.
Make sure that any advertising you do is accurate.

seamless care for the woman in the episode that you are aware of? Identify where you think events did not work as they should have. Can you identify possible reasons for the difficulties encountered?

Example

A woman who was 26 weeks pregnant was diagnosed with diabetes. She was referred to the medical team but the midwife responsible for her care was not informed. The woman attended her general practitioner (GP) in a state of distress because of the conflicting advice she was being given over her plans for breastfeeding and her care during labour.

Care pathways

One tool currently used to try and optimise care of women in maternity care (in common with many areas of health and social care) is a care pathway. The aim of a care pathway is to support the standardisation of care processes a woman may require so that there is decreased variability in care provided and the outcome is optimised. The multidisciplinary element (and interprofessional working) has to be implicit within any care pathway. Using care pathways helps to ensure that a specific group of service users are on a structured, organised and efficient clinical course which has their needs at the centre of care. Care pathways allow room for planning so that any interventions needed can be defined, used to the best effect and used at the right time.

Midwifery wisdom

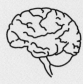

One of the most significant aims is to ensure that the focus remains on the woman and her care rather than on the specialisms providing that care.

Case study 6.1

Paramedics are called to a shopping centre in a large city. A young woman has collapsed while browsing in the shops. Shop assistants have given basic first aid and the woman is now conscious but obviously unable to speak any English. The woman is taken to the nearest accident and emergency department where she is examined and noted to have a low Body Mass Index (BMI) and to be in the middle trimester of pregnancy.

Consider the scenario highlighted in Case study 6.1. How many of the professionals mentioned in Table 6.1 are likely to be involved in the care of this woman? What are their roles? Using a care pathway (based on the National Service Framework), draw a likely path for this woman through the variety of services that she may need to access. Make sure that the woman and her child are at the centre of the process. Use arrows to show how information is shared. You can use a variety of arrow formats to show how well the

Table 6.1 Professionals who may be involved (in alphabetical order)

Professional	Role
Adult nurse	
Diagnostic radiographer (sonographer)	
Dietician	
Health visitor	
Interpreter	
General practitioner	
Government agencies	
Midwife	
Obstetrician	
Paramedic	
Social worker	

different agencies work together (e.g. bold arrows for established partners and interrupted arrows for liaisons that are more challenging). Retain your diagram so that you can review it after the next section.

Barriers to and opportunities for collaborative working

Collaborative working is so fundamental to the concept of interprofessional working that it is important to take some time to examine it in depth. We should start by being sure of what we mean by collaboration.

The definition below is appropriate for our purposes in this text:

> *an active and ongoing partnership, often between people from diverse backgrounds, who work together to solve problems or provide services*

(Barr et al. 2005).

Language

We will start by considering the use of language when we are working with other professionals to provide a high-quality service to women and their families. If we take a moment to consider how we learned language as small children, we can see that some language is learned formally and some informally. As children, we began by hearing conversations around us, and being spoken to directly (informal learning). A more formal approach to learning language began when we started school. Here, we were asked to read, write and learn spellings. As we grew up, these different ways of learning language merged and we became able to put the informal and formal learning together.

There are very clear parallels with learning our own profession-specific language during higher education. In the academic environment, lectures, tutorials and textbooks are all used for formal learning of our new professions and the required language. This learning is then compounded, and sometimes confused, with informal learning of language in the clinical environment as students. Similarly, as we progressed through our early education, there was a process of socialisation with those we are surrounded by. One consequence of the higher education system for healthcare professions is that this language learning is often going on only in single profession-specific environments. The obvious outcome of all this learning, and the source of difficulties, is that each healthcare profession will have its own jargon (Marshall et al. 2011). Some words, abbreviations and acronyms will be the same, others different, depending on the professional group and scenario being considered. A good example is the acronym 'BM'. Depending on your discipline, it could mean either breast milk or bowel movement. This is a really good illustration of some potential confusion. Can you think of other abbreviations that are likely to result in confusion?

Midwifery wisdom

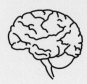

We need to remember not to assume that others interpret jargon in the same way as we do.

We need to think carefully how using our 'own' profession-specific jargon excludes not only other professions but the women and their families for whom we are caring. If women, their families and healthcare professionals are to work together in a truly collaborative manner, use of jargon has to be seen as a potential barrier. How can midwives make sure that language is not a barrier between themselves and the client?

Hierarchy and power

Many authors discuss the hierarchical structure of health and social care. The co-dependent issues of power and hierarchy are often seen as barriers to collaboration in interprofessional teams (Brown et al. 2011, Howkins & Bray 2008, Pollard et al. 2010). Traditionally medicine is seen as a hierarchical structure with the consultant as the leader (Eraut 1994). Other professions have often been regarded as subservient to medicine.

If we consider working within an interprofessional team, an existing hierarchy might have a negative effect. It is possible that the team members believed to be more superior in the hierarchy can be perceived as having a stronger voice. As mentioned above, in midwifery, if the midwife is to be key co-ordinator within the team (DH 2010) then the presupposed hierarchy may need to be reassessed. An interprofessional maternity team should value all opinions equally, with the woman's needs being central. This requires a commitment from all members to value each member and each discipline in the same way. Here lies a challenge for newly qualified midwives as they will need to have the confidence to take their part within this team.

Refer back to your list of professionals involved in the care of the woman in the care pathway. Can you create some examples of where a typical hierarchy might be either useful or an undermining factor?

Attitudes to other professions

If we are honest with ourselves, as we develop human relationships we all experience some degree of prejudgement, prejudice and stereotypical views. Working in an interprofessional team requires us to recognise these views and be aware of how they may affect our judgement in our professional lives. Difficulties arise in team working if we are not aware of how these views may affect our actions. Typically, these prejudices and stereotypes may involve ethnicity, religion, gender, nationality, body habitus, sexual orientation or even hair colour. In addition to these, we can develop similar prejudice and stereotypical views about other professions, e.g. some may believe that all doctors are arrogant and all nurses are caring.

Activity 6.3

 Complete the table below which lists many of the professions that you will encounter in your working life as a midwife. Write an adjective that you think best describes each profession. Then use the third column to suggest an honest reason for your choice of adjective.

Profession	Adjective	Reason
Medical practitioner		
Paramedic		

Profession	Adjective	Reason
Adult nurse		
Paediatric nurse		
Social worker		
Porter		
Midwife		
Radiographer		
Physiotherapist		
Health visitor		

It is important for our practice that we genuinely reflect on our views so that we learn from experiences. Take some time to review your answers in the above table and to consider how this may affect your practice.

Did you include any of the following adjectives: caring, practical, team player, good communicator, intelligent, hard working, unapproachable, inefficient, arrogant, unsupportive, rude, aggressive, bully? (van Rijswijk et al. 2006). Is it acceptable for us to have preconceived ideas about other healthcare professionals if we are to achieve our aim?

Midwifery wisdom

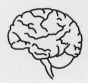
As professionals, we have to give the same standard of care to every service user regardless of our attitudes. Equally, we are obliged to work co-operatively with every other profession in an equal manner.

Communication

For interprofessional teams to work together collaboratively and effectively, each member needs to communicate with each other and the woman they are caring for. Having well-developed capabilities as a communicator is one of the most important skills for a healthcare professional (Brown et al. 2011). There are many facets to effective communication and each of them is important.

The first aspect of effective communication is understanding the role of each of the professional members of the team. We have already mentioned how understanding other professional roles is important. Making assumptions about what others are trying to achieve is not likely to lead to success.

One of the challenges faced by newly qualified members of a profession is having sufficient confidence to check their own understanding. This is not always easy and is likely to be more difficult across members of an interprofessional team. By understanding what others are trying to achieve, and in consultation with the woman in our care, the interprofessional team is able to have a shared, mutually agreed goal. In a team, if every professional's views and knowledge are considered, and each team member is allowed to contribute, there is likely to be consensus. This agreed goal is often crucial to the successful functioning of a team.

This activity needs to extend beyond each team member contributing equally, as the question of information sharing is key here. Information sharing can be considered from two different perspectives. The first is how the information is shared, such as forms, service users' notes, IT systems, email, etc. A difficulty is that it would be possible to list a large number of ways in which information is shared. In tandem with this is making sure that every professional understands the need for appropriate information sharing (Pollard et al. 2010). Understanding each other's roles helps members of the interprofessional team to determine what information needs to be shared.

Using your list compiled earlier in Activity 6.3, carry out some research about the goal of each professional. The key points of the role of the physiotherapist are listed below to help you get started:

- Physiotherapists work with people of all ages who may have physical difficulties which can be associated with illness, accident or ageing.
- Movement is seen as fundamental to recovering or continuing health and well-being of the individual.
- Physiotherapists aim to recognise and exploit movement potential.
- Physiotherapists are involved in health promotion, preventive healthcare, treatment and rehabilitation.
- Techniques used by physiotherapists include manual therapy, therapeutic exercises and application of electrophysical modalities.

Active listening is a term that has become popular in healthcare. It means that you ensure your understanding of what the speaker has said is the same as the speaker's understanding of what was said. There are several strategies involved in active listening. The first is to maintain eye contact with the person speaking. This will let the speaker know that you are listening and assure them that the conversation is focused on them. The second point is to *really listen* to what the person is saying. Whether it is another health professional or a service user, we can often find ourselves concentrating on our answer or other ideas rather than truly listening to the person speaking.

It is always important to clarify your understanding of what is being said to avoid misunderstandings and misconceptions. You can do this in two ways. The first is to mentally repeat what the person is saying inside your head. The second way is by repeating back to the speaker your understanding of the information being given.

One really important point which can often get overlooked, particularly in a busy environment, is that the listener shouldn't interrupt. When listening, we should always try and respect the speaker and avoid being judgemental. To help the person who is speaking (we often need the person we are caring for us to tell us things they may not normally share with others), we can give feedback both verbally, using short expressions of agreement, or by positive body language (see later). These steps will help to stimulate dialogue which ensures both parties know that the correct information has been given and received.

Activity 6.4

Write a brief list of all the points mentioned in the paragraph above and learn them by heart. You can use the mnemonic below: Every Really Caring Individual Feels Rewarded. The next time you have a reasonably long conversation, try and put them all into action. At the end of the conversation. ask the speaker how they felt during the dialogue.

Every	eye contact
Really	really listen
Caring	clarify
Individual	(don't) interrupt
Feels	feedback
Rewarded	respect

As indicated above, listening to what is being said is not sufficient for active listening. We also need to be aware of body language (also called non-verbal communication). Non-verbal communication forms a significant part of personal interactions. Initially, this means observing and considering the speaker's body language but equally important is being aware of our own body language so the person we are talking to receives the signals we intend.

There are many texts, papers and websites offering advice on non-verbal communication. It is important to remember that any source should be used in general terms as there may be multiple interpretations of the same signals. Another cautionary note is that many signals have more than one meaning. Is the person sitting with their arms crossed putting up a barrier to what is being said (boredom or disagreement) or are they merely cold?

For each of the following elements of non-verbal communication, make a note of what you would interpret it as meaning. Would you take it as a positive or negative sign?

- Facial expressions: smiling, tight-lipped, frowning
- Eyes: contact or looking away, focused or glazed, others such as eye rolling
- Head movements: nodding, shaking, looking up or down
- Personal space: the distance may vary from touching to 1 metre or more
- Arms and legs: crossed or held apart
- Hand movements: fingers interlinked, open palm gesture or pointing
- Using props such as a pencil: brandishing or pointing
- The other person mirrors your body position

Look back at your list. Can you now add a second, different interpretation to each element? An example is smiling which can be interpreted as pleasure, and so a positive gesture. However, smiling can also be used as a sign of sarcasm and therefore a negative gesture.

We all learn aspects of non-verbal communication alongside learning verbal communication as a small child. By being more aware and more skilled at interpreting signals, we will become better at understanding what is being communicated, reducing the chances of misunderstandings and miscommunications.

Treating other members of the interprofessional team as partners to support them in developing their own self-confidence will promote the development of mutual trust. This mutual respect will allow each member of the team to build on their strengths. By allowing each individual time to express their views, the interprofessional team will work together better (Pollard et al. 2010).

Team working: Tuckman and Belbin

This chapter started by discussing how professional knowledge is an essential aspect of all qualified professionals. We are all able to recognise that it is not possible for any one professional to have all the knowledge and skills necessary to meet a client's needs (Barrett et al. 2005). The obvious next step is to recognise that in order to provide seamless care, all healthcare professionals need to work in effective teams. Just as understanding other professionals' roles and being aware of different aspects of communication are needed for effective interprofessional working, the same is true of team working.

A team can be defined as a group of people who are concentrating on achieving the same goal. The successful outcome of teamwork relies on sharing responsibilities and productive interaction between team members (Robinson & Cottrell 2005). Interprofessional teamwork in modern healthcare plays an important role in delivering high-quality services to patients and can be described as a dynamic process of collaboration between healthcare professionals with interdependent professional knowledge and backgrounds (Xyrichis & Ream 2008).

The next section of this chapter will address theories and concepts behind good team working. This will not guarantee that any team that you are part of during your professional life will be effective. However, knowing about and understanding relevant theories will help you to understand team-working situations you are involved in. This is important if you are in a team where the functioning is not effective as it could be. Being aware of strategies that can be used to evolve team behaviour is useful. Awareness can help an individual to develop behaviours so that a more positive outcome can be achieved where difficulties and challenges are being experienced.

The first theory of team working we will look at is that proposed by Bruce Tuckman during the 1960s (Tuckman & Jensen 1977). Tuckman's theory is one of the most widely known and accepted. He describes team working as a number of phases in a particular sequence that members of a team will go through when tackling a task. Initially, four phases were proposed: forming, storming, norming and performing. Additional phases (adjourning and transforming) were then proposed and different texts will cite them according to the context being discussed. This chapter will consider the four phases that were initially proposed as these are most relevant to interprofessional working within the healthcare setting.

Forming occurs when a group initially starts to work as a team. There are commonly certain behaviours going on within the team at this stage. Team members may be unclear as to the goals and objectives of the team initially and members will often be mostly self-motivated. Individual roles and responsibilities may be unclear. If there is a leader in the team, it is likely that the other members will be heavily reliant on this person to inform and direct behaviours and tasks. It is at this stage that members of the group may test both each other and the leader.

The second phase is storming. Now the individuals in the team are likely to compete with each other for their positions within the team and subgroups are likely to form. Members of the team are likely to be distracted from the goal and the team's functioning is likely to be poor during this phase.

Team functioning becomes more settled during the third, norming, phase. Individuals' roles and responsibilities are likely to be better defined and team members are usually clear about the common goal. Where there is a leader, the role is likely to be more one of facilitator than actively leading the team. Team members will have developed respect for each other.

During the fourth phase, performing, behaviour will be cohesive and decisions are generally made collaboratively and unanimously. Any disagreements will be resolved in a straightforward manner. The team may develop a social life at this stage.

The benefits of effective interprofessional team working are that individuals will develop mutual trust and respect and they will both understand and value the other members both as individuals and representatives of their professions. In this effective functioning, all members will be making productive contributions towards a common goal, and there is efficient use of resources and useful sharing of information. All of this will lead to positive emotions in the team members, which will help behaviours to be reinforced and reproduced, meaning that the team is likely to continue the effective functioning.

The second theory of team working was developed by Meredith Belbin. He spent years studying team behaviours and his work focused on the roles people play within teams (Belbin 2004). His theory recognises that individuals have different personal characteristics and different strengths and the consequence of this is that we are likely to react differently from others in similar situations. Belbin proposed that for a team to work well, it needs to be balanced in terms of the way individual members react and work. These characteristics are based on personal preferences and tendencies. Currently Belbin has identified nine different roles that describe tendencies demonstrated when working in teams. This theory does not mean that you need nine people to make a successful team, more that people in a successful team need to have complementary characteristics from among the nine roles. Two examples of the roles Belbin has described are the 'monitor-evaluator' and 'completer-finisher'. If we look at these two roles in terms of their characteristics, we can see how the roles would complement each other in successful teamwork.

The monitor-evaluator will have a tendency to be the analytical member of the team. They will naturally be objective in examining problems and complex issues. In teamwork, they will be the member who monitors team progress towards the goal and they will also often be the one whose analysis prevents mistakes.

The completer-finisher is the person who has an eye for detail and is likely to spot mistakes and gaps. This preference for keeping an eye on detail will highlight the quality of the work.

While these roles complement each other and would each add an important dimension to successful teamwork, it is also clear that a team composed of two completer-finishers and two monitor-evaluators is unlikely to be successful.

There are many textbooks and free websites which will allow you to discover your own Belbin role. You may find it a useful exercise to complete a questionnaire from one of them so that you become more aware of your own strengths, preferences and tendencies. The team roles we use are not permanent but may develop as we develop knowledge, skills and expertise. We are also likely to react differently in different situations. An emergency in the clinical environment is likely to cause us to react with a particular set of behaviours compared to a non-urgent situation within our home lives.

Complexity theory: dealing with uncertainty

One only needs to have experienced the NHS as a service user to realise that not only is it an extremely large organisation but it is also very complex. Once you start working within it, the complexities become very apparent and can sometimes seem overwhelming. There are systems within systems, some of which work together and others which operate with complete disregard for others. In addition, the demands on the system are neither stable nor consistent and vary constantly, e.g. day and night, summer and winter. We are able to manage this level of complexity by thinking of the whole system as a number of component parts, e.g. accident and emergency, radiology, outpatients, etc.

Within these subdivisions, many of the professions tend to simplify their own working patterns so that the complexity again becomes manageable. For example, medicine could be described as working on a reductionist approach where health is considered as the absence of disease, and where our understanding of the human body is broken down into specific areas, e.g. anatomy and physiology. This allows us to be comfortable with our specific areas of knowledge as a comprehensive understanding of the whole is not possible. The more you learn about a clinical environment, the more specific areas and subdivisions become apparent.

Within the profession of midwifery (or any other), there is very naturally a tendency to focus on only our own discipline and specialism so that we can function comfortably within our role. This method of dividing the whole into manageable sections makes the task of client-focused care more challenging. We can consider a woman due to give birth to twins as the same as any other woman giving birth to twins but that simple categorisation does not allow us to consider the individual woman's needs, e.g. diabetes, social needs, etc. However, we began this chapter by discussing how, in order to provide seamless care, we need to be able to work collaboratively with a number of different disciplines and agencies. We clearly have a dilemma here, and complexity theory can help us understand how we can resolve it.

By making the care we provide 'patient centred', we can continue to be comfortable making expert decisions within our own area of expertise. It will also help us to recognise when a situation varies from what we are used to. Being comfortable working with a range of different disciplines will support us in attempting to make the care we provide seamless. Working collaboratively with other professions will allow us to consider situations from a variety of perspectives, and solutions that are suited to individual clients may be more easily discovered and put into effect.

Conclusion

The learning in this chapter will be an important factor to help you to build a successful career. In completing the activities and exercises, you will have considered the impact of professional standards from both a midwifery point of view as well as the perspectives of other professionals. For successful interprofessional working, both perspectives are equally important. Using care pathways as a focus helps to demonstrate where interprofessional working has a very real impact on the care we are able to give our clients. This chapter does not describe good interprofessional working as easy, and reflection on both the opportunities and barriers will help any professional develop better practice. Being aware of the theories of team working and roles as well as complexity theory will help make sense of interactions and complex situations that are a daily occurrence in our working lives in providing high-quality maternity care.

Quiz

1. Fill in the blanks in the following statement.

    'The people in your care must be able to trust you with their _____ '

2. Fill in the blanks in the following statement.

    'Interprofessional working occurs when two or more _____ learn with, from and about each other to improve _____ and the_____ '

3. Explain the following midwifery-specific terms to someone outside the profession.

   a. Manual removal of placenta
   b. Lower section caesarean section
   c. Spontaneous rupture of membranes
   d. Postpartum haemorrhage

4. What are the four stages of team work described by Tuckman?
5. Explain what happens during the second phase of Tuckman's model.
6. How many roles are described and explained by Belbin?
7. Explain the likely behaviour of a completer-finisher in a team.
8. Explain the mnemonic that can help you to practise and become an active listener.
9. Explain the following examples of non-verbal communication: tight-lipped, focused eye contact, looking up, personal space less than 20 cm, legs crossed, pointing with finger or pencil, body mirroring.
10. What is the reductionist approach in health?

References

Barr H, Koppel I, Reeves S, Hammick, M, Freeth D (2005) *Effective Interprofessional Education. Argument, assumption and evidence*. Oxford: Blackwell Publishing Ltd.

Barrett G, Sellman D, Thomas J (2005) *Interprofessional Working in Health and Social Care. Professional perspectives*. London: Palgrave Macmillan.

Belbin RM (2004) *Management Teams: why they succeed or fail*, 2nd edn. Oxford: Elsevier Butterworth-Heinemann.

Brown J, Lewis L, Ellis K et al. (2011) Conflict on interprofessional primary health care teams – can it be resolved? *Journal of Interprofessional Care* **25**: 4–10.

Centre for the Advancement of Interprofessional Education (CAIPE) (2002) Available at: www.caipe.org.uk/resources/ (accessed May 2013).

Department of Health (DH) (2010) *Midwifery 2020: delivering expectations*. London: Department of Health.

Eraut M (1994) *Developing Professional Knowledge and Competence*. Oxford: Routledge Falmer.

General Medical Council (GMC) (2009) *Tomorrow's Doctors. Outcomes and standards for undergraduate medical education*. London: General Medical Council.

Health and Care Professions Council (HCPC) (2009) *Standards of Proficiency – Radiographers*. London: Health and Care Professions Council.

Health and Care Professions Council (HCPC) (2012) *Standards of Performance, Conduct and Ethics*. London: Health and Care Professions Council.

Howkins E, Bray J (eds) (2008) *Preparing for Interprofessional Teaching: theory and practice*. Oxford: Radcliffe.

Marshall C, Medves J, Docherty D, Paterson M (2011) Interprofessional jargon: how is it exclusionary? Cultural determinants of language use in health care practice. *Journal of Interprofessional Care* **25**(6): 452–453.

Nursing and Midwifery Council (NMC) (2008) *The Code: atandards of conduct, performance and ethics for nurses and midwives*. London: Nursing and Midwifery Council.

Pollard K, Thomas J, Miers M (2010) *Understanding Interprofessional Working in Health and Social Care*. London: Palgrave Macmillan.

Robinson M, Cottrell D (2005) Health professionals in multi-disciplinary and multi-agency teams: changing professional practice. *Journal of Interprofessional Care* **19**(6): 547–560.

Tuckman BW, Jensen MAC (1977) Stages of small-group development revisited. *Group Organiz Studies* **2**(4): 419–427.

Van Rijswijk W, Haslam S, Ellemers N (2006) Who do we think we are? The effects of social context and social identification on in-group stereotyping. *British Journal of Social Psychology* **45**: 161–174.

Xyrichis A, Ream E (2008) Teamwork: a concept analysis. *Journal of Advanced Nursing* **61**(2): 232–241.

7

Intrapartum Care
Annabel Jay and Cathy Hamilton

Aim

To introduce the student midwife to the principles of supporting a woman during the intrapartum period with a focus on the promotion of a normal birth.

Learning outcomes

By the end of this chapter you will:

1. be able to define 'normality' in relation to labour and childbirth
2. have an understanding of factors which lead to the onset of labour
3. be able to recognise the signs which may Indicate the onset of labour
4. be aware of the different methods of pain relief which may be offered during labour
5. be able to describe methods that a midwife may use when assessing a woman's progress in labour
6. be able to describe the role of the midwife in supporting a woman and her family during childbirth
7. be aware of the importance of practising in a holistic way in order to avoid unnecessary intervention by treating each woman as an individual.

Introduction

The midwife is the expert in normal childbirth. It is her role to promote and support the normal physiology of labour, whilst noting any signs of variations from the norm that might harm the woman or her baby. The *Midwives' Rules and Standards* (NMC 2012) require the midwife to report any deviations from the norm to another suitably qualified health professional (who may be a doctor) with the

The Student's Guide to Becoming a Midwife, Second Edition. Edited by Ian Peate and Cathy Hamilton.
© 2014 John Wiley & Sons, Ltd. Published 2014 by John Wiley & Sons, Ltd.

Box 7.1   Definition of normal birth

- Birth without caesarean section
- Birth without assisted delivery (ventouse or forceps)
- No induction of labour
- No regional anaesthesia (epidural or spinal block)

Source: Maternity Care Working Party (2007).

necessary skills required to manage the situation. In order to do this, the midwife should have a clear understanding of what is meant by a 'normal' labour and birth. The focus of this chapter will be on the midwife's role in the promotion of a normal labour resulting in a safe and memorable childbirth experience for the woman and her family.

Definitions of normality

There is currently no standard or universally acceptable definition of a 'normal' birth. The term has different meanings for obstetricians, midwives and members of the public. Even within the midwifery profession, individuals may hold different definitions, ranging from anything short of a caesarean section at one end of the scale to a totally physiological birth without any intervention at the other. Most people, however, would probably consider normal birth to be somewhere between these two extremes (Mead 2004).

For the purpose of statistics, the government has adopted the definition of normal birth proposed by the Maternity Care Working Party (2007) (see Box 7.1)

The World Health Organization (WHO 1996) advises that interventions to the physiological process of birth should not occur without a clear rationale. Examples of such interventions are induced labour, restriction of a woman's mobility, the use of continuous fetal monitoring, the withholding of food and fluid and the routine use of vaginal examinations to assess labour progress.

Midwifery wisdom

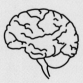
Midwifery is the 'art of doing nothing well' (Kennedy 2000).

Stages of labour

Labour has been traditionally divided into three stages:

1. The onset of labour to the time when the cervix (neck of the womb) is fully opened to allow the fetus to move down into the birth canal.

2. From when the cervix is fully open to the birth of the baby.
3. From when the baby is delivered to the expulsion of the placenta (afterbirth) and membranes from the woman's body.

The organisation of labour into these three stages has been challenged by some writers, who suggest that labour should be considered as a continuum, with physiological, physical and emotional factors playing an integral part in the process (Walsh 2011).

Promoting spontaneous labour: avoiding induction of labour

Over 20% of pregnant women have their labour induced (BirthChoiceUK 2012). In most cases, this is because the pregnancy is prolonged but is otherwise normal. It is current practice in most maternity units to offer routine induction of labour to women whose pregnancy goes beyond 41 weeks (NICE 2008). Whilst there is little argument against induction for serious obstetric complications, it should be remembered that the process is an invasive procedure requiring many interventions.

'Sweeping the membranes'

This process involves the midwife inserting a gloved forefinger through the cervical os and rotating it in a circular fashion to separate the membranes from the lower uterine area. This causes prostaglandins to be released which promote cervical effacement (thinning and stretching) and dilation. Research shows that 'a sweep' increases the chances of labour starting spontaneously within the next 48 hours and can reduce the need for other methods of induction (NICE 2008). It is only possible if the cervix is already open sufficiently to admit a finger. This should never be forced. This process may be carried out in the antenatal clinic or the woman's home and may result in a 'show' (a lightly blood-stained mucous discharge) and some mild cramps afterwards. The current NICE guidelines recommend that a sweep should be offered prior to any induction process (NICE 2008).

Onset of spontaneous labour

The timing of the start of labour in humans is less precise than it is in other species. It is suggested that the average day of onset is 39.6 weeks' gestation (Howie & Rankin 2011a). The underlying mechanism of labour is still not fully understood although the timing of its onset is believed to be related to fetal brain activity. It is suggested that adrenocorticotrophic hormone (ACTH) is released from the fetal pituitary gland which causes the woman's hormone progesterone to be converted to oestrogen. This in turn increases the sensitivity of the uterus to prostaglandins and oxytocin, which are produced by both the mother and the fetus (Howie & Rankin 2011a). These hormones cause the uterine muscle fibres to contract and shorten, so stimulating the beginning of labour. Studies demonstrate that where there is an abnormality in the fetal hypothalamus and pituitary gland, prolonged pregnancy may follow (Johnson & Everitt 2007).

Case study 7.1

Fiona was expecting her first baby and was 3 days overdue. That morning she was very excited when she noticed a small amount of blood in her underwear. She felt sure that she was going into labour and would probably give birth that night. Indeed, as the day went on she began to experience regular contractions, which became more and more painful and that night she was unable to sleep. However, in the morning the contractions subsided and for the rest of the day she felt no further pain. She felt disheartened and wondered if she would ever go into labour.

She spent the rest of the day in bed and slept deeply. At midnight, contractions resumed and became longer, stronger and more frequent. She went into hospital at 0200 hours and eventually gave birth at 1100 hours. This was almost 3 days after she had first noticed the show and to Fiona seemed like a very long time.

Signs that labour is starting

Onset of uterine contractions

As labour begins, the formerly painless uterine tightenings (Braxton Hicks contractions) increase in frequency and the woman starts to feel discomfort with the contractions. This may be felt as pain in the lower abdomen, the lower back or the tops of the legs. The woman will eventually notice that this discomfort coincides with a tightening of her uterus. At first, the uterine contractions occur approximately every 15–20 min and may only last 20–30 seconds. However, as labour progresses they begin to increase in length, strength and frequency, leading to effacement and dilation of the cervix.

Passage of a Mucous 'show'

During pregnancy, the cervical canal contains a plug of mucus (the operculum), which is believed to protect the fetus from infection. As the cervix begins to dilate in early labour, this Mucous plug will often be dislodged and the woman will notice a blood-stained discharge in her underwear or after she has passed urine. This is often the first sign that labour is imminent, although it may still be some hours or days before it begins in earnest. Some women are never aware of the passage of this show.

Spontaneous rupture of the membranes ('the waters breaking')

This may occur before the onset of labour or at any time during labour. It is not a true sign that labour has begun unless it is accompanied by dilation of the cervix.

Spontaneous rupture of the membranes can be recognised by the sudden loss of a significant amount of clear fluid from the vagina. However, for some women this may not be instantly recognisable if only very small amounts of fluid are lost. If the fetal presenting part is engaged deeply in the pelvis then this could well be the case. Small amounts of fluid loss could be mistaken for urinary incontinence, which is common in the latter stages of pregnancy due to excessive pressure of the fetus on the bladder. The midwife will need to take a careful history from the woman. Continued observation of fluid lost from the vagina will usually lead to a definite confirmation that spontaneous rupture of the membranes has occurred. Approximately 60% of women will start to labour spontaneously within 24 hours of their membranes rupturing (NICE 2007).

Other signs

Some women feel nauseous as labour approaches and others experience mild diarrhoea as uterine activity stimulates bowel movement. Some women become preoccupied with cleaning and tidying their homes in preparation for the arrival of the newborn. This is referred to as the 'nesting' instinct (Johnston 2004, Odent 2003).

Midwifery care in early labour

When the midwife receives a call from a woman in early labour, she needs to take a history to ascertain whether the woman should come directly into hospital for assessment or whether she can stay at home and await further events. If the woman has no complications and is in early labour with contractions occurring irregularly and infrequently (maybe every 15–20 min) then it is better if she remains at home. This is known as the latent phase of labour. A significant link between later admission to hospital and a positive birth outcome (for example, a reduced caesarean section rate) has been shown (Ghacero & Enabudosco 2006).

Increased levels of stress which a woman may experience on admission to the unfamiliar environment of the modern labour ward may lead to an increased production of catecholamines. These are the 'fight or flight' hormones (adrenaline and noradrenaline) and they tend to inhibit the production of oxytocin (Peled 1992, Wuitchik et al. 1989). As oxytocin causes contraction of the uterine muscle, it follows that a reduction in oxytocin leads to diminished contractions and a slowing down of the labour process. It is suggested that ensuring that hospital labour wards are kept as calm, peaceful and private as possible will lead to better birth experiences and outcomes (Hodnett et al. 2010).

The midwife could suggest to the woman that she has a warm bath to help her relax, that she tries to get as much rest as possible and that she has a light meal and drinks plenty of fluid in order to prepare herself for the onset of the active phase of labour. Sometimes, however, despite being in early labour, a woman may decide that she wants to go into hospital for reassurance from a midwife that all is progressing normally.

If the woman reports any complications such as vaginal bleeding which appears to be more than a 'show', or if she has any medical disorders such as diabetes, cardiac problems, pregnancy-induced hypertension or a known malpresentation such as breech, she should be asked to come directly to the labour ward. This is in accordance with the *Midwives' Rules and Standards* (NMC 2012), which state that where a deviation from the norm becomes apparent, a practising midwife should inform an appropriately qualified healthcare professional.

Women are also usually asked to come into hospital if they think that their membranes have broken. This is so that the midwife can exclude any signs of infection, such as a raised temperature and pulse rate, as infection poses a risk to the fetus when the protective membranes have ruptured. Women with ruptured membranes: and without signs of infection or fetal compromise are often discharged home to await the onset of labour, once they have been assessed. In 60% of cases, labour will start spontaneously within 24 hours (NICE 2008). If it does not occur spontaneously, then induction of labour may need to be considered (NICE 2008).

Initial examination

On arrival at the labour ward, the woman and her birth partner should be welcomed by the midwife who will be caring for them. In most labour wards today, the woman will not know her midwife and this initial meeting is of great importance.

Pregnancy history

Before examining the woman, the midwife should review her medical records. Most women will bring them to the labour ward on their admission. The progress of the current pregnancy should be ascertained as well as the outcome of any previous pregnancies, as this may have a bearing on the current one. The woman's general health and any medical history of note should also be considered.

Physical examination

The midwife should observe the general condition of the woman. This includes an assessment of how she is coping with the contractions and whether she appears anxious or fearful.

The general colour of the woman should be noted. Extreme pallor, flushed skin or cyanosis could be an indication that there are underlying medical problems, such as anaemia, heart disease or infection, which might affect the management of care. Signs of oedema should also be noted. It is very common for women in the latter stages of pregnancy to have swollen fingers and feet. However, if the oedema is marked, and particularly if it involves the face (the woman's birthing partner could be asked for his or her opinion in relation to this), this may be a sign of pre-eclampsia (also referred to as pregnancy-induced hypertension (PIH)) which could have serious implications for the woman and her baby.

Physical examination includes taking the woman's pulse, blood pressure and temperature. These recordings should be noted in the woman's records as they will act as baseline readings as the labour progresses.

A sample of the woman's urine should be tested on admission and then regularly throughout the labour. If protein is detected, then this may indicate the presence of PIH, although it may also be due to contamination with amniotic fluid if the membranes have broken.

The presence of ketones (ketonuria) suggests that the woman has not eaten for some time or has suffered from excessive vomiting. Ketonuria is an indication that the body is using fat as a major source of energy rather than carbohydrate.

A small amount of ketonuria is to be expected during labour as a physiological response to the increased energy demands within the body at this time. However, if large amounts of ketones are present, this may indicate a severe depletion of the body's energy source which could lead to a reduction in uterine activity and slowing down of the progress of labour.

An abnormality in any of these readings should be reported to the obstetrician as they may indicate an underlying problem with the general health of the woman or with the progress of her labour.

Assessment of the progress of labour

There are many ways of assessing a woman's progress in labour, requiring midwives to draw on their knowledge, skills and experience.

Midwifery wisdom

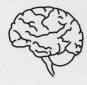

A holistic practitioner will assess progress not only through physical examination but also by observing more subtle outward signs, including the woman's behaviour and psychological state.

Observation of the woman's behaviour

A woman in the latent first stage of labour may not display any outward signs. As cervical dilation advances and the woman enters the active phase of labour, she may become restless and uncomfortable and suffer pain. She will probably want to change position frequently, often finding a mobile, upright or forward-leaning posture more comfortable. It is thought that this instinctive behaviour assists the descent and rotation of the fetus.

Vocal changes are often noted as labour progresses. In early labour, conversation and interaction are usually unhindered, but as the frequency and intensity of contractions increase, women find it increasingly difficult to hold a conversation and will often close their eyes in concentration until the pain passes. The level of breathing changes as contractions intensify: as the second stage approaches, women are often heard to make a deep, slow 'mooing' sound which is associated with the urge to bear down. This may increase in intensity as the fetus is expelled. Women should not be discouraged from vocalising in labour and indeed, it may be unhelpful to attempt to do so (McKay & Roberts 1990, RCM 2012c).

The urge to bear down, or push, is usually automatic and beyond the woman's conscious control. As the second stage intensifies, the urge will become overwhelming and women may briefly hold their breath and bear down, often several times, during the peak of each contraction. However, when the baby is in an occipito-posterior position, this may cause an urge to push well before full cervical dilation. If in doubt, a vaginal examination may be undertaken with the woman's consent to confirm full dilation of the cervix.

Outward signs

Natal line

One non-invasive means of estimating progress is to observe the 'purple line' that slowly ascends from the anal margin to the top of the natal cleft (skin between the buttocks). It is generally supposed that this line moves at roughly the same rate as the cervix dilates, reaching the top of the natal cleft at full dilation.

A recent study (Shepherd et al. 2010) found that the purple line does exist and that there is a medium positive correlation between the length of the line and both cervical dilation and the station of the fetal head. Where the line is visible, it may provide a useful guide for how labour is progressing. However, further research is needed to assess whether measurement of the purple line is acceptable to both labouring women and midwives.

The rhombus of Michaelis

The rhombus of Michaelis is a kite-shaped area over the lower back that includes the lower lumbar vertebrae and sacrum (Figure 7.1). It is believed that this area of bone moves backwards during the second stage of labour, pushing out the wings of the ilea and increasing the pelvic diameter (Wickham & Sutton 2005). This

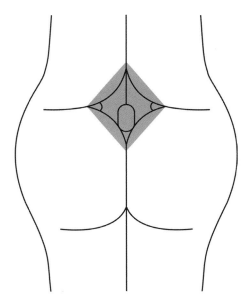

Figure 7.1   Rhombus of Michaelis.

allows more space for the fetus to descend through the pelvis. Sutton notes that when in a forward-leaning posture, a lump appears on the woman's back, at and below waist level. This happens at the start of the second stage. This is thought to be the reason why, if a woman is labouring in a semi-supine position, she may automatically reach up to find something to hold on to and arch her back (Wickham & Sutton 2005).

Anal dilation

As the presenting part reaches the pelvic floor and begins to displace the muscle and tissue, anal dilation may be noted. This is usually a sign that the second stage of labour is reaching its culmination. The woman may pass an involuntary bowel motion at this time if her rectum is full, as the pressure of the presenting part flattens the rectum against the sacral bone, expelling any contents.

However, anal dilation may be caused by deep engagement of the presenting part or early pushing (Howie & Rankin 2011d), so should not be taken as a definitive indicator of progress if no other signs are seen.

Vulval gaping/appearance of the presenting part

As the second stage progresses, the vaginal opening stretches and the perineal body flattens and distends. The presenting part may be visible on parting the labia. This is usually a sure sign of progress when noted for the first time. However, if there is a lot of caput and moulding (swelling and distortion of the fetal skull) this may be misleading, as the bony part of the fetal skull may be much higher in the birth canal than it appears. Caput and moulding may cause the scalp to protrude through the cervix prior to full dilation, as may a breech (Howie & Rankin 2011d).

Spontaneous rupture of membranes

The most common time for the woman's membranes to break *naturally* is at the end of the first stage of labour when the cervix is fully dilated and thus unable to support the forewaters against the force of uterine contractions (Howie & Rankin 2011b).

Observation of woman's psychological state

The transitional phase

The definition of the transitional phase varies but it is commonly used to describe the period from the end of the first stage of labour to full dilation of the cervix (Downe 2011) It is essentially a midwifery observation and relies on the midwife knowing the woman and recognising changes in her behaviour that indicate that birth is imminent.

During the transitional phase, a woman's behaviour and mental state may change and this phase often represents a psychological low point when the woman becomes overwhelmed by both physical and emotional pain (Downe 2011). She may become very agitated and restless, display aggression, irritability and irrational behaviour, such as wanting to go home or demanding a caesarean section. It is important to remember that this phase is temporary and not a reflection of her true personality.

Another manifestation of the transitional phase is an apparent withdrawal of the woman into herself. She may close her eyes, cease talking and appear unaware of what is happening around her. Leap (2000) explains that the woman is subconsciously focusing her energy and concentration in preparation for the supreme effort of giving birth.

Midwifery wisdom

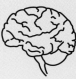

The transitional phase of labour is challenging for both the woman and the midwife who supports her but it is a sign that the end is in sight!

Abdominal palpation and auscultation

The purpose of abdominal palpation during labour is to assess the lie, presentation, position, flexion and descent of the presenting part (usually the head). These findings are significant when done repeatedly over a period of time, as an indicator of how far labour has progressed, and give some indication of how it is likely to continue. Continuity of midwife is preferable as findings may be subjective.

The most common findings of abdominal palpation are a fetus that is in a longitudinal lie, a cephalic (head-down) presentation and a left occipito-anterior (LOA) position. The head is normally flexed and descent is measured in fifths palpable above the symphysis pubis. When 2/5th or less is palpable, the head is said to be engaged. Engagement is defined as the widest part having passed through the pelvic brim (Howie & Rankin 2011b). In primiparous women, the head is normally engaged before labour commences. In multiparous women, the head may still be free at the start of labour. As labour progresses, the fetus will gradually move into a direct occipito-anterior (OA) position and the head will descend further until no fifths are palpable through the abdomen.

Listening to the fetal heart allows the midwife to assess fetal well-being and also enables descent of the fetus to be tracked. The point at which the heart sounds are loudest will gradually change as the fetus rotates and descends. Once deeply engaged, it may be difficult to auscultate the heart sounds with a Pinard stethoscope, due to the positioning of the fetal chest behind the symphysis pubis.

Monitoring of contractions

Contractions generally begin as mild, period-type cramps that are often irregular and intermittent continuing for hours or even days (Walsh 2011). This happens as the cervix is effacing and beginning to dilate. This early period is often referred to as the latent phase and varies in length: many women will not be aware when it began. Indeed, some women may believe that they are in established labour. The midwife will need to give careful explanations to help the woman understand what is actually happening to her body.

Eventually, the latent phase of labour merges into the active phase, and contractions start to become regular and closer together. The active phase of labour is defined as progressive cervical dilation with regular, painful contractions (NICE 2007). In the earlier part of the active phase, contractions may be as little as 2:10 (i.e. twice in 10 minutes), lasting 30 seconds. They gradually increase in length, strength and frequency as labour progresses, up to a maximum of around 5:10 (five times in 10 min), lasting over a minute with little break in between.

The midwife can place her hand on the woman's abdomen at fundal level in order to assess the length and frequency of contractions. It is difficult to assess the strength of a contraction through palpation – the woman herself is a better judge of that.

Some women experience a temporary lull in contractions at the end of the first stage of labour, but prior to the onset of expulsive contractions. This coincides with the presenting part descending and rotating as it reaches the pelvic floor (Howie & Rankin 2011d). This period is sometimes referred to as the latent phase of second stage, before contractions begin to feel expulsive, and it should not be assumed that labour has slowed down or ceased.

Vaginal examination

Some hospitals will have a policy of performing regular vaginal examinations (VE) throughout labour, regardless of the risk status of the woman. Midwives covering homebirths or working in birth centres may take a more relaxed approach, as their clients will by definition be low risk and thus they may only undertake a VE when there is a clear clinical need. In consultant units, however, midwives are increasingly working in an environment in which the evidence from VE supersedes all other indications of progress. There is thus a risk that midwives and students will lose confidence in other means of assessing progress (Sookhoo & Biott 2002).

The first VE is often carried out soon after admission to the delivery suite. However, depending on local policy, the midwife may wait until she is sure that the woman is in active labour. It is common practice to carry out a VE to confirm onset of the second stage of labour, though this may not be necessary if the presenting part is already visible. However, if the woman displays an urge to push when there is doubt about progress in labour, a vaginal examination may be carried out.

Vaginal examination allows the progress of labour to be assessed through a number of indicators.

The state of the cervix

The midwife will assess the position, effacement, consistency and dilation. In early labour, these findings may be expressed using the Bishop's score system, a tabular representation which allocates points to each factor (see Table 7.1). The higher the number of points, the more advanced the state of cervix towards established labour.

Table 7.1   Bishop's score

Parameter	0	1	2	3
Dilation	<1 cm	1–2 cm	3–4 cm	5–6 cm
Length	>4 cm	2–4 cm	1–2 cm	<1 cm
Consistency	Firm	Medium	Soft	–
Position	Posterior	Centre	Anterior	–
Station	–3	–2	–1–0	+1,+2

Adapted from: www.preg.info/BirthNotes/pdf/birth_notes_bookmarked.pdf (accessed May 2013).

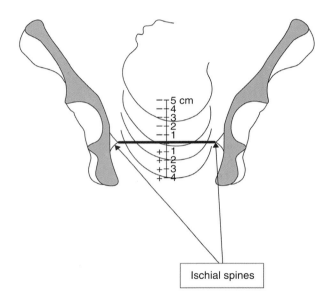

Ischial spines

Figure 7.2   Ischial spines.

The station of the presenting part

Even if the cervix is closed, the midwife will be able to ascertain the descent of the presenting part (PP) through the pelvis. This should have been estimated by abdominal palpation prior to commencing the VE. The PP is measured in relation to the ischial spines (Figure 7.2) and is estimated in centimetres. The ischial spines may be felt as blunt, bony prominences on stretching the examining fingers to the sides of the vaginal wall. Thus a position of 0 means that the PP is level with the ischial spines: minus 1 means 1 cm above the ischial spines; plus 1 means 1 cm below (see Figure 7.2). The midwife would expect the PP to descend steadily throughout labour as the cervix dilates. However, midwives may have difficulty locating the ischial spines in some women if they are not particularly prominent and the use of this landmark is highly subjective and therefore may not always be a very accurate tool for measuring descent of the fetus.

Position of the cervix

Prior to the onset of labour, the cervix points towards the posterior vaginal wall. On VE, it may be very difficult to locate. From the end of pregnancy until the onset of established labour, it gradually becomes central and eventually anterior facing. Thus the ease with which the cervix can be reached is an indicator of progress in the latent or early phase of labour.

The size and shape of the bony pelvis

The midwife conducting the VE will note any unusual findings such as a narrow pubic arch or a prominent sacrum, either of which might impede the progress of labour. A higher than expected PP coupled with an unusual pelvic structure is a likely indicator that labour will not progress to vaginal delivery, regardless of the strength of contractions. This must be reported urgently to the senior obstetrician as a caesarean section is likely to be needed.

The position of the presenting part

If the cervix is sufficiently dilated, it will be possible for the midwife to assess the attitude (flexed or deflexed) of the fetal head by feeling for the fontanelles. A deflexed head at the start of labour would be expected to gradually flex, so that the posterior fontanelle becomes readily palpable. Lack of flexion may be an indicator of poor progress due to an unfavourable fetal position or to inefficient contractions.

The position of the fetus can be determined through palpation of the sutures on the fetal skull. By noting the position and direction of the sutures, the midwife can assess whether the fetus has rotated into a good position for birth. If VEs are repeated over a period of time, the midwife should be able to track the progress of the fetus as it rotates and descends through the birth canal. These are important signs of progress in labour and a lack of rotation, flexion and descent may indicate an obstruction to normal labour.

The partogram

The standard tool in hospitals for assessing the progress of labour is the partogram (sometimes known as the partograph). This maps cervical dilation and descent of the PP along a time-scale, with space to include basic observations such as the fetal heart, length, strength and frequency of contractions, maternal temperature, pulse, urine output and blood pressure (NICE 2008). It is commonly used once a woman is in 'established' labour – local policies may differ in their definition of this term but it usually refers to a state of regular contractions becoming longer, stronger and closer together with progressive dilation of the cervix and descent of the PP.

The partogram requires the midwife to undertake physical observations and document the findings at regular intervals throughout labour. The woman's progress is thus represented in the form of a graph, allowing her carers to see at a glance how she has progressed, which may give an indication of the normality of her labour. However, the value of the partogram depends on an accurate diagnosis of the onset of labour and this is often unknown.

The purpose of a partogram is to detect dysfunctional physical patterns in labour, thereby allowing early intervention before the mother or fetus becomes compromised. Over time, there have been modifications to the use of this assessment tool, including the introduction of an *alert* and an *action* line with the action line being 2 hours to the right of the alert line and meaning that augmentation of the labour is recommended (Church & Hodgson 2011).

Despite its widespread use, the partogram is controversial as it depends on clock-watching and demands regular physical interventions (Figure 7.3). It takes little account of the subtler signs of progress.

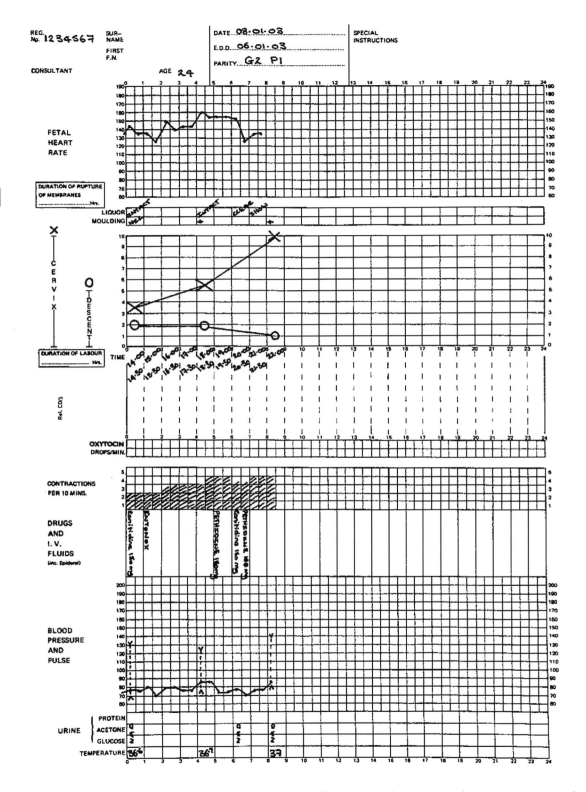

Figure 7.3   A partogram. Reproduced with permission from Symonds M, Symonds IM (2003) *Essential Obstetrics and Gynaecology*, 4th edn. London: Churchill Livingstone.

Medical forms of pain relief

Although labour is a physiological process, many woman feel the need to resort to different methods of pain relief to help them cope with what can be the overwhelming pain of labour.

The exact definition of what constitutes a medical form of pain relief is open to debate. Most practitioners would take it to include all drugs, whether taken orally, by injection, by inhalation or by regional block. Other methods of pain relief are less easy to categorise. These include transcutaneous electronic nerve stimulation (TENS), acupuncture, aromatherapy and other alternative or complementary therapies. It may be argued that any form of pain relief, whether drug related or not, that involves an invasive procedure is 'medical'. However, a woman who is enabled to use her own choice of alternative therapy during labour will probably feel that she has laboured 'naturally' and without medical pain relief.

An analgesic can be defined as a drug which reduces the pain sensation but without causing a loss of consciousness or touch (Howie & Rankin 2011c). The most desirable characteristic of an analgesic given during labour is that it should provide maximum pain relief with minimal adverse effects on the woman and her baby. Unfortunately, as will be seen, the perfect labour analgesic is not currently available!

Nitrous oxide/Entonox

Entonox is a colourless, odourless gas which consists of nitrous oxide and oxygen in equal parts. It is colloquially referred to as 'gas and air' or sometimes 'laughing gas'. It is approved for use by midwives and can be used throughout labour, although a woman inhaling it continually throughout a long labour may start to tire and be unable to use it effectively.

Entonox is provided by piped supply directly into the delivery room or stored in portable cylinders which may be carried by midwives and used in the home setting. The gases start to separate if stored at a temperature below 7°C. For this reason it is important that cylinders are stored at a temperature of at least 10°C and inverted several times before use in order to ensure that the gases are adequately mixed (Howie & Rankin 2011c).

Women inhale the gas by breathing it in via a mouthpiece or a facemask. As the analgesic effect of the gas does not take effect until after about 20 seconds, the woman should be encouraged to start inhaling as soon as she feels the contraction beginning. In this way, the maximum effect of the analgesic will coincide with the peak of the contraction.

The midwife can assist the woman by helping her to breathe the gas effectively. It is suggested that taking short panting breaths is not efficient and the woman should be encouraged to take deep breaths at the normal breathing rate (Bartholomew & Yerby 2011). Rapid breathing should be discouraged as it can lead to hyperventilation and less oxygen getting to the baby via the placenta.

A notable advantage of Entonox during labour is that it is excreted rapidly via the maternal lungs so that toxic levels do not accumulate and affect the fetus adversely. If a woman does not like the sensations evoked by using the gas, she simply stops inhaling it and the effect is soon lost. Some women report feeling dizzy and nauseous while inhaling Entonox, although the majority find that the sense of euphoria evoked, coupled with the lessened pain sensation, make it a popular pain-relieving choice.

Entonox is not, however, the perfect analgesia for labour in that while it helps many women cope with the pain of the contractions, it does not take away the pain sensations completely and in this sense is not a true analgesic (Bartholomew & Yerby 2011).

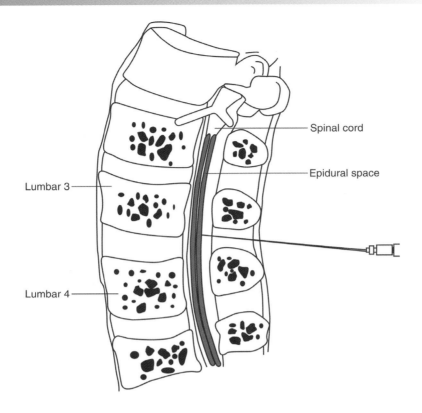

Figure 7.4   The epidural space.

Epidural analgesia

Epidural analgesia involves the introduction of a local anaesthetic into the epidural space around the spinal cord. Drugs which have been used include opiates such as diamorphine, morphine and fentanyl. It has been found that mixing an opiate with a local anaesthetic gives longer, more effective pain relief with less loss of movement in the lower limbs (Collis et al. 1993). This is known as the 'mobile epidural' and it means that potentially women are able to walk about as their labour progresses. The initial study used an injection of the combined drugs straight into the cerebrospinal fluid via the subarachnoid space followed by insertion of an epidural catheter. It was also known as a 'combined spinal epidural' (Collis et al. 1993). However, this method has largely been discontinued and anaesthetists tend to use the combined drugs directly into the epidural space with the epidural being maintained by the midwife administering regular bolus top-ups (Collis 2007). The drugs commonly used are bupivacaine (the local anaesthetic) and fentanyl (the opiate).

   The epidural space (Figure 7.4) is approximately 4 mm wide and located around the dura mater (the outermost layer of the meninges surrounding the spinal cord). It contains a number of blood vessels, fatty matter and spinal nerves. During pregnancy and more specifically labour, the size of the space is reduced considerably by the engorgement of the veins which occurs during pregnancy. The local anaesthetic is inserted into the space with the aim of surrounding the fibres of the spinal nerves in order to block the pain sensations. It is usual practice for the lumbar route to be used and usually the anaesthetic is introduced between lumbar vertebrae 3 and 4 or 2 and 3.

An epidural may be indicated in the following situations (Howie & Rankin 2011c):

- It is the woman's choice as an effective method of pain relief.
- During prolonged labour, as this method is usually very effective and will allow an exhausted woman a chance to rest and recuperate.
- A malposition such as occipital-posterior which often leads to severe back pain and an early need to push before the cervix is completely open.
- A malpresentation such as a breech or a multiple pregnancy. In both examples, certain manipulations are likely to be required during the second stage of labour and there is a higher risk that a caesarean section might be indicated.
- A woman who has very high blood pressure. The use of epidural analgesia may lead to a reduction in blood pressure as the local anaesthetic blocks the transmission of both motor and sensory nerves as well as having an effect on the sympathetic nervous system. This will cause dilation of the veins and a subsequent fall in blood pressure.
- For instrumental (forceps and ventouse (suction)) deliveries (caesarean section).

On the other hand, an epidural is not recommended if a woman has chronic backache or a spinal deformity, as this could lead to difficulties during the procedure. If she has a blood clotting disorder this might lead to excessive bleeding around the site where the needle is introduced into the spinal cord. Due to the effect which this type of anaesthesia has on blood pressure, it is not recommended if a woman has low blood pressure or a low blood volume (Howie & Rankin 2011c). In this situation, the woman would be advised to use another method of pain relief such as pethidine or diamorphine.

Administration of epidural anaesthesia: the procedure

The introduction of anaesthesia into the epidural space is a skilled procedure which should only be carried out by a suitably qualified anaesthetist. The role of the midwife in this case is to support the woman in her choice, and to ensure that she has all the information she needs about the risks and disadvantages associated with this method of pain relief. The midwife will also be required to assist the anaesthetist in the preparation of the necessary equipment and drugs, as well as ensuring that the woman is lying in the most appropriate position. The midwife will also need to monitor the condition of the woman and fetus during and following the procedure and report any deviations from the norm to the anaesthetist.

Disadvantages of epidural use

Effect on the progress of labour

The epidural usually gives a high degree of pain relief but research shows that it prolongs the second stage of labour, increases the incidence of fetal malposition, increases the need for oxytocin augmentation of labour and leads to an increased number of instrumental deliveries (Anim-Somuah et al. 2011, Lieberman et al. 2005, O'Hana et al. 2008, Tracy et al. 2007).

Lowering of blood pressure (hypotension)

As epidural anesthesia lowers blood pressure, the woman may feel faint, dizzy and sick as her blood pressure falls. Hypotension can be rectified by ensuring that sufficient intravenous fluids are given.

Inability to pass urine

Women may be unable to pass urine with an epidural in place due to the loss of sensation in the bladder (Anim-Somuah et al. 2011).

A full bladder can lead to a delay in the labour and the possibility that the bladder will be damaged if an instrumental delivery is later required (Bartholomew & Yerby 2011). This could lead to problems such as urinary infection or incontinence in the postnatal period.

The midwife should remind the woman of the need to pass urine regularly at least every 2–3 hours and her abdomen should be palpated at regular intervals to assess for signs of a full bladder. If the woman is unable to pass urine, then the insertion of a urinary catheter may be required.

Dural tap

This complication occurs in approximately 0.5–2% of individuals receiving regional anaesthesia (Bartholomew & Yerby 2011). It occurs when the dura is pierced by the needle and anaesthetic is inadvertently injected into the cerebrospinal fluid (CSF). As the CSF leaks out, it causes a fall in pressure in the brain which results in the woman experiencing a severe headache, which is worse when she sits up. Eventually the dura will heal but this can take several days and may mean that the woman has to lie flat, unable to take care of her baby. An alternative method of treatment is for the anaesthetist to inject 10–20 mL of the woman's own blood back into the epidural space. This will seal over the puncture in the dura and will alleviate the problem (Howie & Rankin 2011c).

Total spinal block

This is a rare but serious complication which is caused by the inadvertent injection of anaesthetic into a vein. This causes a loss of sensation and movement in the upper part of the woman's body and will affect the muscles required for breathing. The midwife needs to be alert to the fact that this has occurred, the first sign being that the woman complains of a slight tingling sensation in her tongue followed by a rapid deterioration in her general condition. Immediate resuscitative steps will be needed urgently in this case.

Long-term backache

Earlier research had shown a higher incidence of backache in women who have received epidural anaesthesia (MacArthur et al. 1990). It is suggested that the loss of sensation during labour results in an unusual strain on the ligaments of the back which can lead to long-term backache. The woman might have been sitting in an awkward position for some time but felt no discomfort and so did not alter her position. However, other studies do not show an increased incidence of backache in women who had received epidurals when compared with women who had not. The latest Cochrane review update (Anim-Somuah et al. 2011) concluded that there was no statistical evidence to suggest that epidurals caused long-term backache.

Research continues but women should be aware that there may be a greater chance of experiencing backache if they have an epidural. This might be particularly relevant to them if they already suffer with back problems.

Opioid analgesia

Opioids (also known as narcotics) are drugs derived from the opium poppy (*Papaver somniferum*). They induce a sense of well-being and drowsiness. Three opioids are commonly used in labour in the UK (Tuckey et al. 2007):

- pethidine
- meptazinol
- diamorphine.

Pethidine

Pethidine is a controlled drug which a midwife can administer intramuscularly without the need for a prescription from a doctor (see Chapter 11). It is a synthetic substance which has pain-relieving and sedative properties. It works by attaching itself to receptor proteins and then diffusing through cell membranes where it affects the central nervous system. It does this by changing the sensitivity of the nerves to pain perception and actually reducing the pain sensation (Bartholomew & Yerby 2011).

Once in the muscle, pethidine has a rapid onset with the effect lasting up to 4 hours. It can also be injected straight into a vein. The dose is usually 50–200 mg depending on the weight of the woman, the progress of her labour, the degree of pain she is experiencing and the route of administration (BNF 2012).

Side-effects include nausea, vomiting, a fall in blood pressure and excessive sweating, and a woman may also feel that she is 'out of control'. Others may be unable to pass urine because the smooth muscle in the bladder sphincter contracts as a result of the drug.

Pethidine can delay stomach emptying which may put women at risk of inhaling their stomach contents (gastric aspiration) if a general anaesthetic is needed.

Another disadvantage of the use of pethidine during labour is that it readily crosses the placenta. Following an intravenous dose of pethidine, it is found in the cord blood within 2 min. After an intramuscular injection, it appears within 30 min (Briggs et al. 2008). Pethidine is broken down in the liver and as the fetal liver is immature, the process takes longer, which makes the fetus even more susceptible to side-effects of the drug (Briggs et al. 2008).

In the fetus, potential side-effects include a change in the heart rate pattern and a loss of the variability of the heart rate. It also affects the respiratory centre in the fetal brain and can lead to a decrease in the respiratory rate at birth. For this reason, it is preferable not to give pethidine if delivery is expected within 2–3 hours. If, however, it is given within 1 hour of the birth or more than 6 hours prior to the birth, the effect on the neonatal respiratory rate is minimal (Howie & Rankin 2011c).

Rosenblatt et al. (1981) observed that babies whose mothers had received pethidine during labour were less alert, quicker to cry and more unsettled up to 7 days after birth. Barrett (1983) noted that these babies were less efficient at attaching to the nipple and suckling.

If a baby does have difficulty breathing at birth, then the antidote to pethidine – naloxone – can be given by intramuscular injection. This has the effect of blocking the protein receptors which pethidine binds to, so stopping the action of the drug and the subsequent effect on respiration. Naloxone can be given in doses of 1 mg per kg of body weight (Bartholomew & Yerby 2011). The effects of naloxone wear off after an hour. For this reason, it is important that the newborn baby is observed carefully as the respiratory depression effect of the pethidine may remain problematic once the naloxone has ceased working (Bartholomew & Yerby 2011).

Although the side-effects of pethidine to both the woman and fetus are noted (Ullman et al. 2010), for some women it is an effective form of pain relief and means that they may not need to resort to the more invasive epidural method. However, it is important that they are aware of the potential difficulties, particularly in relation to breastfeeding, so that they can make an informed choice about what method is most appropriate for them (Wood & Soltani 2005). If pethidine has been used during labour, this should be highlighted by the midwife during the postnatal period so that appropriate support can be given to the mother and baby (Hunt 2002). This may include teaching the woman to hand express her milk and to recognise when a drowsy baby is ready to feed (Hunt 2002).

Meptazinol (Meptid)

Meptazinol is a synthetic substance similar to pethidine (although it is not classified as a controlled drug). It has less effect on the woman's cardiovascular and respiratory functions (Howie & Rankin 2011c). Meptazinol is given intramuscularly and the usual dose is 100–150 mg (BNF 2012). The effect begins approximately 15 min after administration, lasting for about 4 hours. It has been shown that there are no significant differences in the analgesic and side-effects of the two drugs (Howie & Rankin 2011c).

Diamorphine

Diamorphine, another controlled drug, may be given intramuscularly during labour and has similar effects on the woman and her fetus as pethidine (Howie & Rankin 2011c). The suggested dosage is 2.5–7.5 mg (BNF 2012), with the drug taking effect in 5–10 min and lasting around 3 hours. Since 2004, midwives have been able to use it on their own initiative in their professional practice without the need for a prescription from a doctor (see Chapter 11).

Midwifery care in the first and second stages of labour

Avoiding unnecessary time restrictions in labour

Case study 7.2

Jade arrives in the delivery suite in established labour with her first baby. Jade has seen babies being born on television where the woman is lying in bed. On entering the labour room, Jade automatically gets undressed and into the bed. Her partner helps her lie down and arranges pillows around her, as he has seen people do on television. She lies there and waits for the pain.

A few hours later, Jade's contractions are becoming increasingly painful and she is unable to get comfortable. She is thinking about asking for an epidural.

The current practice of timing each stage of labour reflects the dominant medical models of care in operation since the early 20th century. The aim is to reduce adverse outcomes to mother and baby by detecting early signs of deviation from the norm, which may be indicated by an unusually prolonged labour. However, there is no evidence to impose arbitrary time limits on labour or to justify intervention unless there are clear signs of fetal or maternal compromise or a lack of progress (Janni et al. 2002, Myles & Santolaya 2003). There may, however, be an increased risk of maternal morbidity when the second stage of labour exceeds 2 hours (Allen et al. 2009, Janni et al. 2002, Myles & Santolaya 2003). The midwife must decide whether the possible risk to the mother of a prolonged second stage outweighs the possible risks to the mother and baby of a curtailed second stage through the intervention of medical procedures (RCM 2012c).

Guidelines from the National Institute for Health and Clinical Excellence (NICE 2007) advise that normal progress in first-stage labour is identified by cervical dilation of 2 cm or more every 4 hours. Once active second stage has been identified, birth should be expected within 3 hours for primiparous women and 2 hours for multiparous women.

Movement and posture

Women, like most female mammals, are not physiologically designed to give birth in a supine position. Adopting an upright, forward-leaning posture is more natural. Gravity can then assist with the descent and rotation of the PP and pressure is applied on the internal cervical os to promote dilation. Other physiological advantages to adopting an upright posture for labour include a reduction in aortocaval compression, better alignment of the fetus and an increased pelvic outlet (MIDIRS 2008).

When the woman adopts an upright or forward-leaning posture with her legs slightly apart, the ligaments between the sacroiliac joints and the pubic symphisis, already softened by the effects of the hormones progesterone and relaxin, allow the bones of the pelvis to separate slightly. This can create up to 28% more space in the pelvic outlet (Robertson 2001), allowing for an easier birth. When a woman is upright, the natural tilt of the pelvis guides the fetus in a downward direction, whereas a woman in a semi-supine position must push her baby uphill. Postures which interfere with the physiological progress of the fetus through the pelvis are likely to lengthen labour, which in turn may lead to fetal compromise and maternal exhaustion.

A systematic review by Lawrence et al. (2009) concluded that upright positions in labour are associated with a reduction in the length of the first stage of labour and also in the use of epidural analgesia. If a woman adopts an upright position this can also mean less severe pain during the first stage (Miquelutti et al. 2009).

There is little evidence comparing different upright positions during birth itself (as opposed to labour). However, a study by Ragnar et al. (2006) considered sitting and kneeling postures in the second stage of labour. They found that although there was no difference in the length of the second stage, the kneeling position was associated with less pain and a more favourable experience for the woman.

Until the advent of modern obstetric practices, it was normal for women to give birth standing, squatting, on all fours or in some other supported upright posture (Coppen 2005). Twentieth-century hospital practices changed this in order to facilitate the midwife's and obstetrician's role with regard to examinations. Unless the woman has an epidural *in situ* or some other medical impediment, she should be encouraged to move freely and adopt whatever posture is comfortable (NICE 2007, RCM 2012a).

The RCM evidence-based guidelines (RCM 2012a) note that women's choice of position for labour is strongly influenced by what they feel is expected of them. It is therefore incumbent on the midwife to promote the use of different positions. It is not acceptable to impose restrictions based on the midwife's own comfort. Even where continuous fetal monitoring is necessary, the woman need not be restricted to the bed.

Activity 7.1

Take a look around the delivery rooms in the maternity unit you are working in. Think about how easy it would be for women to adopt various postures in labour.

- Could the furniture be adapted or moved to facilitate upright, forward-leaning postures?
- Does the unit supply birthing balls or a birthing stool, and if so, are there any restrictions on their use?

Eating and drinking in labour

Case study 7.3

Jade has been in active labour for several hours. There are no complications. Jade's last full meal was at 7 pm yesterday evening and, after a restless night, she had had only a cup of tea and a small bowl of cereal before coming into hospital 5 hours ago. Jade has been drinking water freely, as the Entonox makes her thirsty. She is now starting to feel very weary and a little dizzy. Her contractions have slowed down and she is beginning to feel discouraged. She asks if she can have something to eat but her midwife appears unsure and is reluctant to give her anything.

The case above is a typical scenario of a labouring woman who needs food. In the latter half of the 20th century, many maternity units in many countries imposed restrictions on eating and drinking during labour (Singata et al. 2010). This practice is based on the principle that reduced gastric motility during labour increases the risk of vomiting. In the event of a caesarean section being required, acid stomach contents could be inhaled, causing a condition known as Mendelsohn's syndrome (Mendelsohn 1946). However, improvements in anaesthesia over the past 50 years have seen this condition almost eradicated (Parsons & Nagy 2006). There is currently no good evidence to support the restriction of food and drink in labour in order to prevent this condition (RCM 2012b). The aspiration of undiluted, acidic gastric fluids is actually more dangerous than when diluted by food or drink (Parsons & Nagy 2006).

It is also common practice on labour wards to give antacids such as ranitidine to all labouring women in order to increase the pH of the stomach contents. However, as Walsh (2011) points out, there is no strong evidence to suggest that this has any effect on maternal mortality and morbidity. It is really only appropriate for women at high risk of emergency procedures and should not be used for women in normal labour.

If food is restricted during labour, a woman's blood glucose level will fall, leading to ketosis which, combined with fatigue, may lead to reduced uterine action and the increased likelihood of medical intervention. Hunger may also adversely affect the woman's sense of well-being. Current evidence suggests that labouring women who feel hungry should be encouraged to eat as they wish providing they are not at increased risk of needing general anaesthesia (Singata et al. 2010).

The only exception to this is when a woman receives a narcotic for pain relief (such as pethidine or diamorphine). This is known to reduce gastric emptying so once narcotics are administered, oral intake should cease (NICE 2007).

Tranmer et al. (2005) undertook a study allowing unrestricted eating and drinking for women during labour. They found that when women choose when and what to eat during labour, they tend to eat small amounts and often only in the earlier part of labour before the onset of strong contractions. Examples of suitable foods and drinks which a woman might choose during labour include low-residue, low-fat, easily absorbed foods such as bananas, smoothies, cereal bars, toast, yogurts or isotonic sports drinks. Foods which are high in fat or energy content tend to slow gastric emptying (and may increase nausea) (Micklewright & Champion 2002).

Support in labour

Most women will instinctively seek support and help in labour. In times past, this support was traditionally the role of female attendants such as lay midwives and family members. Since the 1970s, male partners have become commonplace in the birthing room.

It is widely recognised that labouring women perceive a need for empathic companionship and support (RCM 2012c) and that their reactions to labour may be influenced by the support they receive. Midwives are ideally placed to offer support in terms of physical care and information giving and should also be able to offer emotional support and advocacy. Indeed, this is considered one of the core roles of the midwife (DH 2010). All current national intrapartum practice guidance and maternity policies state that one-to-one midwifery care should be provided to all women in established labour (DH 2007, NICE 2007, RCOG 2007).

There is evidence that women who receive continuous support in labour require less pharmacological analgesia, have fewer operative births and are more satisfied with the outcome of their labour (Hodnett et al. 2011), while women who perceive little professional or lay support in labour appear more likely to suffer post-traumatic stress 6 weeks postnatally (Czarnocka & Slade 2000). Spiby et al. (2003) note that women expect midwives to offer coping strategies for pain and that these help to enhance the experience of labour and reduce distress.

Continuity of care and continuous care

There is good evidence that *continuous* support during labour has more of a positive impact on childbirth outcome and on women's perception of labour than *continuity* of support alone (Hodnett et al. 2011). This may include advice, information, physical assistance or emotional support and may be from either a midwife or a layperson, such as a friend or family member. Hodnett et al. (2011) demonstrated that women who have continuous support during labour are less likely to have an operative birth or analgesia or report dissatisfaction with their experience. However, the benefits of continuous support were shown to be greater when the supporter was not a member of the hospital staff.

Pushing in the second stage of labour

Case study 7.4

 The midwife has just examined Jade and found her cervix to be fully dilated. Jade is experiencing frequent, strong contractions and is starting to get an urge to bear down. Darren, Jade's partner, wants to know what he should do – should he encourage her to push? The midwife explains that it is preferable to leave Jade to find her most comfortable position and then to support her as she pushes in the way she wants to.

Darren is confused as he has seen birth partners and midwives on TV shouting at women to push and he thought that this was the most important part of his role during the delivery. He wants to do all he can to support Jade but now wonders how best to help her.

A typical childbirth scene as portrayed by the media includes a doctor or midwife urging a labouring woman to take a deep breath, hold it as long as possible and push with all her might. This was once common practice in the UK but there is no current evidence to support it. Indeed, this Valsalva manoeuvre, as it is known, is now associated with fetal compromise due to the reduction in oxygenated maternal blood crossing the placenta during the manoeuvre and long-term effects on the woman's urinary tract (Prins et al. 2011). Current evidence suggests that instinctive, physiological pushing behaviour is less harmful to the fetus and the woman (Prins et al. 2011).

The role of the midwife and the woman's partner in this scenario is to be supportive rather than directive of her pushing efforts. It is suggested that only if the woman specifically asks for help with her pushing should instructions be given, otherwise she should be encouraged to listen to her own instinctive urges and push as she feels the need to (Prins et al. 2011).

Midwifery care in the third stage of labour

Activity 7.2

Sita had a managed third stage following the birth of her first baby 3 years ago. She has requested a physiological third stage this time as the oxytocic drugs she received made her extremely nauseous and she had severe after-pains for some hours after the birth. This had made her feel so unwell that she had struggled to establish breastfeeding.

What information can the midwife give Sita in order to help her make an informed decision about the third stage of labour?

As the term implies, physiological management of the third stage of labour relies on the normal physiological processes within the body to facilitate expulsion of the placenta and membranes. The woman takes an active role in this process with the midwife observing her condition and providing support and encouragement as required. The midwife is also required to maintain her records in relation to time of delivery of the placenta and condition of the woman throughout. Harris (2011) describes the 'watchful anticipation' approach which a midwife adopts during physiological or expectant management of the third stage.

Midwifery Wisdom

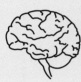

The main principle of physiological management is that there is no intervention on the part of the midwife unless the woman begins bleeding heavily or the baby needs urgent separation from its mother for resuscitation.

The process can take up to an hour although research suggests that an average time is about 15 min (Harris 2011). However long the process takes, if the woman's condition remains stable and she does not begin to bleed heavily, there is no cause for concern.

There is some debate about when is the exact timing of the cutting of the umbilical cord is the subject of current debate, however, as Inch argues, in keeping with the principles of expectant management, the cord should not be clamped and cut until after the placenta and membranes have been expelled. It has been shown that there are benefits to doing this in relation to the baby continuing to receive oxygenated blood via the cord (Hutchon 2006). This is of particular importance if the baby is born prematurely (Kinmond et al. 1993).

However, if the cord is particularly short, then not cutting it means that the woman is unable to hold her baby. Or the cord may be long enough but the woman may want to change her position and move around which might be awkward if the cord is still intact and attached to the baby. A compromise in these situations is for the midwife to help the mother get as comfortable as possible with her baby, wait for a short period until the cord has stopped pulsating (usually after 5–10 min) and then clamp and cut it (Harris 2011).

The woman should be encouraged to breastfeed her baby as soon as possible while waiting for the placenta to be delivered as the natural oxytocin released as the baby sucks will stimulate contraction of the uterine muscle.

The maternal end of the cord should not be clamped but should be left to drain into a suitable receptacle. The blood draining from the placenta will then reduce its overall size which will further help to facilitate delivery (Johnson & Taylor 2010). However, any blood which drains from the placenta should not be included in the final estimate of blood lost during the delivery as it is placental rather than maternal blood (Johnson & Taylor 2010).

When the uterus contacts, the woman may feel some abdominal pain and will then have an urge to bear down. She should be encouraged to do this and she may want to move into a more upright position (standing or squatting) so that gravity can assist the process (Harris 2011). A rush of blood will be seen and the cord may appear to lengthen as the placenta moves into the vagina. The woman will then spontaneously push the placenta out.

Active management of the third stage of labour

Active management of the third stage of labour includes giving the woman an oxytocic drug, the early clamping and cutting of the umbilical cord and controlled cord traction (Harris 2011).

The latest systematic review comparing active and expectant management of the third stage of labour (Begley et al. 2011) concluded that in all the studies reviewed, the active management option did indeed reduce bleeding and anaemia, but also led to an increase in blood pressure, more severe 'after-pains', nausea, vomiting and the increased need for pain-relieving drugs. More women required readmission to hospital with vaginal bleeding. The analysis of the women identified as being at low risk of bleeding demonstrated similar results although there was no statistically significant difference in the risk of severe bleeding (more than 1000 mL blood lost) between the two management options. It is suggested that in the developed world, a healthy woman can cope with a blood loss up to 1000 mL without detriment (RCOG 2009).

The midwife must ensure that women know what options are available to them in relation to the third stage of labour and that this information is presented in a clear, unbiased way so that they can make an informed decision. The choice of whether to have a physiological third stage may be the only one left to a woman who has had to abandon her ideal birth options. For example, a woman may have hoped for a homebirth but due to slow progress in labour may have been transferred to a hospital unit. Other women may be concerned about the unpleasant side-effects of the oxytocic drugs and for this reason would prefer to avoid them.

As Soltani (2008) argues, advising routine active management of the third stage of labour with the specific aim of reducing blood loss is debatable in the Western world where on the whole women are healthy and well nourished and able to withstand significant blood loss during childbirth. Instead, incorporating expectant management with skin-to-skin contact, early breastfeeding and upright posture may also expedite expulsion of the placenta, reduce the length of the third stage and reduce the amount of blood loss. The midwife sharing this kind of information with women will empower them to make an informed choice about the management approach they wish to have.

Syntometrine (1 mL) is an oxytocic drug often used in active management of the third stage. It contains 500 mg of ergometrine and 5 units of oxytocin. The oxytocic component of the drug induces a strong contraction of the upper uterine segment after approximately 2–3 min of administration. This effect lasts 5–15 min (Baskett 2004). In contrast, the ergometrine component induces a strong sustained contraction of the uterine muscle 6–8 min after administration (Sorbe 1978). This effect lasts for approximately 60–90 min.

If a woman is known to have raised blood pressure or cardiac problems, then Syntocinon is the drug of choice as it does not cause sustained contraction of muscle fibres in the way that the ergometrine component of Syntometrine does. If a woman with raised blood pressure is given oxytocin-containing ergometrine, then contraction of muscles within her blood vessels will lead to her blood pressure being raised even more. Syntocinon can be given either intravenously (5 iu) or intramuscularly (5–15 iu). Syntocinon also has fewer side-effects such as the nausea and vomiting associated with Syntometrine.

Due to the various side-effects of Syntometrine (namely increased blood pressure, nausea vomiting and severe after-pains), NICE (2007) recommends that Syntocinon is the drug of choice for an actively managed third stage of labour. Rogers et al. (2011) undertook a retrospective study as a result of concerns expressed by many midwives that the use of Syntocinon during active management was leading to increased blood loss and increased need for blood transfusions. Their study demonstrated a statistically significant increase in the amount of estimated blood loss (more than 1000 mL) but no increase in the number of blood transfusions. The authors of this paper argue that their results do not suggest that there should be a move back to using Syntometrine as the drug of choice for an actively managed third stage.

However, they, along with other authors (Mcdonald & Middleton 2009), call for more studies investigating the issue of which oxytocic drug is most appropriate to use during active management of the third stage.

If a woman is to have an active management of the third stage, the oxytocic drug is traditionally administered intramuscularly by the midwife as the baby's anterior shoulder delivers or following the birth of the baby if the midwife is working alone during the birth. It is important that the oxytocic should always be given following the delivery of the baby's shoulder to ensure that shoulder dystocia (the shoulders trapped behind the woman's pubic bone) is not a possibility (Harris 2011).

The umbilical cord should be clamped using specially designed umbilical clamps. Delayed cord clamping by approximately 2–3 min after the delivery of the baby is currently the recommended practice. It has been shown to benefit the baby by improving iron levels for up to 6 months, albeit with an associated risk of neonatal jaundice needing phototherapy treatment. However, this is not considered to be significant enough to warrant immediate cord clamping unless the baby requires urgent resuscitative measures (McDonald & Middleton 2009, Mercer et al. 2007, Resuscitation Council 2011, WHO 2007).

The woman's partner may ask to cut the cord and this request can usually be facilitated with the support of the midwife.

Following clamping and cutting of the cord, the midwife should place her hand on the woman's abdomen and wait for signs that the uterus has contracted. She will feel that this has occurred when the uterus hardens underneath her hand; it will feel like a smooth, hard, cricket ball. It is important at this time that the midwife avoids so-called 'fundal fiddling' (that is, unnecessary touching of the uterus) which may lead to the placenta only partially separating from the uterine wall (Johnson & Taylor 2010), which may in turn be a cause of excessive bleeding and postpartum haemorrhage. Historically, it was suggested that controlled cord traction (CCT) should be commenced as soon as the uterus contracts and this was a traditional aspect of an actively managed third stage (Spencer 1962). However, a study carried out by Levy & Moore (1985) found that it is preferable to wait for further signs that placental separation has occurred.

Signs of separation include the rising of the fundus and the hardening of the uterus as described above, coupled with a gush of blood from the vagina and lengthening of the umbilical cord. Levy & Moore (1985) found no significant difference in the incidence of postpartum haemorrhage (PPH) or the length of the third stage between those who commenced CCT immediately they felt the uterus contract and those who waited for signs of separation. However, the incidence of PPH did increase significantly when the midwife unsuccessfully applied CCT without waiting for signs of placental separation.

Controlled cord traction involves the midwife either wrapping the cord around her fingers or using a clamp to apply downward, sustained pressure until the placenta becomes visible at the vulva. Once the placenta can be seen, the traction is applied upwards to follow the curve of the vagina. The placenta is then delivered into a bowl. Care should be taken of any trailing membranes and the midwife may need to use forceps to gently tease the membranes out of the vagina. Alternatively, twisting the trailing membranes into a rope may be useful and some midwives ask the woman to cough gently to assist this process.

Midwifery care after birth

Following delivery of the placenta, the midwife documents how long it took. She should also palpate the uterus to ensure that it remains contracted and the amount of vaginal blood loss is estimated and recorded. The placenta and membranes should be examined carefully to ascertain that they are complete and look healthy.

The woman's vagina and external genitalia should then be examined under a good light for signs of trauma. A decision needs to be made as to whether suturing of the area is required. This is often an uncomfortable examination and the midwife should make sure that the woman has Entonox to use if required.

Conclusion

This chapter has focused on the physiological aspects of labour with an emphasis on the role of the midwife in promoting normality. The role of the midwife in empowering the woman to cope with the tremendous physical and emotional demands of childbirth has also been highlighted. It is acknowledged that labour is a complex, multifaceted process with physical, psychosocial and emotional elements underpinning it. As the *Midwives' Rules and Standards* (NMC 2012) emphasise, childbirth is much more than simply the act of giving birth. It is a continuous process from conception, through pregnancy, labour, birth and beyond. Many factors unique to the individual woman will impact on the process and it is essential that midwives are competent to provide effective and appropriate care during this time.

Quiz

Please answer these 'true or false' questions to test your knowledge.

1. It is believed that a trigger in the fetal brain causes labour to begin.
2. It is recommended that midwives offer women the option of a 'membrane sweep' if they go beyond their due date.
3. Syntometrine is currently the oxytocic drug recommended for use during an actively managed third stage of labour.
4. Entonox is the same as nitrous oxide.
5. Opioids given to the woman during labour do not cross the placenta.
6. The Valsalva manoeuvre is the same as the lithotomy position.
7. An actively managed third stage leads to less bleeding during the delivery of the placenta.
8. There is no such thing as the 'purple line' when assessing a woman's progress in labour.
9. Women in the later stages of labour tend to decline food.
10. The umbilical cord should be cut straight away as soon as the baby is born.
11. Epidural anaesthesia does have an effect on the progress of labour.
12. If a midwife notices any deviation from the norm when caring for a woman in labour, she must report this to another healthcare professional.

References

Allen VM, Baskett TF, O'Connell C et al. (2009) Maternal and perinatal outcomes with increasing duration of the second stage of labor. *American Journal of Obstetrics and Gynecology* **113**(6): 1248–1258.

Anim-Somuah M, Smyth RMD, Jones L (2011) Epidural versus non-epidural or no analgesia for pain relief in labour. *Cochrane Database of Systematic Reviews* (**12**): CD000331.

Barrett JWH (1983) Prenatal influences on adaptation in the newborn. In: Stratton P (ed) *Psychobiology of the Human Newborn*. Chichester: John Wiley & Sons, Ltd.

Bartholomew C, Yerby M (2011) Pain, labour and women's choice of pain relief. In: Macdonald S, Magill-Cuerden J (eds) *Mayes' Midwifery: a textbook for midwives*, 14th edn. London: BaillièreTindall, pp521–533.

Baskett TE (2004) *Essential Management of Obstetric Emergencies*, 4th edn. Bristol: Clinical Press.

Begley CM, Gyte GML, Murphy DJ et al. (2011) Active versus expectant management for women in the third stage of labour. *Cochrane Database of Systematic Reviews* (11): CD007412.

BirthChoice UK. (2012) *Induction Rates*. Available at: www.birthchoiceuk.com/Professionals/index.html (accessed May 2013).

British National Formulary (BNF) (2012) *British National Formulary No 64*. London: British Medical Association and British Pharmaceutical Society of Great Britain.

Briggs GG, Freeman RK, Yaffe SJ (eds) (2008) *Drugs in Pregnancy and Lactation*, 8th edn. Philadelphia: Lippincott, Williams and Wilkins.

Church S, Hodgson T (2011) Rhythmic variations of labour. In: Macdonald S, Magill-Cuerden J (eds) *Mayes' Midwifery: a textbook for midwives*, 14th edn. London: BaillièreTindall, pp 861–867.

Collis RE (2007) Analgesia in labour: induction and maintenance. *Anaesthesia and Intensive Care Medicine* **8**(7): 273–275.

Collis RE, Baxendall ML, Srikantharajah ID et al. (1993) Mobility during labour with combined analgesia. *Lancet* **341**(8847): 767–768.

Coppen R (2005) *Birthing Position: do midwives know best?* London: Quay Books.

Czarnocka J, Slade P (2000) Prevalence and predictors of post-traumatic stress symptoms following childbirth. *British Journal of Clinical Psychology* **39**: 35–51.

Department of Health (DH) (2007) *Maternity Matters: choice, access and continuity of care in a safe service*. London: Department of Health.

Department of Health (DH) (2010) *Midwifery 2020: delivering expectations*. London: Department of Health.

Downe S (2011) Care in the second stage of labour. In: Macdonald S, Magill-Cuerden J (eds) *Mayes' Midwifery: a textbook for midwives*, 14th edn. London: BaillièreTindall, pp 509–520.

Ghacero EP, Enabudosco E (2006) Labor management: an appraisal of the role of false labor and the latent phase on the delivery mode. *Journal of Obstetrics and Gynecology* **26**(6): 534–537.

Harris T (2011) Care in the third stage of labour. In: Macdonald S, Magill-Cuerden J (eds) *Mayes' Midwifery: a textbook for midwives*, 14th edn. London: BaillièreTindall, pp 535–550.

Hodnett ED, Downe S, Walsh D, Weston J (2010) Alternative versus conventional institutional settings for birth. *Cochrane Database of Systematic Reviews* (**9**): CD000012.

Hodnett ED, Gates S, Hofmeyr GJ et al. (2011) Continuous support for women during childbirth. *Cochrane Database of Systematic Reviews* (**2**): CD003766.

Howie L, Rankin J (2011a) The onset of labour. In: Stables D, Rankin J (eds) *Physiology in Childbearing with Anatomy and Related Biosciences*, 3rd edn. London: Elsevier, p487.

Howie L, Rankin J (2011b) The first stage of labour. In: Stables D, Rankin J (eds) *Physiology in Childbearing with Anatomy and Related Biosciences*, 3rd edn. London: Elsevier, p 497.

Howie L, Rankin J (2011c) Pain relief in labour. In: Stables D, Rankin J (eds) *Physiology in Childbearing with Anatomy and Related Biosciences*, 3rd edn. London: Elsevier, p 517.

Howie L, Rankin J (2011d) The second stage of labour. In: Stables D, Rankin J (eds) *Physiology in Childbearing with Anatomy and Related Biosciences*, 3rd edn. London: Elsevier, p533.

Hunt S (2002) Pethidine: love it or hate it? *MIDIRS Midwifery Digest* **12**(3): 363–365.

Hutchon DJR (2006) Delayed cord clamping may be beneficial in rich settings. *British Medical Journal* **333**(7577): 1073.

Inch S (1985) Management of the third stage of labour – another cascade of intervention. *Midwifery* **1**(2): 114–122.

Janni W, Schiessl B, Peschers U et al. (2002) The prognostic impact of a prolonged second stage and the effects on perinatal and maternal outcomes. *Acta Obstetrica Gynaecologica Scandinavica* **81**: 214–221.

Johnson MH, Everitt BJ (2007) *Essential Reproduction*, 6th edn. Oxford: Blackwell Publishing Ltd.

Johnson R, Taylor W (2010) *Skills for Midwifery Practice*, 3rdedn. London: Elsevier.

Johnston J (2004) The nesting instinct. *Birth Matters* **8**(2): 21–22.

Kennedy HP (2000) A model of exemplary midwifery practice: results of a Delphi study. *Journal of Midwifery and Women's Health* **45**(1): 4–18.

Kinmond S, Aitchison TC, Holland BM et al. (1993) Umbilical cord clamping and preterm infants: a randomised trial. *British Medical Journal* **306**(6871): 172–175.

Lawrence A, Lewis L, Hofmeyr GJ et al. (2009) Maternal positions and mobility during first stage labour. *Cochrane Database of Systematic Reviews* (**2**): CD003934.

Leap N (2000) Pain in labour: towards a midwifery perspective. *MIDIRS Midwifery Digest* **10**(1): 49–53.

Levy V, Moore J (1985) The midwife's management of the third stage of labour. *Nursing Times* **81**(39): 47–50.

Lieberman E, Davidson K, Lee-Parritz A, Shearer A (2005) Changes in fetal position during labour and their association with epidural analgesia. *Obstetrics and Gynecology* **105**(5): 974–982.

MacArthur C, Lewis M, Knox EG et al. (1990) Epidural and long-term backache after childbirth. *British Medical Journal* **301**(6742): 9–12.

Maternity Care Working Party (2007) *Making Normal Birth a Reality: Consensus Statement*. Available at: www.rcog.org.uk/womens-health/clinical-guidance/making-normal-birth-reality (accessed May 2013).

McDonald SJ, Middleton P (2009) Effect of timing of umbilical cord clamping of term infants on maternal and neonatal outcomes. *Cochrane Database of Systematic Reviews* (**2**): CD004074.

McKay S, Roberts J (1990) Obstetrics by ear: maternal and caregiver perceptions of the meaning of maternal sounds during second stage of labour. *Journal of Nurse-Midwifery* **35**: 266–273.

Mead M (2004) Midwives' practices in 11 UK maternity units. In: Downe S (ed) *Normal Childbirth: evidence and debate*. Edinburgh: Churchill Livingstone.

Mendelsohn CL (1946) The aspiration of stomach contents. Cited in: Parsons M, Nagy S (2006) Anaesthetist's perspective on oral intake for women in labour. *British Journal of Midwifery* **14**(8): 488–491.

Mercer JS, Erickson-Owens DA, Graves B, Haley M (2007) Evidence-based practices for the fetal to newborn transition. *Journal of Midwifery and Women's Health* **52**(3): 262–272.

Micklewright A, Champion P (2002) Labouring over food: the dietician's view. In: Champion P, Cormick C (eds) *Eating and Drinking in Labour*. Oxford: Books for Midwives.

MIDIRS (2008) Positions in labour and delivery. Informed choice for professionals – leaflet. Bristol: MIDIRS.

Miquelutti MA, Cecatti JG, Morais S, Makuch M (2009) The vertical position during labor: pain and satisfaction. *Revista Brasileira de Saúde Materno Infantil* **9**: 393–398.

Myles T, Santolaya J (2003) Maternal and neonatal outcomes in patients with a prolonged second stage of labour. *Obstetrics and Gynaecology* **102**: 52–58.

National Institute for Health and Clinical Excellence (NICE) (2007) *Intrapartum Care: care of healthy women and their babies during childbirth*. Clinical Guideline 55. London: National Institute for Health and Clinical Excellence.

National Institute for Health and Clinical Excellence (NICE) (2008) *Induction of Labour*. Clinical Guideline CG70. London: National Institute for Health and Clinical Excellence. Available at: www.nice.org.uk/CG70 (accessed May 2013).

Nursing and Midwifery Council (NMC) (2012) *Midwives' Rules and Standards*. London: Nursing and Midwifery Council.

Odent M (2003) Preparing the nest. *Midwifery Today* **68**: 13–14.

O'Hana H, Levy A, Rozen A et al. (2008) The effect of epidural analgesia on labor progress and outcome in nulliparous women. *Journal of Maternal-Fetal Neonatal Medicine* **21**(8): 517–521.

Parsons M, Nagy S (2006) Anaesthetists' perspective on oral intake for women in labour. *British Journal of Midwifery* **14**(8): 488–491.

Peled G (1992) Birth and the Gulf War. *MIDIRS Midwifery Digest* **3**(1): 54.

Prins M, Boxem J, Lucas C, Hutton E (2011) Effect of spontaneous pushing versus Valsalva pushing in the second stage of labour on mother and fetus: a systematic review of randomised trials. *British Journal of Obstetrics and Gynaecology* **116**(6): 662–670.

Ragnar I, Altman D, Tyden T, Olsson SE (2006) Comparison of the maternal experience and duration of labour in two upright delivery positions – a randomized controlled trial. *British Journal of Obstetrics and Gynaecology* **113**: 165–170.

Resuscitation Council (UK) (2011) *Newborn Life Support: resuscitation at birth*, 3rd edn. London: Resuscitation Council.

Robertson A (2001) Skills for Childbirth Educators. Volume 1: learning about the pelvis (video). Australia: Birth International.

129

Rogers C, Villar R, Pisal P et al. (2011) Effects of Syntocinon use in active management of third stage of labour. *British Journal of Midwifery* **19**(6): 371–378.

Rosenblatt D, Belsey EM, Lieberman L et al. (1981) The influence of maternal analgesia on neonatal behaviour. *British Journal of Obstetrics and Gynaecology* **88**(4): 407–413.

Royal College of Midwives (RCM) (2012a) Positions for labour and birth practice points. In: *Evidence-based Guidelines for Midwifery-led Care in Labour*. London: Royal College of Midwives.

Royal College of Midwives (RCM) (2012b) Nutrition in labour. In: *Evidence-based Guidelines for Midwifery-led Care in Labour*. London: Royal College of Midwives.

Royal College of Midwives (RCM) (2012c) Second stage of labour. In: *Evidence-based Guidelines for Midwifery-led Care in Labour*. London: Royal College of Midwives.

Royal College of Obstetricians and Gynaecologists (RCOG) (2007) *Safer Childbirth. Minimum standards for the organisation and delivery of care in labour*. London: RCOG Press.

Royal College of Obstetricians and Gynaecologists (RCOG) (2009) *Prevention and Management of Postpartum Haemorrhage*. Available at: www.rcog.org.uk/womens-health/clinical-guidance/prevention-and-management-postpartum-haemorrhage-green-top-52 (accessed May 2013).

Shepherd A, Cheyne H , Kennedy S et al. (2010) The purple line as a measure of labour progress: a longitudinal study. *BMC Pregnancy and Childbirth* **10**: 54. Available at: www.biomedcentral.com/1471-2393/10/54 (accessed May 2013).

Singata M, Tranmer J, Gyte G (2010) Restricting oral fluid and food intake during labour. *Cochrane Database of Systematic Reviews* (**1**): CD003930.

Soltani H (2008) Global implications of evidence 'biased' practice: management of the third stage of labour. *Midwifery* **24**(2): 138–142.

Sookhoo ML, Biott C (2002) Learning at work: midwives judging progress in labour. *Learning in Health and Social Care* **1**(2): 75–85.

Sorbe B (1978) Active pharmacologic management of the third stage of labour. *Obstetrics and Gynaecology* **52**(6): 694–697.

Spencer PM (1962) Controlled cord traction in management of the third stage of labour. *British Medical Journal* **1**(5294): 1728–1732.

Spiby H, Slade P, Escott D et al. (2003) Selected coping strategies in labour: an investigation of women's experience. *Birth* **30**: 189–194.

Tracy S, Sullivan E, Wang Y et al. (2007) Birth outcomes associated with interventions in labour amongst low risk women: a population-based study. *Women and Birth* **20**: 41–48.

Tranmer J, Hodnett E, Hannah M et al. (2005) The effect of unrestricted oral carbohydrate on labor progress. *Journal of Obsteric, Gynaecological and Neonatal Nursing* **34**(3): 319–328.

Tuckey JP, Prout RE, Wee MY (2007) Prescribing intramuscular opioids for labour analgesia in consultant-led maternity units: a survey of UK practice. *International Journal of Obstetric Anaesthesia* **17**(1): 3–8.

Ullman R, Smith L, Burns E et al. (2010) Parenteral opioids for maternal pain relief in labour. *Cochrane Database of Systematic Reviews* (**9**): CD007396.

Walsh D (2011) Care in the first stage of labour. In: Macdonald S, Magill-Cuerden J (eds) *Mayes' Midwifery: a textbook for midwives*, 14th edn. London: Baillière Tindall.

Wickham S, Sutton J (2005) The rhombus of Michaelis. In: Wickham S (ed) *Midwifery Best Practice*, vol 3. Edinburgh: Books for Midwives Press/Elsevier Butterworth Heinemann.

Wood C, Soltani H (2005) Does pethidine relieve pain? *Practising Midwife* **8**(7): 17–25.

World Health Organization (WHO) (1996) *Care in Normal Birth: practical guide*. Available at: www.who.int/reproductivehealth/publications/maternal_perinatal_health/MSM_96_24_/en/index.html (accessed May 2013).

World Health Organization (WHO) (2007) *Recommendations for the Prevention of Postpartum Haemorrhage*. Available at: www.who.int/making_pregnancy_safer/publications/WHORecommendationsforPPHaemorrhage.pdf (accessed May 2013).

Wuitchik M, Kakal D, and Lipshitz J (1989) The clinical significance of pain and cognitive activity in latent labour. *Obstetrics and Gynaecology* **73**(1): 35–42.

8

Effective Emergency Care
Caroline Duncombe

Aim

This chapter aims to provide readers with evidence-based knowledge to strengthen the skills required in emergency situations.

Learning outcomes

It is expected that at the end of this chapter you will:

1. understand how your responsibilities when providing emergency care are supported by the Nursing and Midwifery Council
2. be familiar with the skills and drills required to manage emergencies in childbirth
3. be aware of the importance of comprehensive record keeping.

Introduction

Rule 5 of the *Midwives' Rules and Standards* (NMC 2012) identifies midwives' obligations and scope of practice. The standard that accompanies this rule states that in an emergency situation or where there is a deviation from the norm, the midwife must refer to another healthcare professional who is expected to have the required skills and experience to assist in providing care (NMC 2012).

The Clinical Negligence Scheme for Trusts (CNST) was set up by the NHS Litigation Authority to handle clinical negligence claims against member NHS bodies. The CNST requires annual multidisciplinary practice sessions or 'drills' so that staff members can practise their specific roles in an emergency situation.

The Student's Guide to Becoming a Midwife, Second Edition. Edited by Ian Peate and Cathy Hamilton.
© 2014 John Wiley & Sons, Ltd. Published 2014 by John Wiley & Sons, Ltd.

Midwifery wisdom

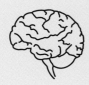

Keep your emergency skills and knowledge up to date.

The emergency situations to be discussed are those identified in the *Standards for Pre-registration Midwifery Education* (NMC 2009), NHSLA (2012) and *Saving Mothers' Lives* (CMACE 2011). They are:

- maternal resuscitation
- neonatal resuscitation
- shoulder dystocia
- vaginal breech delivery
- manual removal of the placenta
- manual examination of the uterus
- management of postpartum haemorrhage
- management of an eclamptic seizure.

With each of these emergency situations, factors that increase the risk of occurrence will be identified. This will facilitate anticipation of problems that might affect delivery.

Maternal resuscitation

Incidence

Cardiac arrest is estimated to occur in 1:30,000 late pregnancies (Morris & Stacey 2003). However, in the 2006–2008 triennium the maternal mortality rate was 11.39 per 100,000 maternities which is equal to 1:8779 women from pregnancy to 1 year after the birth (CMACE 2011).

Risk factors

The most common cause of maternal cardiac arrest, regardless of aetiology, is hypovolaemia and hypotension (Morris & Stacey 2003).

The factors that increase the requirement for maternal resuscitation vary but include those identified by CMACE (2011) as being the leading causes of direct maternal death (due to pregnancy), shown in Figure 8.1.

Certain physiological changes that occur in pregnancy may have an impact on maternal resuscitation:

- *Increase in cardiac output by 30–40%*: this starts as early as 4 weeks' gestation to promote maternal adaptation to pregnancy, as well as the blood supply to the enlarging uterus.
- *Increase in blood volume by up to 50%*: the uterine blood flow increases from 100 mL/min at the end of the first trimester to 500 mL/min by term (Heideman 2005). It results in a fall of haemoglobin due to the effect of haemodilution.

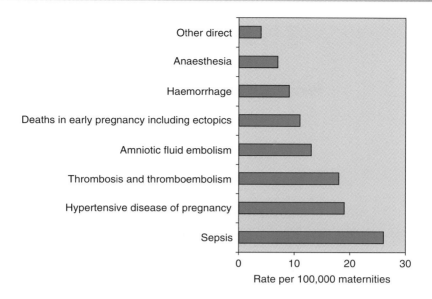

Figure 8.1   Mortality rates per million maternities of leading causes of direct deaths: United Kingdom 2006–2008 (CMACE 2011).

- *Increased oxygen consumption of 20%.*
- *Decreased peripheral* resistance: this is due to both development of the uteroplacental circulation and relaxation of the peripheral vascular tone.
- *Decreased residual capacity of the lungs of 25%.*
- *Delayed emptying of stomach contents*: this leads to an increase in volume and acidity of the gastric contents.
- *The weight of the pregnant uterus*: this can lead to aortocaval compression when a woman is lying in a supine position, particularly after 20 weeks' gestation. The weight presses on the aorta and vena cava, restricting blood flow to vital organs such as the brain and heart, causing a reduction in cardiac output and hypotension.

The Resuscitation Council (UK) currently sets the standard for maternal resuscitation and produces training aids and literature. Figure 8.2 shows the algorithm for basic adult resuscitation.

In pregnancy, physiological changes can complicate the resuscitation procedure and particular attention should be paid to minimising aortocaval compression. The uterus needs to be tilted to the left by 25–30º. This can be achieved by:

- using a firm triangular wedge present in many maternity units, or a pillow
- using a human wedge, i.e. knees
- using a tipped-up chair
- performing manual uterine displacement. This is when an attendant manually lifts the weight of the uterus to the left, off the woman. Aortocaval compression will be relieved by this method and cardiac output increased by 20–25%, but it may interfere with effective chest compressions. Cardiac output is reduced to approximately 30% of normal during effective cardiopulmonary resuscitation and its effectiveness depends on the efficacy of external chest compressions (Lee et al. 1986, Resuscitation Council UK 2010a, Ueland et al. 1972).

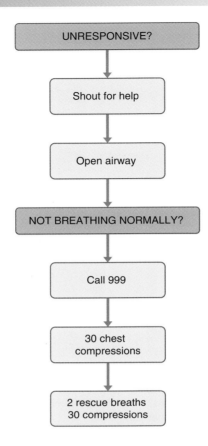

Figure 8.2 Algorithm for basic adult resuscitation. Reproduced by kind permission of the Resuscitation Council UK (2010a).

Perimortem (at or near the time of death) caesarean section may have to be undertaken early in the resuscitation attempt in order to relieve aortocaval compression, increase venous return and increase cardiac output. If it is done within 4–5 min of the cardiac arrest, the likelihood of maternal and neonatal survival is increased.

In all cases it is imperative that staff with the appropriate experience are present when dealing with a cardiac arrest in a pregnant woman. These are an obstetrician, anaesthetist and neonatologist. Particular attention should be paid to effective cardiac compressions. A rate of 30 compressions to two breaths is recommended.

Once expert help arrives:

- incorporate early advanced airway intervention
- apply pressure to the cricoid cartilage to occlude the upper end of the oesophagus against the vertebrae and prevent the acid gastric contents from being aspirated
- treat causative factors such as hypovolaemia or toxicity.

If the situation occurs in an out-of-hospital setting, then the emergency services need to be mobilised and basic resuscitation must continue with the woman tilted to the left until expert help is available.

Neonatal resuscitation

Incidence

A large study in Sweden indicated that 10 per 1000 babies over 2.5 kg required either mask inflation or intubation. Of these, eight per 1000 responded to mask inflation and two per 1000 required intubation (Palme-Kilander 1992). There is no corresponding information available for the UK.

Risk factors

The factors that increase the requirement for neonatal resuscitation vary and it is not easy to predict which babies will require resuscitation at birth. Therefore, everyone who attends births should be trained in newborn life support.

Babies who require resuscitation do so for different reasons from an adult. Physiologically, a newborn baby is prepared to withstand a lack of oxygen for periods during labour and birth. Generally, they are born with strong hearts, and the initial help they need is with respiration. Their lungs are filled with fluid at birth so to resuscitate a newborn baby, it is usually sufficient to inflate the lungs with air or oxygen. The heart will normally still be pumping and so will bring oxygenated blood back to the heart from the lungs, leading to recovery. Rarely, the heart may need to be 'bump' started (defibrillated). Figure 8.3 shows the algorithm for newborn life support.

Newborn life support consists of the following.

Drying and covering the baby to conserve heat

Drying the baby will provide stimulation and allow time for assessment of colour, tone, breathing and heart rate. Babies who become cold following birth are less able to maintain oxygen levels and become hypoglycaemic. The use of food-grade plastic wrapping is recommended by the Resuscitation Council UK (2010b) to maintain body temperature in significantly preterm babies.

Assessing the need for any intervention

Most babies when dried and kept warm will spontaneously start to breathe within 60–90 seconds of birth. A normal heart rate is 120–150 beats/min. This is best judged by listening with a stethoscope.

If *meconium* is present, do not aspirate it from the nose and mouth while the head is on the perineum as it is of no benefit and does not prevent meconium aspiration syndrome. Do not remove meconium from the airways of crying babies for the same reason. However, if babies are not crying at birth and meconium is seen in the oropharynx, this can be cleared with the use of a stiff Yankauer sucker, although there is no evidence of the efficacy of this practice.

Opening the airway

The baby should be placed on its back with its head in the neutral position, i.e. with the neck neither flexed nor extended. A folded towel may be placed under the shoulders to aid positioning if the baby has a prominent occiput (back of head). However, it is important to ensure the neck is not overextended when doing this. If the baby's tone is very poor, it may also be necessary to apply a chin lift or jaw thrust. This may be enough to enable air to enter the lungs to initiate the process of life.

136

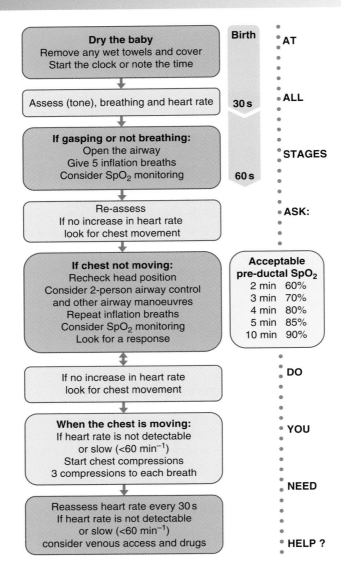

Figure 8.3   Newborn life support. Reproduced by kind permission of the Resuscitation Council UK (2010b).

Breathing

If a newborn does not make an effort to breathe, it will be appropriate to assist the process by giving up to five *inflation breaths* which need to last for 2–3 seconds each to be effective. This is because there may be no or limited chest movement for the first 2–3 inflations due to the movement of fluid from the lungs or poor positioning of the mask.

Midwifery wisdom

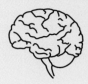 Ensure the baby's lungs are inflating before continuing with resuscitation.

Aerating the lungs triggers the neural centres in the brain responsible for normal breathing to function and the majority of newborns will recover. Air may be used initially, although oxygen should be available in case there is no rapid improvement in the newborn baby's condition.

If the baby's heart rate increases but spontaneous breathing is not initiated, then regular breaths should be provided at a rate of approximately 30–40/min until the baby starts to breathe on its own.

If there is no evidence of lung inflation, consider the following:

- Is the baby's head in the neutral position?
- Do you need jaw thrust?
- Do you need a longer inflation time?
- Do you need a second person's help with the airway?
- Do you need to remove an obstruction in the airway using a laryngoscope and wide-bore suction?
- What about an oropharyngeal (Guedel) airway?

There is no point in progressing until there is evidence that air is entering the lungs, so repeat the inflation breaths.

Chest compression

In a few cases, the cardiac function will have deteriorated so that oxygenated blood is not transferred from the aerated lungs to the heart. If the heart rate remains below 60 beats/min following effective inflation breaths, chest compressions will be required.

The recommended method of delivering chest compressions is to grip the chest with both hands so that the two thumbs can press on the lower third of the sternum, with the fingers over the spine at the back. The chest should be compressed quickly and firmly by about one-third of the depth at a ratio of 3:1 compressions to inflations. A rate of 90–120 compressions/min should be aimed for. The aim is to move oxygenated blood from the lungs back to the heart. It is important to allow enough time during the relaxation phase of each compression cycle for the heart to refill with blood.

Administration of drugs (rare)

In the rare event that lung inflation and chest compressions are insufficient, drugs may be required to restore the circulation. The outlook for this group of babies is poor.

Stopping resuscitation

The Resuscitation Council UK (2010b) states that 'In a newly-born baby with no detectable cardiac activity, and with cardiac activity that remains undetectable for 10 min, it is appropriate to consider stopping resuscitation'. However, the midwife's responsibility is to continue resuscitation until care is transferred to an appropriate practitioner (NMC 2012).

Shoulder dystocia

While caring for mothers in labour, midwives are constantly monitoring progress in order to predict and react to unfolding events. The rate of progress in labour and particularly the second stage is predictive of the possibility of obstruction during the delivery. Shoulder dystocia is one such delay.

Definition

Shoulder dystocia is best defined as an impaction of the anterior shoulder of the fetus against the maternal symphysis pubis after the fetal head has been delivered. Any measures aimed at expediting delivery concentrate on changing the relationship between the two bony parts. Gibb (1995) described three types of shoulder dystocia, increasing in severity:

1. A tight fit when delivering a big baby.
2. A unilateral dystocia, where the anterior shoulder becomes impacted above the maternal symphysis pubis.
3. A bilateral dystocia, where both the shoulders have become arrested above the pelvic brim.

Incidence

The incidence of shoulder dystocia is generally agreed to be 0.6–0.7% (RCOG 2012).

Risk factors

Before labour, a history of the following features is known to increase the risk of shoulder dystocia:

- Previous shoulder dystocia.
- Macrosomic baby (estimated >4.5 kg).
- Diabetes mellitus.
- Maternal Body Mass Index (>30 kg/m^2).
- Induction of labour.

During labour, the following scenarios also indicate an increased risk of shoulder dystocia:

- A prolonged first or second stage of labour.
- A secondary arrest of labour requiring oxytocin augmentation.
- An assisted vaginal delivery.

Although these risk factors are commonly cited, they are of reasonably poor predictive value and it is important to remain vigilant in all cases (AAFP 2000, RCOG 2012).

Management

The manoeuvres described here are currently recommended to assist practitioners to relieve a shoulder dystocia. They are described from the simple to the more complex, but this order is not prescriptive. Organisations such as ALSO (AAFP 2000) recommend the use of the mnemonic HELPERR:

- **H**elp
- **E**valuate for episiotomy
- **L**egs (McRoberts manoeuvre)
- **P**ressure (suprapubic)
- **E**nter (for manoeuvres)
- **R**emove (the posterior arm)
- **R**oll (the patient either into all-fours or through 360°)

Each manoeuvre should take a maximum of 1–2 min and if unsuccessful, it is important to move on to another.

Help

The first action of the midwife is to confidently diagnose a shoulder dystocia and call for help. Once help is on its way, the measures described below should be commenced. In a community setting, help will be requested from the paramedics by dialling 999. Simple measures may be worth considering in the first instance, such as rolling the mother onto all-fours or, in a birthing pool, encouraging her to stand up and place one foot on the edge of the pool to assist delivery.

Midwifery wisdom

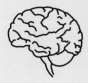

Make sure somebody is stationed at the ward doors to let the emergency team in.

Evaluate for episiotomy

It is widely accepted that in the event of a shoulder dystocia occurring, an episiotomy is desirable to prevent further damage to the mother's pelvic floor and to provide space for the 'enter' manoeuvres. However, once the baby's head has delivered, it is technically very difficult to ensure that the procedure does not damage the baby.

Legs (McRoberts manoeuvre)

This involves placing the mother flat on her back and putting her knees on her chest. Once she is in this position, attempts should be made to deliver the baby. The manoeuvre is aiming to:

- rotate the symphysis pubis anteriorly
- push the posterior shoulder over the sacrum
- open the pelvic inlet to its full capacity

- correct any maternal lordosis
- remove the sacral promontory as an obstruction.

If the manoeuvre is unsuccessful it is suggested that it is repeated before moving on to another. The McRoberts position is a relatively safe intervention with a good rate of success of 40–50%.

Pressure (suprapubic)

The aim of applying suprapubic pressure is to displace the anterior shoulder from the symphysis pubis and allow it to enter the pelvis. This action is sometimes referred to as Rubins 1 and is undertaken as follows:

- Pressure is applied by the midwife or an assistant to the mother's abdomen, above the baby's back, in a downward direction towards the side of the mother that the baby is facing.
- Whilst this pressure is applied, the delivering midwife will continue to try to deliver the baby with *gentle* traction. The pressure should initially be continuous. If unsuccessful, the assistant can be asked to provide suprapubic pressure as a rocking movement.

These manoeuvres have been shown to be effective in 67% of cases of shoulder dystocia cases (Luria et al. 1994).

Enter (for manoeuvres)

The 'enter' manoeuvres aim to rotate the shoulders. They are also known as Rubins 2 and the wood screw manoeuvres and are often combined to expedite delivery.

- *Rubins 2*: working from behind the baby, the anterior shoulder is located with the fingers and pushed into the oblique. This aims to reduce the diameter of the shoulders.
- *Wood screw manoeuvre*: at the same time, the fingers of the other hand can be used to add pressure to the front of the posterior shoulder to aid rotation of the shoulders into the oblique diameter. **If at any time during the manoeuvre it is seen that the baby has moved, an attempt to deliver should be made**.
- *Reverse wood screw*: if no movement is achieved, the fingers from in front of the posterior shoulder should be removed and the fingers behind the anterior shoulder can be slid down to behind the posterior shoulder and pressure applied in the opposite direction to rotate the baby.

For the 'enter' manoeuvres, the mother should be placed in the lithotomy position or, if at home, the McRoberts position. Suprapubic pressure can also be continued.

Remove (the posterior arm)

If the previous endeavours have been unsuccessful the last of the 'enter' manoeuvres is when an attempt to deliver the posterior arm is made. The midwife enters her fingers in front of the baby's body and locates the lower arm. Pressure is exerted on the elbow to try to make the lower arm raise; this is then grasped and gently pulled across the baby's face in a 'cat lick' motion, thereby delivering the posterior shoulder

Roll (the patient either onto all-fours or through 360º)

This position optimises the sacral curve and is in effect a McRoberts manoeuvre upside down. With the mother on all-fours, she can be encouraged to rock, thereby mimicking the movement of the legs when in the McRoberts position. This is therefore a useful tool when delivering in a birth centre or in the mother's home.

If these manoeuvres are unsuccessful, the whole round of procedures should be performed again. It is recommended that this is undertaken by another midwife or obstetrician if available.

Activity 8.1

Following a case involving a shoulder dystocia in your unit, ask if you can look at how the incident was managed and documented. Reflect on whether the records meet the recommendations.

Vaginal breech delivery

Incidence

Babies present by the breech in 15% of pregnancies at 29–32 weeks and 3–4% at term (Enkin et al. 2000). The later they stay breech, the less likely they are to turn spontaneously.

Risk factors

In many cases there is no explanation of why a baby presents by the breech, but it may be due to maternal reasons, such as:

- uterine malformation, e.g. bicornuate uterus (a uterus with a division down the middle), fibroids or tumours
- placenta praevia (when the placenta is situated in the lower uterine segment)
- oligohydramnios (reduced amount of amniotic fluid) – restricting movement
- polyhydramnios (increased amount of amniotic fluid) – providing plenty of space for movement
- multiple pregnancy
- contracted pelvis
- primigravid woman (expecting her first baby) with firm uterine and abdominal muscles
- grand multiparous woman (expecting her fifth or subsequent baby) with lax uterine and abdominal muscles,

or for fetal reasons, such as:

- anomalies, such as anencephaly (partially formed brain)
- short umbilical cord
- prematurity
- lack of tone such as fetal death *in utero*.

A breech is defined when the fetus is lying in a longitudinal position with the buttocks presenting. It may be described in the following ways:

- *Extended or frank breech* (70% of breech presentations): the hips are flexed and the knees extended so that the feet are near the head. This is more common in primigravid women with firm uterine and abdominal tone. It is also the most difficult to diagnose as the buttocks may be deeply engaged on abdominal palpation.
- *Flexed or complete breech*: the legs are bent at the hips and knees so the baby is sitting cross-legged. This is more common in a multiparous woman or when there is polyhydramnios.
- *Footling breech*: the foot or feet present before the buttocks. This is rare, but more common in premature gestations.
- *Kneeling breech*: this is very rare, and is described when the baby is in a kneeling position.

142

A breech is identified by the following methods:

- *Abdominal palpation*: the presenting part will be firm but not hard and smooth, although this might be difficult to identify if it is deeply engaged. The head may be ballotable (moveable) in the fundus, and the fetal heart may be auscultated above the level of the umbilicus, but again, this may be lower if the breech is deeply engaged.
- *Vaginal examination*: the presenting part may be higher in the pelvis prior to labour than when cephalic (head down).
- *Ultrasound scan*.

If a baby is known to be presenting by the breech prior to labour, there are a variety of methods which can be used to try to turn the baby, including visualisation techniques, breech tilt exercises, massage, homeopathy, hypnosis, acupuncture, acupressure, moxibustion, chiropractic adjustments and external cephalic version (Banks 1998). If the baby does not turn, it has been recent practice for a caesarean section to be recommended (Hannah et al. 2000) but discussion concerning this is beyond the scope of this chapter.

It is commonly thought that the baby's bottom is smaller than the diameter of the head and may pass through a cervix that is not fully dilated. The concern is that the larger head may become trapped behind the cervix. However, this is more likely with preterm infants. For a term infant presenting in a frank breech position, the bottom will be the same size as the head (Banks 1998).

If a woman presents in established labour and a breech presentation is diagnosed, the following procedures will help to promote a safe outcome:

- Use of ultrasound facilities if available to confirm the presentation of the baby and to identify whether any obstruction is present such as placenta praevia or a fibroid.
- A comfortable position to labour in.
  - On hands and knees is a good posture to adopt (Cronk 1998).
  - Lying prone or semi-recumbent works against the normal physiology of birth. If the woman is semi-recumbent, her legs should be in a lithotomy position and an episiotomy is generally recommended when the buttocks distend the perineum, especially if it is the woman's first birth.
  - There is a concern that if an upright position is used in the second stage, the placenta may separate from the uterus too quickly because of traction on the cord/placenta just after the birth due to gravity and in the absence of a contraction (Cronk 1998).
- Hands should be kept off the breech that is birthing spontaneously. Excessive handling may cause the baby to extend its arm above its head and lead to more complications.

- The fetal back needs to rotate anteriorly to the woman. If it is necessary to assist this process, the baby should be supported by the hips. It is not safe to hold the abdomen as damage can occur to the kidneys and adrenal glands.
- If required, a finger may be used to flex the knee and abduct the thigh to deliver the legs. They should not be pulled out.
- A loop of umbilical cord can be gently pulled down to release traction, but be careful that it does not go into spasm.
- If necessary, once the tip of the scapula is visible, the attendant can splint the baby's upper arm between the index and middle finger, then flex it and bring it down over its face, like a cat washing its face. If the arms are extended or nuchal (around the nape of the neck), it may help to undertake a modified Lovsett's manoeuvre. For this, the baby is first rotated by holding the hips and using downward traction, so the posterior arm is brought into an anterior position and then released as described above. If necessary, the procedure can be repeated for the second arm by rotating the baby back through a semi-circle, ensuring the back remains anterior. This manoeuvre is more likely to be required if the woman is lying on her back. It is rarely needed when an upright position is adopted (Banks 1998).
- Once the nape of the neck is visible, the woman should lean forward if she has been upright. A modified Mauriceau–Smellie–Veit grip may be used to assist the birth of the head, which should be born slowly (see Figure 8.4). The procedure is as follows.
  - Rest the baby with its face and body over your hand and arm with legs either side.
  - Place the first and third fingers of this hand on the baby's cheekbones to encourage flexion of the head. Current advice is to avoid placing a finger in the baby's mouth as this can damage the jaw. An assistant could be asked to push above the mother's pubic bone as the head delivers, to keep the head flexed.
  - Use the other hand to grasp the baby's shoulders and flex the baby's head towards its chest, while applying downward pressure to gently deliver the head (WHO 2003).
- Some breech babies will be slow to breathe spontaneously at birth, usually due to shock. It is important to have resuscitation equipment available and ready, and that the parents are aware that this may be required (Cronk 1998).

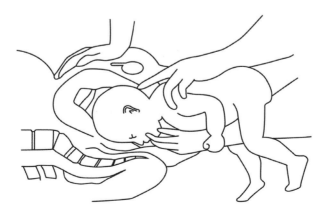

Figure 8.4   Breech presentation.

143

Activity 8.2

 Speak to some experienced midwives and ask them what experience they have of delivering breech babies.

144

Manual removal of the placenta

Incidence

The incidence is approximately 3% of all births (Titiz et al. 2001).

If the third stage is managed physiologically, up to 1 hour may pass before considering the procedure to be prolonged. With active management, it is expected that the placenta and membranes should be expelled by controlled cord traction within 30 min. If the placenta is not delivered within an hour, it should be removed manually. More complications occur in both physiological and active management if delivery of the placenta is delayed beyond 75 min. Forceful cord traction and fundal pressure should be avoided as they may cause uterine inversion.

If the placenta is retained, it may either be separated or partially separated but trapped, or it may be morbidly adherent (see Risk factors) to the uterine wall.

Risk factors

If the placenta is separated or partially separated but trapped, bleeding is more likely as the uterus cannot contract adequately to seal the vessels from the placental site. Risk factors include:

- the cervix reforming
- full bladder
- mismanagement of third stage, i.e. performing controlled cord traction or fundal pressure without giving oxytocin
- formation of a constriction ring or spasm between the upper and lower uterine segments
- uterine abnormality, e.g. bicornuate uterus.

If the placenta is morbidly adherent and there is no separation, bleeding may not occur. Risk factors for this include:

- previous caesarean section
- previous placenta praevia
- previous retained placenta
- high parity.

An adherent placenta occurs when there is a scanty or absent layer of decidua basalis (the maternal part of the placenta) at the site of implantation. Types of adherent placenta are as follows:

- *Placenta accreta*: the chorionic villi have adhered to the myometrium
- *Placenta increta*: the chorionic villi invade the myometrium
- *Placenta percreta*: the chorionic villi have penetrated through the myometrium either to or beyond the serosa (outer layer of the uterine wall)

This is a procedure all midwives should be familiar with in case of emergency when there is no appropriate assistance available. The following actions will help to promote a safe outcome:

- Call for help. If at home, this will be a paramedic ambulance by calling 999.
- If the bladder is not empty, catheterisation will be required.
- Oxytocin 10 iu (international units) can be given by intramuscular injection if it has not already done for active management of third stage. Do not give ergometrine as it can cause a tonic uterine contraction, which may delay expulsion.
- An intravenous infusion should be commenced as soon as possible to provide intravenous access and replace fluid loss.
- Analgesia must be given as available. Shock may occur due to pain from the procedure if analgesia is not adequate.
- Full aseptic precautions must be taken to minimise risk of infection.
- The umbilical cord should be made taut and the attendant's leading hand inserted into the vagina and uterus following the direction of the cord. If the cord has separated, this will still need to be done.
- Once the placenta is located, the cord should be released and the fundus supported. This will provide countertraction to prevent inversion of the uterus.
- A separated edge of the placenta should be felt for and the edge of the attendant's hand should be eased between the placenta and the uterine wall (Figure 8.5). A careful slicing motion with the edge of the hand should be used to continue to separate the placenta until it is detached.
- The fundus can then be massaged to assist the hand holding the placenta to be expelled from the uterus, still grasping the placenta.

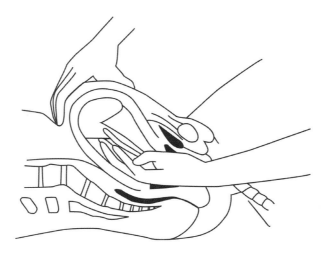

Figure 8.5   Removal of the placenta.

- Following the procedure:
  - the placenta must immediately be inspected for completeness. If any placental lobe or tissue is missing, the uterine cavity must be explored to remove it
  - an assistant should then massage the fundus of the uterus to encourage a tonic uterine contraction
  - an intravenous bolus of oxytocin (10 iu) should be given after successful removal of the placenta, followed by an intravenous infusion of oxytocin.
- Observations should be made for:
  - vital signs (pulse, blood pressure, respirations) at least every 30 min for 6 hours or until the woman is stable
  - uterine contraction: the uterine fundus should be palpated and lochia should be monitored to ensure it is not excessive
  - signs of coagulopathy (the ability of the blood to clot), particularly if bleeding has been excessive
  - signs of infection, i.e. fever or foul-smelling vaginal discharge. Intravenous antibiotics should be given prophylactically, according to local protocols.
- Intravenous fluid administration should be continued and a blood transfusion considered as necessary (WHO 2003).

Potential complications

If the tissue is extremely adherent and cannot be separated easily, heavy bleeding or perforation of the uterus may result. There are two choices:

1. A hysterectomy
2. The placenta can be left *in situ* to be reabsorbed

If the placenta is retained due to a constriction ring, or if hours or days have passed since delivery, it may not be possible to get the entire hand into the uterus. The placenta should be removed in fragments using two fingers, ovum forceps or a wide curette.

Manual examination of the uterus

A manual examination of the uterus will be necessary following manual removal of the placenta. This is because the placenta is likely to be evacuated in pieces and it may be very difficult to ensure it is complete. A careful examination of the uterus will ensure that no remaining fragments of placental tissue are left *in situ*. If placental fragments are retained, there may initially be minimal blood loss from the vagina. However, there is a high risk that bleeding will eventually occur as retained tissue will prevent the uterus from contracting effectively, and also the risk of infection will be increased.

The procedure for manual examination of the uterus is similar to the technique described for manual removal of the placenta. However, it is important to recognise that efforts to extract fragments of placental tissue that do not separate easily may result in heavy bleeding or uterine perforation, which usually requires hysterectomy. This procedure is carried out by a midwife in an emergency only when no obstetric help is available (NMC 2012).

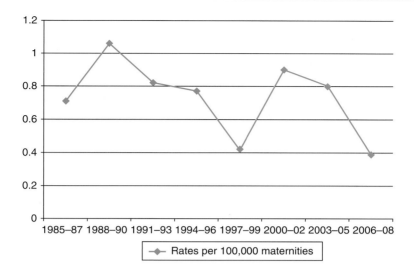

Figure 8.6 Maternal mortality for deaths due to haemorrhage in the UK, 1985–2006 (CMACE 2011).

Management of postpartum haemorrhage

Incidence

A major postpartum haemorrhage occurs in about 3.7 per 1000 births with uterine atony being the primary cause (CMACE 2011). In the triennium 2006–2008, postpartum haemorrhage (PPH) accounted for five out of nine direct maternal deaths from obstetric haemorrhage in the UK, which was the sixth highest cause of maternal death. This is equivalent to 0.39 per 100,000 births. Substandard obstetric care was reported in six (i.e. 66%) of the nine women who died. The figure has dropped and is now at its lowest since reporting began in 1952 (CMACE 2011). Figure 8.6 demonstrates figures since 1985.

The definition of a PPH is a blood loss of 500 mL or more from the genital tract following birth. However, calculation of blood loss is very subjective and is usually underestimated. Emergency treatment should be initiated if the woman becomes symptomatic, or if the blood loss is estimated to be over 1000 mL, which is classified as a major obstetric haemorrhage (RCOG 2009). The ability of a woman to cope with blood loss depends on her general health status. A primary PPH occurs within 24 hours of birth and secondary PPH occurs after this time (WHO 2009). Table 8.1 outlines risk factors for a PPH.

Midwifery wisdom

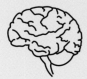 Blood loss is often underestimated.

Table 8.1   Risk factors for postpartum haemorrhage

Antepartum	Intrapartum
Proven abruptio placentae	Delivery by emergency caesarean section
Known placenta praevia	Delivery by elective caesarean section
Multiple pregnancy	Retained placenta
Pre-eclampsia/gestational hypertension	Episiotomy
Nulliparity	Assisted delivery (forceps/vacuum)
Previous PPH	Prolonged third stage (>30 min)
Asian ethnicity	Prolonged labour (>12 hours)
Obesity	Big baby (>4 kg)
Previous caesarean section	Pyrexia in labour
	Augmented labour
	Arrest of descent
	Lacerations (cervical/vaginal/perineal)

Source: Data from Combs & Laros 1991; AAFP 2000

Management

Once a PPH has been identified, four actions need to occur *simultaneously*, but will be addressed individually. They are: communication; resuscitation; monitoring and investigation; and arresting the haemorrhage. These are described by ALSO UK (AAFP 2000).

Communication

HELP IS REQUIRED. An emergency call must always be made to summon senior staff including a midwife, obstetrician and anaesthetist. If the woman becomes symptomatic, or if the blood loss is estimated to be over 1000 mL, a major obstetric haemorrhage call should be put out to summon additional staff to document the events (a scribe), portering staff (to deliver and collect specimens/blood to and from appropriate laboratories) and the haematologist for advice. If a PPH occurs outside the hospital setting, paramedic support will be required.

Substandard care frequently relates to failure to involve appropriate senior professionals at an early stage. The consultant obstetrician and anaesthetist must be alerted if not present.

Midwifery wisdom

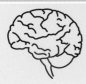

If there is an emergency in the woman's home, use available personnel to call for help.

Resuscitation

- Assess airway, breathing and circulation.
- Give oxygen by mask at 10–15 L/min (RCOG 2009).
- Lie flat/head-down tilt.
- Intravenous access with two large-bore (14–16 gauge) cannulae.
- Commence crystalloid infusion (e.g. Hartmann's solution) (maximum 2 L).
- Alternate with colloid (e.g. gelofusine, Haemaccel, human albumin 4.5%) (maximum 1.5 L).
- Transfuse blood as soon as available (if cross-matched blood is unavailable by the time 3.5 L of clear fluid have been infused, group 'O' rhesus negative or uncross-matched, own group blood may be used).

149

Monitoring and investigation

Blood is taken from the woman and should be sent immediately to the laboratory for:

- cross-matching of 4–6 units
- full blood count
- clotting screen
- renal and liver function tests (for a baseline).

A member of the team observes frequent pulse and blood pressure measurements to monitor the woman's condition, ideally recorded continually. Oxygen saturations are observed; an indwelling urinary catheter is passed in order to monitor urine output and central venous pressure monitoring is carried out to guide fluid volume replacement. Temperature should be measured every 15 min. Observations should be recorded on an obstetric early warning chart (RCOG 2009).

Arresting the haemorrhage

A haemorrhage may occur as a result of one or more of four causes. The AAFP (2000) identifies them as the four Ts, listed in order of frequency, and they all must be considered as the potential cause:

1. *Tone (70%)*: uterine atony is the most common cause of a PPH and should be perceived to be the cause of the bleeding, unless proven otherwise.
2. *Trauma (20%)*: cervical, vaginal and perineal lacerations; ruptured uterus; pelvic haematoma; uterine inversion.
3. *Tissue (10%)*: retained products (placenta, membranes, clots).
4. *Thrombin (1%)*: coagulopathies.

1. Tone

- Rub up a contraction by rubbing up the fundus: this will stimulate the uterus to contract.
- Ensure the bladder is empty. Insert an indwelling catheter and leave *in situ*.
- Bimanual compression of the uterus if atony persists. This is done by inserting one hand into the vagina, then making a fist against the body of the uterus inside. The other hand is placed above the uterus and squeezes against the first hand.
- Give drugs as appropriate.
  - Syntocinon 10 units by slow intravenous (IV) injection or intramuscular (IM) if not already given by this route.
  - Ergometrine 0.5 mg by slow IV injection.

- ○ Syntocinon infusion at 10 iu per hour (e.g. 40 units in 500 mL Hartmann's at 125 mL/hour).
- ○ Carboprost (Haemabate) 0.25 mg IM (repeated at intervals of not less than 15 min to a maximum of eight doses).
- If bleeding persists, transfer to operating theatre and consider the other Ts.

2. Trauma

If bleeding continues, consider the possibility of lacerations, a ruptured or inverted uterus. Continue bimanual compression until appropriate help is available.

3. Tissue

If the placenta is delivered, ensure it is complete. If the placenta is not delivered, a manual removal of placenta or manual examination of the uterus may be indicated as described previously.

4. Thrombin

Coagulation disorders are very rare and are usually identified in the antenatal period. However, a large blood loss from one of the above causes may lead to the blood clotting mechanisms becoming deranged. This is identified through blood clotting studies.

Activity 8.3

Reflect on any cases of postpartum haemorrhage you have been involved with. Can you identify what the cause was? Did it affect the management?

Management of an eclamptic seizure

Eclampsia is defined as one or more convulsions occurring during or immediately after pregnancy, as a complication of pre-eclampsia. Rapid recognition of signs of severe pre-eclampsia and awareness of risk factors may prevent progression to eclampsia.

Incidence

Severe pre-eclampsia/eclampsia is a major factor in maternal and fetal mortality and morbidity. In 2006–2008, CMACE (2011) reported 19 maternal deaths due to pre-eclampsia or eclampsia which is equal to 0.83 per 100,000 maternities. This is compared to 0.66 in the previous report.

Pre/eclampsia/eclampsia remains the second leading cause of maternal deaths in the UK and substandard care is constantly stated as being a major factor in a number of cases.

The midwife is usually the first professional in a position to detect pre-eclampsia and it is vital that she involves the obstetricians immediately so a management plan can be put in place and attempt to prevent progression to eclampsia.

Risk factors

- Age 40 years or above
- First pregnancy
- Pregnancy interval of more than 10 years
- Family history of pre-eclampsia
- Previous history of pre-eclampsia/eclampsia
- Body Mass Index more than 30 at booking
- Pre-existing vascular disease such as hypertension, diabetes, thrombophilias
- Pre-existing renal disease
- Multiple pregnancy
- Abnormal uterine Doppler studies at 18 and 24 weeks of pregnancy (APEC 2005, NICE 2008, Sibai 2003)

Signs and symptoms

Some women who present with eclampsia will have *no* pre-existing signs or symptoms. Therefore, the midwife must be aware of the risk factors of developing pre-eclampsia at booking and refer and monitor closely throughout the pregnancy. Women also need to be informed of symptoms of worsening disease so they are able to alert the midwife if they have any concerns.

Hypertension

Hypertension is said to occur when the diastolic blood pressure (BP) is 90 mmHg or more on two occasions and the systolic BP is 140 mmHg or more. The CEMACH Report (2004) highlighted that whilst diastolic BP is one of the important indices of the severity of pre-eclampsia, it is thought that it is the systolic BP which causes intracerebral haemorrhage. It therefore recommended that antihypertensive treatment should be considered for a systolic BP of 160 mmHg or above. However, if signs of severe disease are present, medication should be commenced at lower levels (RCOG 2011).

However, eclampsia is not always preceded by severe hypertension, with 34% of eclamptic women having a maximum diastolic BP of 100 mmHg or below (Douglas & Redman 1994).

Proteinuria

A dipstick analysis of urine that reveals a 2+ of proteinuria or more should be confirmed by a 24 hours urine collection. A urine protein excretion of 300 mg or more over 24 hours is significant (RCOG 2011).

Severe headaches

These could be a sign of cerebral involvement.

Visual disturbances

Due to papilloedema, this is a swelling of the optic nerve and a sign of increased intracranial pressure.

Vomiting

This is one of the signs of increased intracranial pressure.

Epigastric pain

This is of particular concern and may be associated with vomiting. There will be tenderness on palpation (APEC 2005).

Signs of clonus

Clonus is rapid rhythmic movements and is described as alternate muscle relaxation and contraction resulting in brisk reflexes.

Small for gestational age fetus

This could be one of the first signs of pre-eclampsia and occurs in 30% of pre-eclamptic pregnancies (RCOG,2011). It is important that fundal height is measured, any abnormalities reported and a growth scan arranged if indicated.

Reduced fetal movements

This may indicate fetal compromise due to placental insufficiency.

Management

The first seizure will occur in 44% of women within 48 hours of delivery, 38% in the antenatal period and 18% during labour (APEC 2005).

Help from a senior obstetrician and anaesthetist should be summoned. If in the community, an emergency paramedic ambulance must be summoned and the woman should be protected from injury during the convulsion. Following convulsion, the woman should be placed in a left lateral position and given oxygen. Assessment of the airway, breathing and circulation is required as well as measurement of blood pressure, pulse, temperature and oxygen saturation.

Intravenous access is required if not already instigated. Magnesium sulphate is the anticonvulsant of choice (CEMACH 2004). A loading dose of magnesium sulphate 4 g should be given by infusion pump over 5–10 min, followed by a maintenance dose of 1g/hour for 24 hours after the last seizure. Antihypertensive therapy is required to reduce the BP and this is provided according to local protocol. Blood is obtained for group and save, full blood count, analysis of urea and electrolytes along with tests for liver function and clotting.

A woman suffering from breathing problems with laryngeal oedema or if presenting with status eclampticus (continuous convulsions) will require intubation and ventilation (Arulkumaran et al. 1997).

Fetal monitoring is required to assess fetal well-being if the baby is not already delivered. Delivery should be undertaken as soon as the maternal condition is stable as this is the only definite way to resolve the crisis (Arulkumaran et al. 1997).

Conclusion

Emergency scenarios occur both in and out of hospital. Fortunately, they are relatively uncommon in the community setting where midwives are more likely to be working without close access to obstetric support. However, it is midwives in these settings who will have to be prepared to carry out these procedures should the need arise.

When faced with an emergency situation, the key points are to:

- call for appropriate help – paramedic assistance out of the hospital setting
- deal with the emergency
- work effectively as a team – good communication required
- document the events and action taken clearly – this is a professional requirement (NMC 2012) and helpful for analysis of the event. Remember that if it's not written, it didn't happen! A scribe has a very important role in emergency scenarios and enables accurate, contemporaneous record keeping. Any notes made should be firmly attached to the main record
- report the incident through the incident reporting system
- debrief after the event with colleagues and a supervisor of midwives
- reflect on the event.

If possible, a member of the team should be allocated to remain with the woman and her partner to ensure communication and offer support throughout the emergency situation (NICE 2006).

Quiz

1. What training is a requirement by the CNST?
    a. Regular midwifery 'emergency skills' training
    b. Annual multidisciplinary 'drills' in maternity unit
    c. Annual mandatory assessment on the management of emergency drills
2. How common is cardiac arrest in late pregnancy?
    a. 1:3000
    b. 1:30,000
    c. 1:300,000
3. What is the most common cause of maternal cardiac arrest?
    a. Cardiac arrhythmias
    b. Cardiac disease
    c. Hypovolaemia and hypotension
4. Within what length of time will a newborn baby usually breathe spontaneously?
    a. 30 seconds
    b. One minute
    c. 60–90 seconds
5. What is the most effective way of opening the airway of a newborn baby?
    a. Give baby to Mum to cuddle
    b. Place on back with head in neutral position
    c. Hold upside down
6. What is the incidence of shoulder dystocia?
    a. 1:100
    b. 1:1000
    c. 6–7:1000
7. What is the first thing to do in any emergency?
    a. Ask for a second opinion
    b. Call for help
    c. Ensure documentation is up to date

8. What is the most common presentation for a term breech baby?
    a. Extended breech
    b. Flexed breech
    c. Footling breech

9. What is a good reminder of the possible causes of a postpartum haemorrhage?
    a. 4 As
    b. 4 Cs
    c. 4 Ts

10. If a woman has an eclamptic seizure after 37 weeks' gestation, what should be planned?
    a. The baby should be delivered immediately.
    b. The fits should be stabilised and then the baby should be delivered.
    c. The fits should be stabilised and then spontaneous labour awaited.

References

American Academy of Family Physicians (AAFP) (2000) Advanced life saving. In: *Obstetrics (ALSO) Provider Manual*, 4th edn. Kansas: AAFP.

Action on Pre-Eclampsia (APEC) (2005) PRECOG: The Pre-eclampsia Community Guideline. Available at: www.apec.org.uk/downloads/precog.pdf (accessed May 2013).

Arulkumaran S, Ratnam SS, Bhasker Rao K (1997) *The Management of Labour*. India: Orient Longman.

Banks M (1998) *Breech Birth Woman-wise*. New Zealand: Birthspirit Books.

Centre for Maternal and Child Enquiries (CMACE) (2011) *Saving Mothers' Lives: reviewing maternal deaths to make motherhood safer: 2006–08*. Eighth Report on Confidential Enquiries into Maternal Deaths in the United Kingdom. *British Journal of Obstetrics and Gynaecology* **118**(Suppl. 1): 1–203.

Combs CA, Laros RK (1991) Prolonged third stage of labor: morbidity and risk factors. *Obstetrics and Gynecology* **77**: 863–7.

Confidential Enquiry into Maternal and Child Health (CEMACH) (2004) *Why Mothers Die 2000–2002. The Sixth Report*. London: RCOG Press.

Cronk M (1998) Midwifery skills needed for breech birth. *Midwifery Matters* **Autumn**: **78**.

Douglas KA, Redman CWG (1994) Eclampsia in the United Kingdom. *British Medical Journal* **309**: 1395.

Enkin M, Keirse M, Neilson J et al. (2000) *A Guide to Effective Care in Pregnancy and Childbirth*, 3rd edn. Oxford: Oxford University Press.

Gibb D (1995) Clinical focus: shoulder dystocia. *Clinical Risk* **1**(2): 49–54.

Hannah ME, Hannah WJ, Hewson SA, Hodnett ED, Saigal S, Willan AR (2000) Planned caesarean section versus planned vaginal birth for breech presentation at term: a randomised multicentre trial. *Term Breech Trial Collaborative Group. Lancet* **356**(9239): 1375–1383.

Heideman B (2005) Changes in maternal physiology during pregnancy. *Update in Anaesthesia* **20**: 21–24.

Lee R, Rodgers B, White L (1986) Cardiopulmonary resuscitation of pregnant women. *American Journal of Medicine* **81**: 311–318.

Luria S, Ben-Arie A, Hagay Z (1994) The ABC of shoulder dystocia management. *Asia-Oceania Journal of Obstetrics and Gynaecology* **20**(2): 195–197.

Morris S, Stacey M (2003) ABC of resuscitation. Resuscitation in pregnancy. *British Medical Journal* **327**(7426): 1277–1279.

National Health Service Litigation Authority (NHSLA) (2012) *Clinical Negligence Scheme for Trusts. Maternity. Clinical Risk Management Standards. Version 1. 2012/13*. Available at: www.nhsla.com/safety/Documents/CNST%20Maternity%20Standards%202013-14.pdf (accessed May 2013).

National Institute for Health and Clinical Excellence (NICE) (2006) *Intrapartum Care: care of healthy women and their babies during childbirth*. Draft guideline for consultation. London: National Institute for Health and Clinical Excellence.

National Institute for Health and Clinical Excellence (NICE) (2008) *Antenatal Care: routine care for the healthy pregnant woman*. Clinical Guideline No. 62. London: National Institute for Health and Clinical Excellence.

Nursing and Midwifery Council (NMC) (2009) *Standards for Pre-Registration Midwifery Education*. London: Nursing and Midwifery Council.

Nursing and Midwifery Council (NMC) (2012) *Midwives' Rules and Standards*. London: Nursing and Midwifery Council.

Palme-Kilander C (1992) Methods of resuscitation in low Apgar score in newborn infants – a national survey. *Acta Paediatrica* **81**: 739–744.

Resuscitation Council UK (2010a) *Adult Basic Life Support*. Available at: www.resus.org.uk/pages/blsalgo.pdf (accessed May 2013).

Resuscitation Council UK (2010b) *Newborn Life Support*. Available at: www.resus.org.uk/pages/nlsalgo.pdf (accessed May 2013).

Royal College of Obstetricians and Gynaecologists (RCOG) (2009) *Prevention and Management of Post Partum Haemorrhage*. Green-top Guideline No. 52. London: Royal College of Obstetricians and Gynaecologists.

Royal College of Obstetricians and Gynaecologists (RCOG) (2011) *Hypertension in Pregnancy: the management of hypertensive disorders during pregnancy*. National Collaborating Centre for Women's and Children's Health. London: Royal College of Obstetricians and Gynaecologists.

Royal College of Obstetricians and Gynaecologists (RCOG) (2012). *Shoulder Dystocia*. Green-top Guideline No. 42. Available at: www.rcog.org.uk/files/rcog-corp/GTG%2042_Shoulder%20dystocia%202nd%20edition%202012.pdf (accessed May 2013).

Sibai BM (2003) Diagnosis and management of gestational hypertension and preeclampsia. *Journal of the American College of Obstetricians and Gynecologists* **102**(1): 181–192.

Titiz H, Wallace A, Voaklander DC (2001) Manual removal of the placenta – a case control study. *Australian and New Zealand Journal of Obstetrics and Gynaecology* **41**: 41–44.

Ueland K, Akamatsu TJ, Eng M et al (1972) Maternal cardiovascular dynamics: caesarean section under epidural anaesthesia without epinephrine. *American Journal of Obstetrics and Gynecology* **114**(6): 775–780.

World Health Organization (WHO) (2003) *Managing Complications in Pregnancy and Childbirth: a guide for midwives and doctors*. Geneva: World Health Organization.

World Health Organization (WHO) (2009) *Guidelines for the Management of Postpartum Haemorrhage and Retained Placenta*. Geneva: World Health Organization.

9

Initial Assessment and Examination of the Newborn Baby

Lyn Dolby

Aim

This chapter aims to provide midwifery students with the foundation of knowledge required, first, to complete the initial health assessment and examination of the newborn baby and second, to recognise and/or pre-empt those conditions that may adversely affect neonatal well-being.

Learning outcomes

By the end of this chapter you will be able to:

1. complete the initial health assessment and examination of the newborn baby
2. recognise and/or pre-empt those conditions that may adversely affect neonatal well-being as well as appreciating and understanding the process of transition from fetal to neonatal life and ongoing development
3. understand how the normal parameters of well-being in the newborn are assessed and the features of normal neonatal behaviour and reflexes
4. describe the common but generally benign conditions that may present in the neonate, such as those affecting the skin, minor birth trauma, physiological jaundice
5. outline the common conditions that may adversely affect the health of the newborn
6. value normal parent–child interactions and the importance of health promotion and aiding parents in acquiring the knowledge and skills that will help them to care for their newborn baby.

The Student's Guide to Becoming a Midwife, Second Edition. Edited by Ian Peate and Cathy Hamilton.
© 2014 John Wiley & Sons, Ltd. Published 2014 by John Wiley & Sons, Ltd.

Introduction

The *Midwives' Rules and Standards* (NMC 2012) clearly highlight's a midwife's responsibility within her sphere of practice. Some of the responsibilities and activities from this document are directly related to the recognition of neonatal normality and abnormality as well as the need to refer to the paediatric team and take appropriate emergency action. The midwife's role in aiding the mother to care for her baby, observe and record normal progress and offer information on health issues that may directly or indirectly affect the health of both her and her baby are reflected within the *Standards for Pre-Registration Midwifery Education* (NMC 2009a). The midwife's responsibilities are also referred to in the guidelines *Routine Postnatal Care of Women and their Babies* issued by the National Institute for Health and Clinical Excellence (NICE 2006).

This chapter also provides a foundation for those students who are undertaking their midwifery education within universities that have integrated the 'Physical Examination of the Healthy Newborn' course within their pre-registration midwifery programmes of study.

Midwife's immediate role

The birth of a baby is a significant event in the life of its parents. For many mothers, the minutes after birth are full of many emotions, including concern about the baby's condition. At birth, the midwife's immediate concern is usually related to the baby's ability to accomplish the initial changes that are required in order to adapt and survive outside the uterus, such as the physiological changes in heart function. A midwife's ability and attitude at this time are extremely important in providing the parents with adequate and understandable information.

Conversely, the baby's condition may provoke anxiety at birth or there may be an obvious physical abnormality. Occasionally, an abnormality that was not detected antenatally may present at or soon after birth. For example, the baby may exhibit signs of a chromosomal abnormality, heart conditions or limb abnormality.

The midwife's sensitivity and level of professional experience and the actions that she takes will enable the parents to 'cope' as the initial impact of the issue of concern sinks in. However, it is paramount that the midwife voices her concerns to the parents followed by an explanation regarding the action that she is going to take.

The immediate care and handling of the baby should provide the parents with a professional and appropriate role model at all times; for example, limbs are not handles with which to turn a baby over. However, unswaddling a baby and removing hats when the baby demonstrates good temperature control encourage good role modelling, particularly in relation to the prevention of sudden infant death syndrome. Information and rationales given should be informative and appropriate to the individuals concerned.

The midwife is responsible for the assessment and recording of the initial vital signs of the baby (see sections below entitled 'Assessment at birth', 'Thermoregulation' and 'The chest'), thus providing a comprehensive record of the baby's condition at birth and during the first few hours of life.

The initial introduction of the baby to its parents and when the midwife assists the mother with the baby's first feed are important landmarks. Both these events link with the need to observe the initial parent–baby attachment process. Factors arising before and during pregnancy can affect these processes – for example, maternal abuse, domestic violence, environmental and social concerns (for example, housing and sanitation) or the circumstances under which the pregnancy was conceived. If this initial attachment process is affected, good communication both verbally and in written format with members of the midwifery team and other healthcare providers is paramount, as it enables all professionals involved to be well informed of the situation and assists effective multidisciplinary communication.

Comprehensive record keeping is a necessity if the midwife is to demonstrate that she has acted in accordance with her professional responsibility, local guidelines/procedures and parental wishes (NMC

2009b). The woman's record should provide information regarding an agreed plan of care, midwifery/obstetric and paediatric involvement including actions taken and why, any changes required and the rationale for so doing, maternal consent when required, observations performed and any other information as it arises. Information on both the antenatal and intrapartum periods may relate to the condition of the baby at or soon after birth. Reading previous notes made by other staff and providing comprehensive notes at the time of giving care are not a luxury, they are a professional necessity.

Initial assessment and examination at birth

Assessment at birth

Assessing the condition of the baby at birth is in the first instance by means of the Apgar scoring system (Table 9.1) and secondly by performing a complete physical examination in order to confirm normality and detect any anomalies.

Dr Virginia Apgar devised the Apgar scoring system in the 1950s (AAP/ACOG 2006). It consists of a systematic assessment of five key factors, each significant in determining the health status of the baby. Each factor is given a score (from 0–2), so the overall condition of the baby can be determined by calculating the score out of a total of 10. The Apgar score is usually calculated at 1 min and again at 10 min after birth. A score of 0–3 at 1 min indicates a baby who is in poor condition, requires resuscitation and possibly ventilation, whereas a score of 7–10 at 1 min usually indicates a baby who is in good condition and is able to make the adaptations necessary for extrauterine life. A good account of the Apgar scoring system is contained in Johnson & Taylor (2010).

Examination of the newborn baby

In the UK, each baby within 72 hours of birth is given a comprehensive physiological neonatal examination the standard for which is set by the Newborn and Infant Physical Examination committee (National Screening Committee 2008) by a midwife who holds an additional qualification in the physical examination of the newborn, a paediatrician, general practitioner or specially trained neonatal nurse specialist. This examination involves a more in-depth assessment of neonatal well-being and also incorporates cardiovascular and respiratory assessment, examination of the eyes and testes and assessment of hip stability. However, the initial assessment and examination that is performed by the midwife immediately after birth is paramount in providing information regarding the initial parameters of health and well-being of the baby at birth and highlighting conditions that need urgent management soon after birth or paediatric review postnatally.

Table 9.1   The Apgar scoring system (AAP/ACOG 2006)

Sign	0	1	2
Appearance (colour)	Blue, pale	Body pink, limbs blue	All pink
Apex beat	Absent	Below 100	Above 100
Grimace (response to stimuli)	None	Grimace	Cry
Activity (muscle tone)	Limp	Some limb flexion	Active movements, limbs well flexed
Respiratory effort	None	Slow, irregular	Good, strong cry

Preparation

Under normal circumstances, this initial examination can be performed within the first hour after birth after the parents have had time to look at and cuddle their baby. The process of the examination should be explained to the parents and their consent obtained. The examination should be performed where it can be easily witnessed by the parents and the lighting is good, particularly natural daylight. Hands should be washed and dried prior to the examination and everything required should be close at hand (for example, scales and baby clothes). The examination itself should be performed quickly and comprehensively, only uncovering the part of the baby to be examined and re-covering the baby as soon as practicable.

Before commencing the examination, visually observe the baby, noting:

1. colour
2. activity
3. posture
4. respiratory effort
5. cry.

Address any urgent requirements such as obvious abnormalities or a baby who appears distressed or cyanosed. Continue to observe these five key points during the process of the initial examination in order recognise if the baby's condition changes.

Thermoregulation

A baby emerges from the warm uterine environment (37°C+) to a much lower temperature of approximately 21°C. Loss of body heat can occur quickly, due to the baby's skin being wet, a large ratio of surface area to body mass and the relatively thin layer of insulating subcutaneous fat. A drop of 1–2°C can occur during the immediate postbirth period and if the baby has suffered some form of compromise – such as hypoxia, the baby is small in relation to the gestational age or if infection is present – this can result in a baby who may be unable or slow to regain a normal body temperature. Hypothermia is one of the three major considerations within the energy triangle (Figure 9.1).

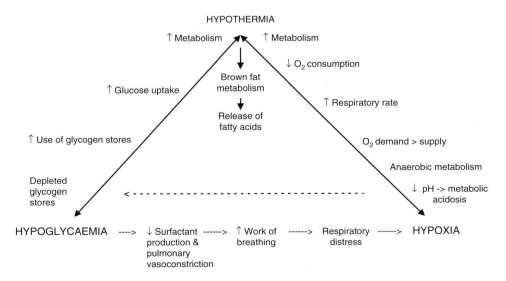

Figure 9.1   The energy triangle. Adapted from Aylott (2006a, b).

Activity 9.1

Read Aylott (2006a, 2006b) Parts 1 and 2, as they provide a good discussion on the interaction between hypothermia, hypoglycaemia and hypoxia.

The close relationship of hypothermia, hypoglycaemia and hypoxia/anoxia must never be underestimated. The midwife needs to be vigilant in facilitating the baby's adaptation to extrauterine life by being aware of the interactions between these three major factors and her role in recognising external factors that may have an adverse impact.

The risk of the baby becoming hypothermic (low body temperature) will increase if the baby has not been dried adequately, is preterm or is less than the expected weight for its gestational age. This is because small and/or preterm babies have less brown fat to utilise for energy/heat production. Brown fat (otherwise known as brown adipose tissue) is present in the body of newborn babies and is used to generate body heat. In terms of the baby's body temperature, one must be aware that the presence of infection may cause the baby's temperature to rise as well as fall.

Activity 9.2

Where on the baby's body is brown fat stored?

As has been discussed, it is important to prevent hypothermia so the room and cot in which the baby is to be examined need to be warm (turn fans off) with no draughts (close windows/doors). It is also good practice to assess the temperature of the baby before commencing the examination and maintain awareness of its temperature during the examination. In some sites, checking the temperature of the baby may not be routine but assessing the warmth of the baby's chest and upper back with the back of the hand during the examination is good practice. It must also be borne in mind that when using thermometers to measure temperature, their accuracy depends on the site and technique used (Johnson & Taylor 2010).

Head

Observe the overall shape and symmetry of the skull, bearing in mind that these factors may be influenced by the presence of moulding or caput succedaneum as described below.

Case study 9.1

 Consider the factors that may arise in the following case:

Baby Stephen was delivered after a difficult labour, possibly experiencing hypoxia. He weighs less than expected for his gestational age and possible antenatal factors may need to be taken into account.

What basic actions could you take in order to further reduce adverse impacts and how might knowledge of the 'energy triangle' assist you?

Possible answers at the end of the chapter!

The suture lines on the skull should be easily palpable and may be found to be overlapping due to the pressures exerted during labour – a process known as 'moulding'. The parents should be reassured and made aware that this will resolve over the next 24–48 hours.

The oedematous area on the fetal scalp in the vicinity of the presenting part of the head is known as caput succedaneum. The oedema can cross suture lines and is more obvious after prolonged labour but will normally only remain evident for a short while, usually disappearing within 48 hours.

Sometimes there is a soft, bruised-looking swelling that is restricted by the bone margins over which it is localised (usually the parietal bones), known as a cephalhaematoma. It is due to a localised subperiosteal haemorrhage, often occurring as the result of no apparent trauma except for the usual pressure that occurs on the presenting part of the fetal head. Parents will need to be reassured that the cephalhaematoma will gradually reabsorb, usually over a period of 3 months. If bilateral cephalhaematomas are present, they may take longer to disappear. In an extremely small proportion of cases, a fracture may be suspected and if present will be seen on an X-ray of the skull.

The cranial fontanelles should be observed for normality. The posterior fontanelle located at the junction of the lambdoid and sagittal sutures is usually triangular and measures approximately 0.5 cm at birth, closing shortly afterwards. The anterior fontanelle measures approximately 3–4 cm at the largest diameter and usually closes between 18 months and 2 years of age.

A large anterior fontanelle may be found in the premature baby or be due to hydrocephalus, while a small one may indicate microcephaly. If the fontanelle appears raised or tense, this may be associated with hydrocephalus or indicate raised intracranial pressure or infection. However, a depressed fontanelle may suggest that the baby is dehydrated but this is very rarely seen at birth and tends to be a 'late' sign of dehydration. Occasionally, there is a third fontanelle to be found between the anterior and posterior fontanelles, the size of which can be variable. It can be indicative of congenital abnormalities (e.g. trisomy 21).

The whole head needs to be examined for the presence of trauma (for example, forceps marks, fetal scalp electrode or amnihook lacerations) or bruising (for example, Kiwi or ventouse cup). In the event of any bruising, the parents should be made aware that the baby is more likely to demonstrate physiological jaundice, due to the increased breakdown of red blood cells.

The occipitofrontal circumference (OFC) is noted and provides a record, for example, in the event of hydrocephalus occurring. Place the centimetre scale of a tape measure 1 cm above the nasal bridge and encircle the largest diameter and note the measurement in the neonatal record. The measurement tends to be more accurate if the baby's head is lifted off the mattress (caput can distort the measurement) or the measurement can be taken when the baby is being held. The degree of moulding can of course affect the measurement noted.

Midwifery wisdom

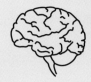

To prevent paper cuts, the tape measure should be shortened and the tape itself not dragged round the head when the measurement has been completed.

Facies

The face should appear relatively symmetrical, with the eyes, nose and mouth lying in a normal relationship to each other. Observation of the face assesses normality and for signs of any dysmorphic features, such as low-set ears (see the section on 'Ears' below).

Midwifery wisdom

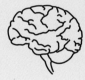

However, make sure that you see both parents before assuming that a certain feature is part of a syndrome – it may be just familial.

Eyes

Check that both eyes are actually present, assessing their size and shape. If both eyes are symmetrically positioned at a slight angle, this may be race orientated (e.g. Chinese) or due to a genetic anomaly (e.g. trisomy 21). Eyelashes should turn outwards and there should be very little discharge to be seen. Features around the eyes such as the epicanthic folds, eyelids and eyebrows should appear normal. The pupil should appear to be round and not cloudy or silvery in appearance – often indicative of neonatal cataracts. Even a baby of even a few hours old is able to fix its eyes on an object or face and follow it as it moves (an ability known as fixation), but sometimes a squint may be seen at this stage due to the immaturity of the muscles controlling the eyeball. The sclera should be white and clear, whereas a yellow discoloration can occur as a result of raised bilirubin levels (jaundice) and a blue sclera can be found in babies with osteogenesis imperfect (brittle bones). Occasionally, a subconjunctival haemorrhage may be present due to pressures exerted during the birth, so reassure the parents that this will disappear over time.

Ears

Correct positioning of the ear can be determined by tracing an imaginary line horizontally across the eyes and when looking straight down at the baby, note if the top of the pinna is positioned above this line. To produce a reasonably true horizontal line, you need to draw an imaginary line between the inner canthi of the eyes and then extend it in your mind. Do not use the outer canthus of the eye as your point of reference, as this can change according to the slant of the eye due to race or anomalies.

Examine the ear and behind it for any skin tags, dimples or periauricular sinuses. At term, the ears should contain enough cartilage to allow them to 'spring' back into position if they are folded over slightly. The pinna should be of normal appearance with well-defined curves in the upper part and the ear lobe should be a normal size and shape. Check that the orifice of each ear is not obviously blocked.

Midwifery wisdom

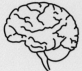

Babies often have ears just like one of its parents or a grandparent so always ask – sensitively!

Nose

Note the shape of the nose and width of the bridge. It is not unusual to find a nose that has been squashed at birth and may not appear straight. However, if the baby is able to breathe easily then it is usually not a problem and it will usually resolve fairly soon. Babies are obligatory nose breathers, so anything obstructing inhalation and exhalation will cause a problem. In respiratory illness, flaring of the nostrils is often observed. Quite often, a baby may sneeze and the parents may need to be reassured that a sneeze is nature's way of blowing their baby's nose.

Lips and mouth

The lips should be complete and symmetrical, as asymmetry may indicate the presence of a facial palsy. The mouth should look in proportion to the face. A small mouth can be due to micrognathia (underdevelopment of the jaw) that is often associated with underlying abnormality.

The presence of a cleft (unilateral or bilateral) in the upper lip should be noted and referred. Internally, the hard and soft palate should also be felt with a finger (noting if the suckle reflex is normal) and by visualising with a light source. Encourage the baby to open its mouth so that you can see and feel for any natal teeth round the alveolar ridges (gums) or other anomalies and inspect the colour of the mucous membranes which should be well perfused. Natal teeth are often removed as they can become loose, so referral to the paediatric team is required.

The presence of one or two harmless white spots or cysts (Epstein's pearls) may be seen, usually on the soft palate. As the baby moves its tongue in the mouth, observe its condition, position, presence of cysts or dimples and the length of the frenulum as a short frenulum may interfere with feeding, a condition known as angyloglossia or tongue tie. The midwife needs to be fully aware of the guidelines and criteria for referral if treatment is required.

Neck

Babies tend to have short necks in proportion and symmetry to their bodies. Observe both physically and visually to determine if there are any swellings that may indicate, for example, a sternomastoid tumour or cystic hygroma. Any signs of webbing or thick/loose skin at the back of the neck should be noted. The former may be associated with Turner's syndrome and the latter may indicate a chromosomal abnormality such as Trisomy 21.

Clavicles

The clavicles, the two bones that run from either side of the sternum (breastbone) to the shoulder, should be examined with the index finger to check that there are no indentations or crepitus to be felt and that they are intact. Babies who may be more at risk of clavicular fracture include those who have had an assisted breech delivery where there was shoulder dystocia at birth or if a palsy (for example, Erb's palsy) is suspected. Do not presume that a baby with a clavicular fracture cannot move its arm or that it will not elicit a Moro reflex. If the bones lie in good apposition to one another, a Moro reflex can still be demonstrated.

Arms and hands

Both arms should be gently straightened and compared for equality of length. Any signs of fracture or bruising should be recorded and referred. The arms should move freely and demonstrate good muscle tone. A baby in the first week of life exhibits a 'closed' posture of flexed arms and closed fists. Within a couple of weeks, the baby adopts a more open posture where the arms are less tightly held to its body.

Activity 9.3

How many creases should there be on the palm of the hand?

Encourage the baby to open its hand by gently tapping on the back of the hand or the inner aspect of the associated wrist.

Midwifery wisdom

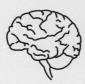

Another method to stimulate the baby to open its hand, is to encourage the baby to grasp your fingers with the opposite hand and let go of the hand that you want it to open.

You need to be able to visualise the palm to check the number of palmar creases as a single crease can suggest a chromosomal abnormality (for example, Trisomy 21). An open palm also enables you to detect any anomalies such as extra digits that may be hidden by a closed fist.

164

Midwifery wisdom

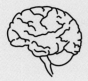

Be aware that a small proportion of the population only have one palmar crease on one hand and a lower number will have this phenomenon in both hands.

The digits of the hand should be counted and the nails visualised for any sign of paronychia (inflammation of the folds of skin surrounding the fingernail) as infection may occur as a consequence. Any polydactyly (extra digits) or syndactyly (webbed fingers) should be noted and referred. Both of these conditions can be associated with particular syndromes such as trisomy 21 or be familial in origin.

Chest

The general appearance of the chest should be noted for colour, shape and birthmarks or skin tags.

Movement on respiration should be symmetrical and the heartbeat should not be clearly visible or easily felt on the skin surface. The respiratory rate can be easily counted and should be approximately 20 breaths per minute during sleep and 30–60 breaths per minute when awake. Any signs of respiratory distress, characterised by intercostal and sternal recession (where the chest wall is pulled inwards), tachypnoea, grunting on expiration, cyanosis (where the baby's colour changes), nasal flaring or periods of apnoea (greater than 20 seconds) should be referred to a paediatrician immediately. These factors can be indicative of respiratory disease but it is not unusual for the baby born by caesarean section to demonstrate a transient tachypnoea, as the pressure exerted on the baby that aids removal of excess fluids during a vaginal delivery has not occurred and therefore it takes longer to resolve post birth.

If necessary, the apex beat can be counted by putting a stethoscope over the heart (fourth intercostal space, midclavicular line), noting the rate and rhythm. Normal heart rate usually falls within the range of 110–160 beats per minute, but can be extremely variable over the first 48 hours of life. During sleep, the heart rate will slow (sometimes to 90 beats per minute) but will rise in direct relation to an increase in the level of consciousness and activity.

In the term baby, the nipples and areolae should be well formed and aligned symmetrically on the chest. If the nipples are wide spaced (distance between is greater than 25% of the chest circumference), this may indicate the presence of a congenital disorder such as Turner's syndrome. Accessory (or supernumerary) nipples should be noted and the parents made aware of their presence. Accessory nipples can be found anywhere from the breast to the groin. Usually there is little or no breast tissue underlying the accessory nipple, particularly the further away from the breast that they are found.

Abdomen

The abdomen should appear relatively smooth and rounded, slightly pot-bellied and move in synchrony with respiratory effort. Refer to the paediatrician if there are any birthmarks or obvious swellings.

Check that the umbilical cord is securely clamped and that the clamp itself is not too near to the skin at the base of the cord as this can cause abrasion and encourage infection. It must be remembered that if not properly cared for, the cord can provide an entry site for bacteria, straight to some of the major organs of the body. Therefore, assessing the base of the cord for inflammation, haemorrhage and signs of infection and discussing with the parents how to cleanse the area is a necessary part of care.

Male genitalia

Overall appearance should be assessed, noting any general deviations from the normal. The penis should be at least 2.5 cm in length but sometimes it may appear short due to a swollen scrotum and therefore the base of the penis will need to be located in order to determine its true length. Rarely, a baby will be found to have a micro-penis which measures less than 2.5 cm and paediatric referral is required.

The urethral meatus should lie centrally at the tip of the penis and when the baby passes urine, a good 'flow' should be seen. Referral to a paediatrician should be made if hypospadias or epispadias is found as a malpositioned meatus may be associated with abnormalities of the urethra and kidneys. In some cases, surgery may be necessary and therefore parents need to be aware that circumcision is not advisable in case part of the glans penis is required to affect a good repair.

The foreskin is adherent to the glans penis until the child is between 3 and 10 years of age. Therefore, no attempt should be made to make the foreskin retract as this can lead to phimosis, inflammation and infection.

The scrotal sac should be palpated on both sides in order to palpate each individual testis. The testes in most babies will have descended by 40 weeks' gestation. However, in a small number of babies one testis may not yet have descended and this should be recorded and is usually followed up by the GP at the 6–8-week examination. In a few cases, both testes may be found to be undescended and referral to the paediatrician must be made as further investigation may be required in relation to ambiguous genitalia and prevention of torsion and later sterility.

The colour of the scrotal sac may be darker depending on cultural heredity (e.g. Asian or black parents) or may appear bruised or swollen due to trauma during delivery. However, a hydrocoele or a scrotum that appears very swollen (and/or discoloured) needs referral for further assessment in case of hernia, haematoma or torsion of the testis.

Female genitalia

Parents often question if the genitalia of their baby girl is normal. This is because in relation to a woman, the labia majora are relatively large, covering the labia minora and have not yet been influenced by the hormones arising during puberty.

As with the male infant, the labia can appear bruised or swollen due to the pressures exerted during birth. The labia can also be pigmented if the child is born to non-Caucasian parents, but it can also be an early finding in congenital adrenal hyperplasia.

The vaginal orifice should be clearly visualised and the hymen may be clearly observed. Occasionally, it may be perceived that the hymen is imperforate as it may bulge slightly. It is also possible to mistake a bulging hymen for an enlarged Bartholin gland. Vaginal skin tags may also be present; most will disappear but some may require treatment so their presence should be discussed with a paediatrician.

Soon after birth, a creamy white discharge which may appear slightly blood-stained may appear from the baby's vagina, but parents should be reassured that this is a normal occurrence due to the withdrawal of maternal hormones after birth. Rarely, this 'pseudo-menstruation' can present as a mini period, but the duration of the blood loss should not be overly prolonged or excessive.

The clitoris can appear overly large in small-for-dates and preterm babies, but its size needs to be assessed in comparison to other associated structures. Paediatric referral should always be sought if the possibility of indeterminate sex is suspected.

The urethral meatus is more difficult to locate in the female baby, but it should lie in a normal position between the clitoris and the vaginal orifice. When the urinary stream is observed, the flow should be good.

Anus

The position of the anal opening is best assessed in relation to its distance from the coccyx and other structures such as the base of the scrotum in males and the posterior fourchette in females. An anteriorly positioned anus may be associated with conditions such as malformation of the rectum and constipation in later life. It is necessary to visualise the anus clearly, as it is possible to mistake a large fistula for the anal opening.

The first stool to be passed from the bowel is known as meconium. On close inspection, it can be observed that meconium is actually a dark green colour and not black as it is often perceived. The anus can only be referred to as 'patent' when meconium has actually been seen to pass through the anal orifice. It is possible for meconium to emerge from the urethra of the vaginal orifice via a fistula arising between the rectum and the vagina.

Legs and feet

As with the arms, the legs should be assessed for symmetry, equality of length, muscle tone and flexion. It should be remembered that newborns have a natural stricture behind the knees and therefore forcibly straightening them causes discomfort. Putting knees together with the feet placed flat on the cot mattress usually provides a good method for assessing leg length. Run the fingers down the major bones of the legs in order to assess for fractures or malformations.

The dorsal (upper) part of the foot should easily line up with the anterior (front) aspect of the shin. Sometimes the line of the foot is off-set, a condition known as talipes, where the foot lies in an inwards, outwards, upwards or downwards position. If the foot can be easily moved into alignment with the shin, the condition is known as positional talipes and occurs due to the squashed position of the feet *in utero*. However, in fixed talipes, the foot cannot easily be manipulated into alignment and referral for treatment is required.

An abnormal shape to the foot (e.g. 'rocker bottom' which is an abnormality of the foot in which the soles curve outwards, rather than inward, giving them the appearance of a rocker) or signs of oedema should be noted and the baby referred to a paediatrician. The number of toes must be counted and the toes separated to check for the presence of webbing between them. Polydactyly and syndactyly should be noted and referred.

Activity 9.4

Look at the STEPS website for further information about lower limb abnormalities and treatment (www.steps-charity.org.uk).

Spine

The spine is best examined by turning the baby over so it straddles your hand. In this position, the baby curls comfortably over your hand, opening the vertebrae slightly so that anomalies can be more easily visualised.

Examine the back, making sure that you can see both sides adequately. Run your finger down the spine from just into the hairline at the back of the head, all the way down to the sacral area, checking for integrity. The presence of hair tufts, dimples or sinuses may indicate involvement with the spinal cord and referral to a paediatrician is paramount. Gently part the cleft of the buttocks, checking the anal sphincter (this time from a different angle) and the presence of any hidden dimples or sinuses. Quite often, you may find a dimple just where the cleft of the buttocks begins and you need to ascertain if you can easily see the end of it; if not, refer to a paediatrician.

Midwifery wisdom

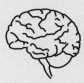

Use a good light source (such as an ophthalmoscope) to check that you can see the base of the dimple. If necessary, cleanse the dimple with a damp piece of cotton wool to remove meconium or products arising from birth.

Skin

Throughout the examination, the condition of the skin needs to be checked. Observe for colour, birthmarks and where they are placed, rashes (not usually common at birth), bruising, cuts and abrasions, referring as necessary. The most common birthmarks that do not require referral to a paediatrician include naevus simplex (salmon patch) and the Mongolian blue spot.

Usually the naevus simplex appears as a reddened 'patch' on the brow between the eyes, over the brows themselves and/or within the hairline at the back of the head. The former gradually fade over time and the latter may fade, but heat and anger may make them appear more prominent again.

The Mongolian blue spot usually appear as a bruised-looking area over one or both buttocks, but can also appear on the legs and arms. It is important that the parents are aware that the size and position of each one have been documented to prevent confusion in the future where a case of non-accidental injury is suspected. The role of the midwife in cases of child abuse should not be underestimated and she needs to be conversant with routes of referral (Powell 2011).

Weight and length

The baby should be weighed at the beginning or end of the examination as long as the baby remains warm. The weight should be recorded in kilograms. Many units do not routinely measure the baby's length due to the logistics of ensuring the accuracy of the measurement. However, it may be prudent for those babies who are small for gestational age, have obvious skeletal dysplasias or may have a possible thyroid instability (due to maternal history) to note the length measurement for future follow-up (Hall & Elliman 2006).

Completion of the initial examination

Once the physical examination is completed, any drugs (e.g. vitamin K) can be given if parental consent has been obtained. The baby can then be dressed or given to the mother for skin-to-skin contact.

If not already explained during the examination, the findings should be discussed with the parents and they should be asked if they have any further questions. Make sure that the baby is still warm and content or give the mother assistance if the baby wishes to feed.

Appropriate paediatric referrals can be made if necessary and the examination completed by documenting the findings in the baby's notes.

Conclusion

This chapter has highlighted the role and responsibilities of the midwife in relation to the initial assessment and examination of the newborn baby. The midwife can help to facilitate the bonding process between the parents and their baby by answering their questions and giving them support and guidance as they start to get to know each other. The examination at birth also acts as a baseline so that the initial assessment can inform future care and management, particularly if deviations from the normal are noticed. In this case, referral to the appropriate healthcare professional (usually the paediatrician) is required as stipulated in the *Midwives' Rules and Standards* (NMC 2012). Appropriate communication with the parents and accurate and contemporaneous record keeping are also highlighted as important elements in the examination of the newborn baby.

169

Case study 9.2

You should have taken into account the lower birth weight and therefore the fact that Stephen's level of brown fat is reduced. Stephen will need to be dried quickly and kept warm (skin to skin would be good) and early feeding would also be appropriate. Record Stephen's temperature and take appropriate action if it is low. You also need to take into account any sign of infection or any antenatal factors that may cause further compromise. Relating the risk factors for Stephen with your knowledge of the energy triangle should help you to prevent hypothermia and hypoglycaemia and thus reduce the impact of hypoxia if it occurred.

References

Aylott M (2006a) The neonatal energy triangle. Part 1: metabolic adaptation. *Paediatric Nursing* **18**(6), 38–42.

Aylott M (2006b) The neonatal energy triangle. Part 2: thermoregulatory and respiratory adaptation. *Paediatric Nursing* **18**(7), 38–42.

Hall D, Elliman D (2006) *Health for All Children*, 4th edn rev. Oxford: Oxford University Press.

Johnson R, Taylor W (2010) *Skills for Midwifery Practice*, 3rd edn. Edinburgh: Churchill Livingstone.

National Institute for Health and Clinical Excellence (NICE) (2006) *Postnatal Care of Mothers and Babies*. London: National Institute for Health and Clinical Excellence.

National Screening Committee (2008) *Newborn and Infant Physical Examination: standards and competencies*. London: National Screening Committee.

Nursing and Midwifery Council (NMC) (2009a) *Standards for Pre-Registration Midwifery Education*. London: Nursing and Midwifery Council.

Nursing and Midwifery Council (NMC) (2009b) *Guidelines on Record Keeping*. London: Nursing and Midwifery Council.

Nursing and Midwifery Council (NMC) (2012) *Midwives' Rules and Standards*. London: Nursing and Midwifery Council.

Powell C (2011) *Safeguarding and Child Protection for Nurses, Midwives and Health Visitors: a practical guide*. Maidenhead: Open University Press.

Neonatal crossword challenge

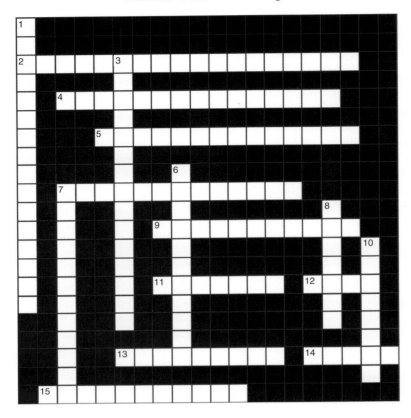

Clues

Across		Down	
2	The slightly blood-stained vaginal loss in the neonate (18)	1	Soft oedematous patch found on the neonatal head after birth (5,11)
4	A type of haemorrhage caused by the pressure of labour that may be seen in the sclera of the neonatal eye (15)	3	The name of the head circumference measurement (9,7)
5	Small, white spots or cysts found on the soft palate or penis of the neonate (8,6)	6	When the urethral opening is found on the underside of the penis (11)
7	The result of low blood sugar (13)	7	Newborn and Infant Physical Examination (NIPE) highlights four particular areas for the physical examination of the newborn: cardiac, eyes and testes, what is the fourth area? (12)

Across		Down	
9	When the hand has more than five digits (11)	8	What does the brain need to work effectively? (7)
11	A foot deformity that can be classed as 'positional' or 'fixed' (7)	10	What does the neonate metabolise for glucose/heat production? (5,3)
12	Reflex where the hands/arms extend outwards and then make a slight movement inwards (4)		
13	A genetic abnormality that may portray one palmar crease (7,2)		
14	The scoring system used to assess neonatal well-being soon after birth (5)		
15	A cold baby is suffering from ... (11)		

10

Effective Postnatal Care
Annabel Jay and Marianne Peace

Aim

To explain the midwife's role in caring for the woman and baby from birth onwards.

Learning outcomes

By the end of this chapter this chapter you will be able to:

1. appreciate the importance of individualised, woman-centred care in the postnatal period
2. describe the key factors which a midwife will take into account when giving postnatal care in hospital and in the community
3. understand the principles of perineal repair and care
4. describe the key elements of care following a caesarean section
5. understand the principles behind the UNICEF Baby Friendly Initiative standards and how these can be applied in practice
6. identify the key indicators of a normal, healthy neonate.

Introduction

The *Midwives' Rules and Standards* (NMC 2012) describe the postnatal period as:

> the period after the end of labour during which the attendance of a midwife upon a woman and baby is required, being not less than 10 days and for such longer period as the midwife considers necessary.

The Student's Guide to Becoming a Midwife, Second Edition. Edited by Ian Peate and Cathy Hamilton.
© 2014 John Wiley & Sons, Ltd. Published 2014 by John Wiley & Sons, Ltd.

This chapter focuses on the essential care that each woman and her baby should receive from the midwife during the postnatal period. Particular reference will be made to current guidelines issued by the National Institute for Health and Clinical Excellence (NICE) on postnatal care of women and babies (NICE 2006). In this chapter the baby will be assumed to be male, to reduce confusion when referring to both woman and baby.

Principles of postnatal care

The postnatal period is a time of change and adjustment for the woman and those close to her. The focus of attention is no longer on the woman alone but on her baby too; therefore the midwife's role is not only to care for them both (NMC 2012) but also to empower the mother to provide the best care for her baby (NMC 2009).

The NICE guideline 37 (NICE 2006) stresses that women should at all times be treated with dignity, kindness and respect. Women should be encouraged to become fully involved in the planning of their postnatal care, which should centre on their individual needs rather than on routine patterns of care. There are many factors which influence the decision on how to plan the woman's postnatal care. These include the state of the mother and baby's health, whether or not the mother has had other children before, her chosen method of infant feeding, her ability to understand and assimilate information, her domestic background and her psychological state. The woman's cultural and family background should always be taken into consideration when planning postnatal care (NICE 2006).

Advice and support should build on women's existing knowledge, responding to their individual needs; a new mother may welcome advice on basic matters such as how to hold her baby, whereas an experienced mother may find such advice patronising, thus building barriers to further communication.

Case study 10.1

 Kelly and her husband arrived home from hospital yesterday with their newborn baby. Kelly's mother-in-law is visiting from Poland. Kelly bottle fed her two older children but has decided to breastfeed baby Michael. The community midwife who visited the family today assumed that as Kelly was an experienced mother and had good family support, she would not need much advice. After making sure that both Kelly and Michael were physically well, the midwife left Kelly some breastfeeding information leaflets and promised to call back in a few days' time.

- Why might the midwife's assumption be wrong?
- List ways in which Kelly's postnatal care could be individualised.

Plan of care

Each woman should have 'a documented, individualised care plan' which should be reviewed regularly (NICE 2006). The usual place to document this is in the woman's hand-held maternity notes. This allows the woman to read it whenever she wishes and to add to it or alter it as necessary. She should be advised to discuss any changes with her community midwife in case there is any conflict with other aspects of her care plan. It is vital that the information, advice and care given to women and their babies in the postnatal period are consistent, as they may be cared for by many different midwives and other health profession-als. Any symptoms, tests performed, deviations from the norm or referral to other professionals should be discussed with the woman and meticulously followed up and documented so that progress can be continuously mapped (NICE 2006).

Immediate postbirth care of the woman: physical assessment and care

Before leaving the new family alone for some private bonding time, the midwife must undertake some basic observations to ensure that the woman's health is not at immediate risk.

Observation and estimation of blood loss

The volume of blood loss is estimated following delivery of the placenta and then observed frequently in the early postnatal period. The midwife will be observing for any signs of postpartum haemorrhage (PPH), a potentially life-threatening condition which is more common if the woman has had a prolonged or complicated labour or birth.

A blood loss of 500 mL or more at or around the time of birth is classed as a 'primary PPH'. However, this figure is not a good indicator of maternal well-being: some women can withstand a blood loss of 500 mL or more with little or no detriment to their health, whilst others will show symptoms of hypovolaemia (low blood volume) well before 500 mL has been lost. The midwife must call for urgent medical assis-tance if PPH occurs or is suspected or if the woman is showing signs of hypovolaemia (raised pulse, drop in blood pressure, dizziness, fainting) regardless of the volume of blood lost. Assessing blood loss is not easy: blood is soaked up by pads, bedding and clothing and is often clotted or mixed with amniotic fluid.

Activity 10.1

Fill a large measuring jug with water and colour it red using food dye. Gather several bowls of varying sizes and place inside them an assortment of absorbent items. To each bowl, add a measured amount of liquid and allow the contents to soak it up. Ask other people to estimate the volume of liquid in each bowl.

How many got it right?

Observation of fundal tone and position

Poor uterine tone following delivery of the baby and placenta may lead to excessive bleeding. The mid-wife should gently palpate the fundus, which should feel very firm and central, just below the level of the umbilicus. If the uterus feels soft and broad, it is likely to be poorly contracted and the midwife will 'rub up' a contraction until the uterus feels firm. If the woman is well enough, putting the baby to the breast may also help, as this stimulates the release of the hormone oxytocin, which helps the uterus contract.

A full bladder may displace the uterus, causing it to feel higher than expected or deviated to one side. If the woman is unable to pass urine, it may be necessary to empty the bladder using a catheter, as a full bladder may impede involution of the uterus, leading to excessive blood loss. Subsequent midwives will then need to monitor the woman's urine output so that any continuing disturbance to normal bladder function can be investigated and treated promptly.

Vital signs

Observation of vital signs (blood pressure, temperature, pulse, respirations) is undertaken shortly after completion of the third stage of labour and thereafter may be repeated on a regular basis according to local policy or the woman's state of health. Any unexpected changes should be immediately investigated as these may be indicators of potentially life-threatening conditions such as PPH, pre-eclampsia or infection. In the homebirth setting, any deviations from the norm that do not quickly resolve may require the woman and baby to be transferred swiftly into hospital for further observation and treatment. Women who have had complications or health problems in the antenatal period or during labour will require more frequent monitoring of vital signs and the midwife will liaise closely with the obstetric team in accordance with the care plan or as necessary.

Inspection of the perineum and vagina

Following a normal vaginal birth, the midwife will inspect the woman's perineum and vagina to assess the following:

- The presence of any trauma to the tissues.
- The extent of any trauma.
- Whether or not suturing is required.
- Whether or not referral to an obstetrician is required.

The procedure must be carefully explained to the woman and verbal consent obtained prior to commencing.

Examination of the placenta

A full examination of the placenta, cord and membranes should be undertaken as soon as possible after the birth to enable the midwife to assess whether any part has been retained. Retained placental products are a potential cause of PPH, as their presence may prevent full involution of the uterus. If not passed, they may also provide a route for pathogens, leading to infection (Johnson & Taylor 2010).

If there is any suspicion that part of the placenta or membranes have been retained, the midwife must refer to an obstetrician without delay. It may be necessary to evacuate the uterus under epidural or general anaesthetic. All findings must be documented in the woman's notes.

Before wrapping and disposing of the placenta, the midwife should check whether the woman or her family wish to see it or even take it home. Some cultures object to the usual hospital practice of incineration and prefer to bury the placenta privately (Johnson & Taylor 2010).

Perineal repair

The majority of women suffer some degree of perineal damage during a vaginal birth (Steen 2012). The aim of perineal repair is to restore the integrity of the perineum and surrounding tissues and to reduce bleeding and risk of infection (Johnson & Taylor 2010). Learning to identify the extent of any perineal trauma is an important midwifery skill and failure to do so correctly may have serious long-term consequences for the woman (Steen 2010, 2012). Evidence suggests an association between the skill of the person carrying out the repair and subsequent perineal pain and healing (Kettle et al. 2010). The repair of any perineal trauma is normally the responsibility of the person who assists at the birth; however,

Table 10.1   Degrees of perineal trauma (data from RCOG 2007)

Degree	Trauma involves...
First degree	The skin of the perineum only
Second degree	Perineal skin, posterior vaginal wall mucosa and the muscle layers of the perineum, but *not* the anal sphincter
Third degree: 3a 3b 3c	 Less than 50% of the thickness of the external anal sphincter is damaged More than 50% of the external anal sphincter is damaged There is damage to both external and internal anal sphincter
Fourth degree	Trauma to the anal sphincter extending to the anal epithelium

some degrees of trauma may be beyond the midwife's level of skill or the scope of her practice, so the ability to recognise when to refer to a senior colleague or obstetrician is paramount.

Degrees of perineal trauma

The Royal College of Obstetricians and Gynaecologists' (RCOG) definition of the degrees of perineal trauma is summarized in Table 10.1.

Suitably trained and experienced midwives may repair first- and second-degree tears, episiotomies and straightforward labial tears if they feel it is within their competence to do so, but third- and fourth-degree trauma must *always* be repaired by an obstetrician. If the woman has given birth at home or in a stand-alone birth centre, she will need to be transferred to hospital for repair of a third- or fourth-degree tear. This is traumatic for the whole family and will require particularly sensitive care. Trauma to other parts of the genital tract (e.g. the clitoris, urethra, anterior vaginal wall) should always be referred to the obstetric registrar. Any bilateral labial grazes that are in apposition during normal postures should be sutured to avoid the risk of the labia healing together (Johnson & Taylor 2010).

Indications for repair of first- and second-degree trauma

It is usual practice to suture all episiotomies, regardless of their extent. The issue of when to suture first- and second-degree tears is contentious, but NICE (2007b) recommends that all second-degree tears should be sutured, plus those first-degree tears where the sides of the wound are not in direct apposition.

For further information about current practice in perineal repair, the Royal College of Midwives (RCM 2012) has an up-to-date practice guideline on suturing the perineum available online at: www.rcm.org.uk/college/policy-practice/guidelines/practice-guidelines/.

General well-being of the woman

Soiled bedding and pads will need to be changed and the woman assisted into a comfortable position. A bath or shower should be offered. The midwife should not leave the birthing room until she is satisfied that the woman's condition is stable. She must ensure that the woman is aware of the danger signs that

Table 10.2   Signs and symptoms of potentially life-threatening conditions in the puerperium (adapted from NICE 2006)

Condition	Signs and symptoms
Postpartum haemorrhage	Sudden and profuse vaginal bleeding or an increase in bleeding which does not settle Feeling faint, dizzy or experiencing palpitations
Pre-eclampsia	Headache plus one or more of the following: • visual disturbances • nausea • vomiting (within 72 hours of birth)
Infection	Fever, shivering, abdominal pain, may be accompanied by offensive vaginal loss
Thromboembolism	Pain, redness or swelling in one calf Shortness of breath or chest pain

might indicate potentially life-threatening puerperal disorders (see Table 10.2) and has the means to call for help if necessary (NICE 2006).

Bladder care

The bladder and urethra sit interiorly to the uterus and are therefore vulnerable to damage during labour, particularly when labour has been prolonged or when forceps have been used. To prevent the risk of a full bladder obstructing uterine involution, the woman should be encouraged to pass urine soon after birth. However, where the bladder has been emptied using a temporary catheter shortly before the birth or during the third stage of labour, a woman may not feel the urge to pass urine until some hours later.

Reference should be made in the notes of the time that urine was passed and, if measured, the volume should be recorded. NICE (2006) recommends that all urine passed within 6 hours of labour should be documented, so that possible urinary retention may be detected and treated early. If no urine has been passed 6 hours after the birth, extra efforts should be made to encourage micturition: some women find it easier to pass urine in a warm bath or shower, if they find this aesthetically acceptable. If all efforts fail, catheterisation should be urgently considered (NICE 2006) as untreated urinary retention and bladder distension may lead to long-term problems with bladder function as well as impeding normal involution of the uterus.

Activity 10.2

Psychological factors also affect the ability to pass urine. Can you think of any psychological reasons why it may be difficult for a woman to pass urine in the first few hours after giving birth?

How might a midwife help a woman overcome these?

Initiating breastfeeding

Maternity service providers which strive to promote excellence in evidence-based care in relation to infant feeding will in the past have based their care on the '10 Steps to Successful Breastfeeding'. These have now been superseded by the Baby Friendly Initiative standards (UNICEF UK BFI 2012). For a downloadable copy of these, go to: www.unicef.org.uk/BabyFriendly/Health-Professionals/New-Baby-Friendly-Standards/.

According to the standards, maternity care providers should:

- support all mothers and babies to initiate a close relationship and feeding soon after birth
- enable mothers to get breastfeeding off to a good start
- support parents to have a close and loving relationship with their baby (UNICEF UK BFI 2012, p3).

Prior to the birth, the midwife will have established from the woman whether she wants her baby to be given straight to her for immediate skin-to-skin contact. This is recommended for the following reasons:

- It helps the baby to maintain his body temperature.
- It promotes bonding and attachment.
- It facilitates early breastfeeding.

For evidence supporting the benefits of skin-to-skin contact, go to the following link: www.unicef.org.uk/BabyFriendly/News-and-Research/Research/Skin-to-skin-contact.

As long as both woman and baby are well, skin-to-skin contact should be initiated immediately after birth (or as soon as possible) and should continue uninterrupted at least until after the first feed and for as long as desired afterwards (UNICEF UK BFI 2012). It is quite possible for the midwife to undertake most if not all the necessary observations and procedures without separating the mother/baby pair. Healthy babies are usually alert and receptive to feeding in the first hour following birth, so the midwife should encourage the woman to take advantage of this opportunity to initiate breastfeeding, adopting a hands-off approach wherever possible.

Midwifery wisdom

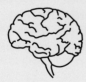

A good first feed not only benefits the baby, but boosts the mother's confidence in her ability to breastfeed successfully in future.

Care after caesarean section

Rising rates of caesarean section across the UK mean that the postoperative care of women is becoming an increasingly large part of the hospital midwife's workload. The woman recovering from a caesarean section requires particular care and attention, not just to her physical well-being but also her state of mind; she has had major surgery as well as giving birth, both of which are major life events (Johnson & Taylor 2010).

> **Box 10.1   Postoperative observations (adapted from Johnson & Taylor 2010)**
>
> - Airway, respirations, heart rate, blood pressure and temperature
> - Oxygen saturation
> - Level of consciousness
> - Control of pain
> - Care of IV infusions and maintenance of fluid balance
> - Care of wound
> - Observation of blood loss per vaginam
> - Care of urinary catheter/observation of urine output
> - Observation for return of sensation following spinal or epidural anaesthesia
> - General comfort, including posture and care of pressure areas
> - General well-being, e.g. nausea, thirst

Care in the recovery area

The immediate postoperative care takes place in the recovery area of the operating theatre, where emergency equipment is on hand. The anaesthetist will hand over care to a midwife, who should remain constantly with the woman until she is fit to be moved to the postnatal ward.

Observations

The woman will have intravenous (IV) infusions running plus an indwelling catheter. Observation of vital signs should be undertaken at 5-min intervals initially until the woman's condition stabilises, then half-hourly for at least 2 hours and thereafter hourly until within satisfactory parameters. Where opioids have been administered, respiratory rate, sedation and pain levels should be monitored hourly for a minimum of 2 hours after treatment is discontinued (NICE 2011).

Routine assessments include those listed in Box 10.1. All observations should be carefully documented and any cause for concern reported immediately to the anaesthetist or obstetrician.

As well as caring for the mother, the midwife must also observe the baby to ensure that he is adapting normally to extrauterine life. Recovery areas may be quite cool and babies born by caesarean are more likely to have a lower temperature (NICE 2011) so the midwife should ensure that the baby does not become chilled, especially as babies born following caesarean section are at greater risk of respiratory distress (Johnson & Taylor 2010). The initial examination for the newborn should be carried out, if not done previously in theatre, and vitamin K administered in accordance with the parents' wishes.

Activity 10.3

 A midwife is caring for a woman alone in the recovery area. The woman's partner is present. What should the midwife do in the following events?

- Her pen runs out of ink whilst completing her records.
- The woman complains of increasing pain.
- The woman asks for help to sit up.

Care of the woman on the postnatal ward following caesarean section

The midwife who has cared for the woman in the recovery area should give a detailed handover to staff on the postnatal ward, including explanation of the documented care plan.

Psychological adjustment in the early postnatal period can be difficult for women who have undergone operative births: as well as physical discomfort, they may feel frustrated by their lack of mobility and their need to seek help with basic baby cares (Johnson & Taylor 2010). Seeing other women around them who need no assistance may increase their sense of inadequacy. The midwife will liaise with the multidisciplinary team, including nursery nurses to help with baby care, maternity care assistants (MCAs) to help with basic observations and hygiene needs and breastfeeding support workers to help establish feeding. The midwife will need to ensure that the woman receives the care and support she needs to develop independence and autonomy in caring for herself and for her baby.

Midwifery wisdom

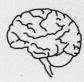

Following a caesarean section, a woman will have very limited mobility for several hours. Once on the postnatal ward she should not be left alone without a call-bell to hand; neither should she be left alone with the baby in her arms unless she is able to place him in the cot safely without assistance.

Pain management

Patient-controlled analgesia (PCA) using opioids is the recommended method of pain control in the immediate postoperative period (NICE 2011). This is set up by the anaesthetist in theatre or the recovery area and will continue in accordance with local protocol.

Non-steroidal anti-inflammatory drugs (NSAIDs) may be used in conjunction with a PCA (NICE 2011) if prescribed. Once the PCA has been discontinued, women should be offered regular analgesia, depending on the level of pain. Gas in the gut (flatus) and constipation are common causes of abdominal pain in the early days following a caesarean section and may be confused with normal 'after-pains' (Marchant 2009a). 'After-pains' are discussed in more detail further on in this chapter. If pain relief is unsatisfactory, the obstetrician should be contacted to review the woman's drug regime.

Hygiene and wound care

The day after her operation, the woman should be offered assistance to take a shower, following which the midwife should help her to remove her wound dressing. The wound site should be inspected to ensure that there is no bleeding or signs of infection and that the suture or staples remain intact. The wound is usually left uncovered by dressings and if non-dissolving sutures or staples have been used, these will be removed by the midwife when local policy dictates. The midwife may take this opportunity to outline the healing process and what to expect in the coming weeks. She can also remind the woman about wearing loose clothing for comfort and advise her on the signs of infection, such as fever, redness, pain, abnormal lochia or wound discharge (NICE 2011).

Fluid balance and diet

The urinary catheter may be removed once a woman is mobile, but should remain *in situ* for at least 12 hours after the last epidural top-up (NICE 2011). Once the catheter is removed, the woman should be encouraged to pass urine frequently. It is important for urine output to be monitored to ensure return to normal bladder function.

Prevention of thromboembolism

Thromboembolism is one of the leading causes of maternal death in the UK (CMACE 2011). All women should be assessed for risk of venous thromboembolism (VTE) in early pregnancy, on admission to hospital for any reason and after delivery (RCOG 2009).This is particularly important for women undergoing caesarean section, as this increases the risk of VTE. Other postnatal risk factors for VTE are listed in Box 10.2.

All women who have had a caesarean section should be encouraged to mobilise as soon as they are able and to remain well hydrated (RCOG 2009). Women who are considered to be at high or intermediate risk of VTE will be given prophylactic anticoagulants in the form of low molecular weight

---

Box 10.2   Postnatal risk factors for venous thromboembolism (VTE) (adapted from RCOG 2009)

High risk:
- Previous VTE
- Caesarean section in labour

Intermediate risk:
- Asymptomatic thrombophilia
- Prolonged hospital admission
- Existing medical conditions such as heart or lung disease, sickle cell disease
- Intravenous drug user

Intermediate risk if two or more factors present:
- Age >35 years
- Obesity
- Parity ≥3
- Smoker
- Elective caesarean section
- Any surgical procedure in the puerperium
- Gross varicose veins
- Current systemic infection
- Immobility, e.g. paraplegia,
- Pre-eclampsia
- Midcavity rotational forceps delivery
- Prolonged labour (>24 hours)
- Postpartum haemorrhage >1 L or blood transfusion

heparin (LMWH) according to current guidelines.Women with three or more persisting risk factors listed in Box 10.2 should be given graduated compression stockings to promote venous return from the lower limbs (RCOG 2009).

Case study 10.2

Tanya gave birth yesterday by emergency caesarean section. Tanya is 41 years old and had a Body Mass Index (BMI) of 35 before becoming pregnant. She feels well but does not want to get out of bed. She has refused a shower. Tanya is eating and drinking normally and her urine output is good. Her catheter is still *in situ*.

- What might be the cause of Tanya's reluctance to get up?
- What risks does Tanya face by refusing to mobilise?

Supporting breastfeeding

A woman who has given birth by caesarean section may be unable to sit upright initially and have difficulty finding a comfortable position in which to hold her baby. Some women find it easier to breastfeed lying on one side or while holding the baby in the underarm position, with a pillow supporting his body. Patience is needed to help the woman find the most comfortable position.

Daily care in hospital for all women

Midwifery wisdom

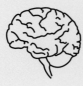

The midwife who helped a woman birth her baby should (if possible) visit her the next day to check on her well-being and answer any questions she may have about events during her labour.

Observations

Within the first 24 hours of giving birth, women should be informed of what to expect during the normal recovery process (NICE 2006). It is no longer considered necessary to complete a daily 'tick-box' list of observations in healthy women unless there is a clear need to do so. One of the essential skills of a midwife is to decide which observations are appropriate (Marchant 2009a).

It is normal for women to pass copious amounts of urine in the first couple of days after giving birth, as the increased blood volume of pregnancy is gradually excreted. It is important that women are made aware of this, so that any difficulty in passing urine can be investigated.

Many women suffer swollen lower legs and feet after giving birth and some may be unable to wear their normal shoes for the first few days. The midwife should explain that this will gradually resolve as the excess fluid from pregnancy is excreted over the following days. Provided swelling is bilateral and there are no other symptoms (e.g. pain, pyrexia or signs of pre-eclampsia), it is not a cause for concern (Marchant 2009b).

The midwife will be alert to the signs and symptoms of the four major life-threatening conditions of the puerperium (see page 177) and should not hesitate to refer to another professional if necessary.

Baby care needs

The midwife will support the woman and her partner to undertake all baby care themselves. However, this does not mean they should simply be 'left to get on with it'. The midwife caring for the woman will check on her progress, offering advice and support as necessary.

Case study 10.3

 Eva had a straightforward birth of a healthy baby boy yesterday. Eva and baby Louis are both healthy and have already enjoyed several good breastfeeds. However, Eva is worried; she tells the midwife that she is getting strong, period-type pains which are worse when Louis is feeding. She has also noticed that her blood loss is heavier when he is on the breast. Her antenatal classes did not mention this and she is afraid something is wrong.

How should the midwife advise Eva?

So-called 'after-pains' are common, particularly among multiparous women. These are caused by the normal contractions of the uterus during involution and are stimulated by oxytocin release, hence their association with breastfeeding. Women should be advised that they may notice a heavier blood loss whilst breastfeeding, due to the effect of oxytocin, and reassured that this is normal (Marchant 2009a). In some cases, 'after-pains' may be almost as strong as labour pains and should never be dismissed as trivial (Marchant 2009a). Prescribed analgesia should be offered and reassurance given about the cause and likely duration of the pain.

Going home

The length of a woman's stay in hospital will depend on many factors, such as her physical recovery, her baby's health and her confidence in her ability to cope at home. Many women choose to go home after just a few hours if all is well and the birth was uncomplicated (Marchant 2009a). Those who have had a caesarean section or difficult forceps delivery may need to remain in hospital for around 3 days.

A woman who has had surgery should have an opportunity to speak with the doctor who performed the operation, and he or she should be satisfied with her recovery. The midwife must follow up any blood tests or other samples sent for analysis and ensure that any prescribed drugs are available for the woman to take home.

Prior to discharge from hospital, the midwife has a duty to ensure that she has discussed the following with the woman and, if appropriate, her partner:

- The continuing plan of postnatal care, including details of any follow-up appointments for mother or baby
- The normal physiological process of recovery from birth and how to seek help in the event of illness of mother or baby
- Emotional well-being and social support at home

- Contact details of local breastfeeding support groups
- Contraception and the return of fertility
- How to reduce the risk of sudden infant death syndrome (SIDS)
- Pelvic floor exercises
- Information on registering the birth
- Information on sterilising bottles and making up feeds if the woman has chosen to bottle feed

Individual hospitals or trusts may issue a 'discharge pack' of information leaflets for each woman. This should not be used as a substitute for a full verbal explanation and the chance for the woman and her partner to ask questions.

Activity 10.4

As can be seen from the list above, midwives are expected to give a lot of information to women prior to discharge home.

- What factors might affect women's ability to take in this information?
- What can the midwife do to facilitate the woman's understanding?

Continuing successful breastfeeding

In order to optimise the chances of the mother and baby successfully continuing with breastfeeding over the coming months, it is important that women are advised on the following:

- How to recognise their baby's feeding cues
- Ways to encourage their baby to open his mouth widely
- The importance of unrestricted duration and frequency of breastfeeds
- The need to offer the second breast if the baby appears hungry after feeding from the first breast
- The fact that transient discomfort at the start of each feed is not abnormal in the early days
- How to recognise good attachment and effective feeding from the breast
  (UNICEF UK BFI 2010a)

The NICE clinical guideline on postnatal care (NICE 2006) recommends that all breastfeeding women be shown how to hand-express milk and be taught how to safely store and use it. The midwife should discuss and assess the woman's experience of breastfeeding at each postnatal contact. Findings should be documented in the relevant notes.

Activity 10.5

Follow this link to NHS Choices, a website providing information on how to express and store breastmilk:
    www.nhs.uk/conditions/pregnancy-and-baby/pages/expressing-storing-breast-milk.aspx

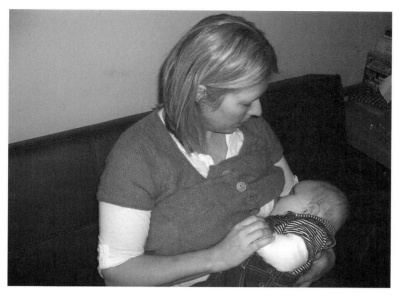

Figure 10.1   Breastfeeding positions: sitting up.

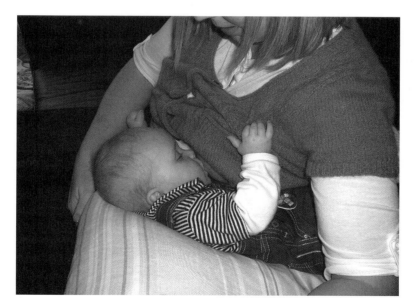

Figure 10.2   Breastfeeding positions: underarm (rugby ball).

The woman should be helped to adopt the position that feels most comfortable to her and her baby. See Figures 10.1, 10.2 and 10.3 for examples of different breastfeeding positions. It is often helpful for the mother to demonstrate the position she has been using so that the health professional may build on that. It is important that a 'hands-off' approach is used (Dyson et al. 2006) and the mother is guided

186

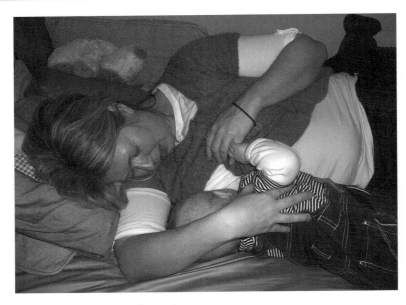

Figure 10.3   Breastfeeding positions: lying down.

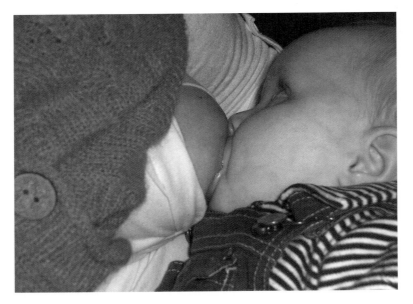

Figure 10.4   Effective breastfeeding.

to position her baby herself, as this will enable her to learn much more effectively how to do this when she is alone.

Once the baby has been positioned, the mother should be advised on how to assess whether the positioning and attachment are good and that the baby is breastfeeding successfully; some of the main signs are illustrated in Figure 10.4. A partner, family member or friend can also help the woman to see if the baby is positioned correctly.

Midwifery wisdom

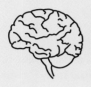

Crying is a late sign that a baby wants to feed; observe for early feeding cues and attempt to position the baby to the breast before he gets to the crying stage (UNICEF UK BFI 2010a).

Activity 10.6

Follow the link again for the UNICEF UK Baby Friendly website: www.unicef.org.uk/babyfriendly/. You will find further information about breastfeeding, including the standards to support breastfeeding in the practice area.

Find out about any local breastfeeding support groups that you have in your own area. Make a list of these for your future reference.

Other methods of infant feeding

If a baby is unable to take the breast for any reason, his mother can be shown how to feed him expressed milk using a cup, spoon or syringe. The latter is ideal in the first 2–3 days when the woman is producing colostrum. The very small volume makes it difficult to collect in a pump; therefore, the midwife should show the woman how to hand-express her colostrum while the midwife or the woman's partner collects it in a small, sterile syringe. This can then be fed directly to the baby.

The cup or spoon method is more suitable once the woman's milk has 'come in', i.e. from about day 3–4 postnatally. In either case equipment must be sterilised before use and strict hand hygiene observed. All methods of expressing and feeding expressed milk are time-consuming, requiring skill and patience.

All women should be offered information about breastfeeding support groups in their area and those who are experiencing difficulty will require additional support from either the community midwife or a specially trained support worker.

Supporting women who choose to bottle feed

The midwife has a duty to support all women in their chosen method of infant feeding. Although midwives should advise women of the benefits of breastfeeding for both mother and baby, the woman is free to make her own decision and should not be made to feel guilty or inferior if, for whatever reason, she chooses not to breastfeed. Parents who choose to use formula milk should receive appropriate support so that they feel confident with how to feed their baby safely (UNICEF UK BFI 2010b). The woman or couple should also be shown how to clean and sterilise feeding equipment in line with the manufacturer's instructions. Ideally, this should be done using the family's own sterilising equipment rather than hospital equipment. The UNICEF UK BFI and Department of Health (DH) (2012) have collaborated to produce a leaflet on bottle feeding, with the aim of ensuring safe bottle-feeding practices. This should be given to parents to reinforce verbal information.

Regardless of feeding practices, promoting methods such as skin to skin and keeping the baby close to the mother will aid bonding and future infant development (Gerhardt 2004; UNICEF UK BFI 2012).

Midwifery care in the community

Once the new family has returned to their home, the community midwife will visit. It is usual to visit the woman on the day after her discharge from hospital and thereafter according to her and her baby's needs.

If the visiting midwife has not met the woman before, she will need to take some time building a rapport with her and gaining her trust. On the first visit, it is important to note the woman's history and any documented care plan, to assist the midwife in planning appropriate future care. The community midwife should inform the parents that they may view the Department of Health booklet *Birth to Five* online (DH 2009a). She should ensure that they have received a copy of their child's personal health record (the 'Red Book') and that the purpose of this has been clearly explained.

Physical assessment of the woman

Before any physical contact with the woman, the midwife will assess her general health and well-being by asking how she is feeling. This may give further clues to any problems or unexpected needs. Any examination of the woman or her baby should only take place following full verbal consent and thorough hand washing. The midwife must assess whether it is appropriate to conduct any physical examination in a communal area of the home where friends and family may be present, or whether she and the woman should move to a more private area, such as a bedroom. Full account should be taken of the woman's cultural and religious background.

Vital signs observations

Providing that there is no history of abnormal vital signs in the postnatal period and the woman is generally well, vital signs need not be repeated unless her condition gives rise to concern. Any unusual findings should be closely observed and referred promptly to the GP if they do not resolve.

Common breast conditions

Regardless of whether or not the woman has chosen to breastfeed her baby, the midwife should enquire about the comfort of the woman's breasts at every visit. Women should be warned about what to expect when the milk 'comes in' on day 3 or thereabouts and that milk may leak from their nipples between feeds. Bras or tops should fit comfortably and not 'dig in'. Women who have chosen not to breastfeed should be given appropriate advice on suppressing lactation. This will include minimal handling of the breasts to avoid stimulating lactation and taking paracetamol to relieve discomfort.

Breast engorgement around day 3 is not uncommon whether or not the woman is breastfeeding, so appropriate, evidence-based advice should be given. Gentle hand expression may relieve engorgement around the areola and help the baby to attach to the breast.

Breastfeeding women should be asked whether they are experiencing any nipple pain and if so, the midwife should ask to examine the nipples. If trauma is evident, appropriate advice should be offered and the breasts re-examined the following day and thereafter until they are healing satisfactorily. In most cases, sore or cracked nipples are the result of incorrect positioning of the baby at the breast, so the midwife must make time to support and advise on correct positioning and attachment. She may refer the mother to a local breastfeeding support group for further assistance.

The woman should be advised on current evidence about nipple preparations to treat or prevent soreness. If the nipple is cracked, UNICEF UK BFI (2010c) currently suggests the use of purified lanolin to aid moist wound healing or a small amount of expressed breastmilk rubbed on the area after a feed. Some women may wish to use nipple shields and whilst there has been much debate regarding their effectiveness (Pollard 2012), the use of ultra-thin nipple shields as a short-term measure only may be of benefit (Chertok 2009). However, assistance to correctly position and attach the baby to the breast should always be the first strategy used to attempt to solve the problem.

Women should be advised on how to recognise signs of mastitis and to report any symptoms to the visiting midwife (NICE 2006). Mastitis is most likely to be caused by a blocked milk duct. The midwife should show the woman how to relieve it by massaging from the affected area towards the nipple during feeding or hand expression. If there is no improvement after a few hours, the woman should be advised to contact her midwife again and may need to be referred to her GP for antibiotic treatment (NICE 2006). However, if the woman is obviously unwell, the midwife may decide to refer to a GP straight away. Advice on continuing to feed the baby and the use of simple analgesia should also be given.

189

Midwifery wisdom

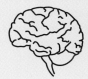 Poor positioning and attachment of the baby to the breast are often the main cause of nipple pain and damage. It is therefore important to observe a full feed so that appropriate advice may be given.

The lochia and uterine involution

The midwife will need to enquire about the woman's lochia (the discharge consisting of blood, epithelial cells and remaining decidua from the uterus). This is a subject some women would rather discuss in private and the midwife needs to be aware of cultural and individual sensitivities when raising this subject.

The woman should be informed of the changing volume of the lochia during the postnatal period. She should be alerted to the fact that the lochia may temporarily increase once she becomes more active, but the overall trend should be a general decrease in volume over the coming 2–3 weeks and a gradual change in colour from bright red to pinkish-brown. Women may pass the occasional small clot, but providing there are no other symptoms, they can be reassured that this is normal. The midwife should, however, advise the woman and her partner to be alert to any sudden or profuse loss, especially if accompanied by symptoms of shock. This requires emergency action (NICE 2006).

The process of involution, by which the uterus returns to its pre-pregnant shape and position, continues until the end of the puerperium. However, most of the reduction in size will have occurred by day 10 postnatally (Johnson & Taylor 2010). Until recently, it was common practice to palpate the woman's abdomen to monitor involution at every postnatal contact. However, current guidelines state that this is unnecessary unless the lochia is abnormal (NICE 2006).

If the woman reports excessive or offensive-smelling lochia, large clots, abdominal tenderness or fever, the midwife should gently palpate her uterus. Any abnormalities in the size, tone or position need urgent investigation or medical referral. However, simple explanations such as a full bladder or rectum should first be ruled out. Unless the woman has recently had a caesarean section, there should be no uterine tenderness on palpation (Johnson & Taylor 2010).

Case study 10.4

A woman who was discharged home yesterday rings the ward in a state of panic. It is day 3 and she has just passed a large clot of blood. The woman had a normal vaginal delivery with no apparent complications.

- What questions do you need to ask the woman?
- Assuming there is no immediate cause for concern, how would you advise the woman?

Perineal care

At each visit, the woman should be asked how her perineum feels and, if there has been any degree of perineal trauma, whether she has any concerns about the healing process (NICE 2006). If the woman reports any pain, offensive odour or dysuria (pain on urinating), the midwife should offer to look at her perineum and assess any changes. Signs of infection such as offensive smell or wound breakdown should be reported urgently (NICE 2006) to the GP so that antibiotic treatment may be commenced. In the event of a severe wound breakdown, it may be necessary to refer the woman back to hospital for obstetric review. The midwife may advise paracetamol and/or cool gel pads to relieve discomfort while healing occurs (NICE 2006). The woman should be informed about perineal hygiene and pelvic floor exercises to promote wound healing and be reminded to wear loose clothing in natural fibres for comfort.

Elimination

The midwife will ask the woman whether her bowel and bladder functions have returned to normal or whether she is experiencing any difficulties. Some women experience haemorrhoids and constipation for which over-the-counter remedies are available. Dietary advice should also be given and if the problem does not resolve, the woman should be referred to her GP.

Minor stress incontinence is not uncommon, especially following an assisted delivery or prolonged labour. Pelvic floor exercises will help regain the tone of the perineal muscles (NICE 2006). If incontinence persists, the woman should be referred for specialist investigation. Faecal incontinence sometimes occurs following a third- or fourth-degree tear and a woman should be offered counselling and appropriate follow-up care in relation to this (RCOG 2007).

Headache

The current NICE guidelines on postnatal care recommend that all women should be asked about headache symptoms at each postnatal contact (NICE 2006). Special vigilance is needed when women who have a history of pre-eclampsia report a severe headache in the first 72 hours after giving birth, especially if accompanied by visual disturbances, nausea or vomiting. These may be symptoms of worsening pre-eclampsia or an impending eclamptic seizure and warrant urgent referral plus blood pressure monitoring. Even where there is no history of pre-eclampsia, women with a severe or persistent headache should be evaluated and referred for urgent medical attention (NICE 2006).

Legs

At every visit, the midwife will ask the woman whether she has any leg pains. This is due to the increased risk of thromboembolic disorders following childbirth. Women should be encouraged to mobilise, building up their physical activity gradually without becoming too tired. Any unilateral calf pain, redness or swelling should be treated as suspicious and evaluated for deep vein thrombosis (DVT) (NICE 2006). This requires immediate medical attention.

Sexual health and contraception

At some point the midwife must introduce the subject of resuming sexual intercourse and contraception, as detailed within the competencies set by the NMC (NMC 2009). The woman should first be asked if she wishes to discuss this and her wishes respected (Hall 2005). All advice should be tailored to the couple's needs and where possible, supported with written information leaflets in the couple's first language. The couple may appreciate having contact details for expert advice (NICE 2006).

Immunisations (NICE 2006)

Women who are rhesus negative should be offered anti-D immunoglobulin within 72 hours of the birth of a rhesus-positive baby. Due to early discharge from hospital, many women now receive their anti-D at home via the community midwife. Women who screened negative for rubella antibodies antenatally should be offered the MMR vaccination prior to leaving hospital. The person who gives the vaccination should advise the woman to avoid pregnancy for 1 month afterwards. Breastfeeding is not contraindicated.

Assessment of the woman's psychological well-being

The arrival of a new baby can be a time of major psychological upheaval for a woman and her family. It is normal for women to feel very tired following the birth, and this may be simply due to the demands of a newborn baby; however, a woman who is persistently tired warrants further investigation for conditions such as anaemia (NICE 2006). On the other hand, there may be a psychological cause.

Case study 10.5

Leo's partner, Shannice, gave birth to their first baby 3 weeks ago. At first, all seemed well, but now Leo is concerned that Shannice seems tired all the time and has little enthusiasm for anything. He has suggested getting a babysitter and going out for a meal, but Shannice is not interested. Shannice has refused visits and offers of help from her family and friends and is often tearful and moody.

- What do you think might be happening to Shannice?
- Find out about sources of help in your area that Leo could refer to.

At each postnatal visit, the midwife should ask the woman about her emotional well-being and whether she has any family or social support network (NICE 2006). Women and their partners should be encouraged to inform their midwife of any concerns about mood changes or uncharacteristic behaviour. Midwives should inform the woman's GP if they suspect a mental health disorder or if they uncover a previously unreported history of mental health problems.

Mental distress during or shortly after pregnancy is common and affects around one woman in six (Wooster 2007). Those who have a history of mental health problems are at high risk of symptoms occurring again following childbirth (RCP 2012a, b) and therefore, the midwife should carefully read the woman's antenatal notes for any indications about previous mental health issues. Some women may be very traumatised by events surrounding the birth, especially if this differed greatly from their expectation. Such women may benefit from referral to an independent support group such as the Birth Trauma Association: www.birthtraumaassociation.org.uk/.

It is not uncommon for women to experience 'baby blues' on or around the third day postnatally. It is thought that this is due to changes in the levels of oestrogen, progesterone and prolactin, causing a temporary alteration in the woman's emotional well-being (Raynor & Oates 2009). This is often compounded by discomfort at the milk 'coming in' and possibly by the transition from hospital to home. 'Baby blues' are often characterised by unexpected tearfulness and anxiety, which may take both the woman and her partner by surprise. If the woman has been warned of this in the antenatal period, she may be better able to accept these feelings and await their natural passing. If not, the midwife should gently explain why she is feeling this way, advise her that it is quite normal and observe her carefully over the next day or so to ensure that her mood returns to normal. This transient period of low mood is not a predictor of future mental health problems. If the symptoms of the 'baby blues' have not resolved by days 10–14, an assessment for postnatal depression should be undertaken (NICE 2006).

Postnatal depression affects 10–15% of mothers (NICE 2006). It is characterised by persistent low mood, loss of interest or pleasure in everyday life, persistent fatigue, loss of self-confidence, poor concentration, despair or even suicidal thoughts (Gutteridge 2007, Wooster 2007). As depression in a mother could also have a significant impact on her child's well-being, particularly in the first 5 years of age (Davies & Ward 2012), it is essential she receives the right amount of care and support early on. Women can be encouraged to look after their mental health by taking exercise, getting sufficient rest, getting help with baby care and talking to an understanding person about their feelings. Social isolation is a known risk factor for postnatal depression, so access to social support networks may be a lifeline (NICE 2006). Women and their partners should be given information on how to recognise the signs of postnatal depression and contact numbers of where to seek help.

Women with mental health problems, whether new or pre-existing, should be offered a longer period of midwifery support with continuity of care, in line with NMC guidance (NMC 2009, 2012) and Midwifery 2020 (DH 2010). This may go beyond the period of physical recovery and may involve other professionals, such as the health visitor.

Puerperal psychosis is an acute condition affecting women after childbirth which causes sudden and dramatic changes of behaviour (Wooster 2007). Although this condition is rare (McGowan et al. 2007), it is often associated with thoughts of suicide or suicide attempts. CMACE recommends that priority is given to the referral of women for urgent specialist care, up to 6 weeks post partum (CMACE 2011). Further information about the management of mental health during pregnancy and the postnatal period can be found in NICE Clinical Guideline 45 (NICE 2007a).

Care of the baby in the community

The purpose of examining the baby is to monitor daily changes and detect any signs of deviation from the expected norm. When visiting a woman in her home or meeting her at a postnatal clinic, the midwife will offer information and advice to enable her to:

- assess her baby's general health
- recognise signs of ill health
- contact the relevant health professional or emergency service if necessary.

Detailed and accurate records must be maintained to enable continuity of care.

It is important that the midwife sees both mother and baby at each postnatal contact so that emotional attachment can be assessed (NICE 2006) and any barriers to this detected as early as possible. This presents a good opportunity for the midwife to explain to both parents and/or other family members the baby's social capabilities and changing needs. Questions from the family should be actively encouraged and information or reassurance offered as required.

When assessing the baby's health and development, the midwife may begin by asking the woman about his well-being. It may not be necessary to undress and physically examine a baby at every visit. However, if the midwife has concerns about the baby's health or about his parents' ability to care for him, this might form part of the overall assessment.

As part of the assessment of the baby, the midwife will ask about and observe the following:

- Feeding: interest in feeding, method, frequency and (if bottle fed) volume
- Elimination: frequency of urination and defaecation, changing stools, signs of constipation or diarrhoea
- Muscle tone, posture
- Behaviour: including ability to settle between feeds, sleep patterns, response to stimuli, response to handling
- Crying: pitch and duration, response to comforting
- Temperature: it is not necessary to measure temperature with a thermometer unless the baby appears unwell
- Skin: colour, condition, lesions or trauma, rashes, spots, signs of non-accidental injury
- Umbilicus: signs of separation of cord stump, signs of possible infection
- Resolution of any birth trauma such as caput and moulding
- Eyes: any discharge is noted
- Mouth: any signs of thrush are noted

The midwife will monitor and record any jaundice until it has resolved, ensuring appropriate referral to a paediatrician if it does not resolve normally or if there are concerns about its effects on the baby. Parents should be advised on how to recognise signs of worsening jaundice and related symptoms and how to seek help (NICE 2006). A mother who is breastfeeding may need particular reassurance and support at this time. Further information on neonatal jaundice can be found in NICE guideline 98 (NICE 2010).

Skin care

Parents should be advised on the daily hygiene needs of the baby and the avoidance of unnecessary cleaning agents and toiletries (NICE 2006). The nappy area may be inspected to observe for soreness, thrush or nappy rash and appropriate treatment recommended.

Colic

If the baby shows signs of colic he should first be assessed to rule out other underlying conditions. The midwife will need to take a detailed history from the parents about the nature, onset and duration of symptoms. There is no medical treatment for colic, but parents should be given sensitive reassurance and advice on ways to position and hold their baby to minimise his discomfort (NICE 2006).

Weighing

Most babies lose anything up to 10% of their birth weight in the first few days of life, but normally regain it by around day 10. Babies are routinely weighed on day 5 to detect any abnormal weight loss so that the underlying cause may be investigated and treated. Other than this, regular weighing of babies is not done routinely unless there is a particular cause for concern.

Newborn blood spot screening

The midwife will undertake the newborn blood spot sampling to screen for certain genetic and metabolic anomalies between days 5 and 8, but ideally on day 5 (counting the birth date as day 0) (UK Newborn Screening Programme Centre 2012). Fully informed parental consent is required, so the midwife must ensure that parents have had time to consider their options beforehand, preferably with access to written information. The midwife must ensure that parents know when and how the results of the test will be conveyed to them.

Activity 10.7

The UK National Screening Committee has produced a free Antenatal and Newborn Screening eLearning Module for health professionals (including students). Follow this link which will take you there:http://cpd.screening.nhs.uk/elearning.

On completing and passing this module, you will receive certification which you will be able to add to your own professional portfolio.

Safety issues

When conducting home visits, health professionals should take the opportunity to assess and advise on relevant safety issues including baby equipment, the home environment, smoking, safe sleeping and the avoidance of sudden infant death (DH 2009b, NICE 2006).

Activity 10.8

A leaflet on safe sleeping can be downloaded from the Lullaby Trust via the following link: www.lullabytrust.org.uk/document.doc?id=295.

Any health professional involved with a family must remain alert to the signs and symptoms of child abuse, and be aware of the consequences of maltreatment on a child's development (Davies & Ward 2012). Midwives should know the route for referral according to local child protection policies and be ready to use them if they suspect abuse.

Ongoing advice and care

During the course of her postnatal visits to the woman's home, the midwife will take the opportunity to inform women and their families about sources of continuing care and local support networks. These are important not just for the woman's and baby's physical well-being, but also to help the family to adjust to their new role and access means of social support if necessary (NICE 2006).

Activity 10.9

- Identify three networks of support for new parents in your area.
- Identify the aims of these organisations and note whether they are targeted at any particular types of parents.

Conclusion

The birth of a baby is a life-changing event, having physical, social and psychological consequences for the woman. Most women adapt well to these changes and become happy and confident mothers. A few succumb to the physical or emotional stresses that this time brings and need ongoing support and care. The midwife has an important role not only in preparing women for birth and motherhood, but also in supporting them through this transition stage and identifying their changing needs. Both woman and baby deserve the best possible care at this crucial time.

Quiz

Answer 'true' or 'false' to the following questions.

1. NICE (2006) recommends that if the 'baby blues' have not resolved by day 5 then the woman must be assessed for postnatal depression.
2. A second-degree tear should not involve the anal sphincter.
3. A medical condition such as lung disease is one of the risk factors for venous thromboembolism.
4. It is common for vaginal blood loss to be heavier during breastfeeding.
5. Crying is an early sign that a baby is ready to feed.
6. If a mother is experiencing sore nipples, assistance to correctly position and attach the baby to the breast should be the first strategy used to attempt to solve the problem.
7. Involution is the process of breastmilk production following delivery.
8. If a woman requires anti-D immunoglobulin, this must be given within 92 hours following delivery.

Word search

How can a woman tell that her baby is *well attached* to her breast and breastfeeding successfully? Locate six key signs in this word search.

```
O D T F Q V C D G E S M Q U W V O S S Q
K G L L T A E P Q P X B L I A O T E W T
R S L G X C J S Y W W E D B B U R I A W
X Z P A D S L R S L H E E E O M D P L H
L G J B O Q E X W R O K L D M D L P L K
U V R Z M V T X P P B Q E S Y D J A O B
T L N O N L N Q E H I L R V U T W N W E
I Y F V O Z C N E P R P L B N Q H Y I Z
W M J B Q D M K X U L A E T U O B T N A
V L U W D O W P C K Z E H Q Q Q Y R G Y
B M N B U Q J P Y P Q W L P H E Y I H W
R H Y T H M I C A L S U C K I N G D E N
N W H P A L D E N B A Q V E U J X D A P
R L W I R V D O D Z B T A I Q P T N R I
A J Y E K Y J B G C B U U O S U E A D R
Y M W E E R F N I A P D Z T G P M T R U
P O D F T A T Q T K X W I B D T J E G P
L H Y C V S W Y O C F W G S J Q M W N V
T Q T F S C Z C O H G R W N O H R I O H
X W L I X Y H N E R L G S E D B A N O Q
```

References

Chertok IRA (2009) Reexamination of ultra-thin nipple shield use, infant growth and maternal satisfaction. *Journal of Clinical Nursing* 18: 2949–2955.

Centre for Maternal and Child Enquiries (CMACE) (2011) *Saving Mothers' Lives: reviewing maternal deaths to make motherhood safer 2006–2008*. The Eighth Report of the Confidential Enquiries into Maternal Deaths in the United Kingdom. *British Journal of Obstetrics and Gynaecology* 118(Suppl. 1): 1–203.

Davies C, Ward H (2012) *Safeguarding Children Across Services: messages from research*. London: Jessica Kingsley Publishers.

Department of Health (DH) (2009a) *Birth to Five*. Available at: http://webarchive.nationalarchives.gov.uk/+/www.dh.gov.uk/en/Publicationsandstatistics/Publications/PublicationsPolicyAndGuidance/DH_107303 (accessed May 2013).

Department of Health (DH) (2009b) *Reduce the Risk of Cot Death*. London: Department of Health.

Department of Health (DH) (2010) *Midwifery 2020: delivering expectations*. London: Department of Health.

Dyson L, Renfrew M, McFadden A, McCormick F, Herbert G, Thomas J (2006) *Promotion of Breastfeeding Initiation and Duration: evidence into practice briefing*. Public Health Collaborating Centre on Maternal and Child Nutrition on behalf of the Health Development Agency. London: National Institute for Health and Clinical Excellence.

Gerhardt S (2004) *Why Love Matters: how affection shapes a baby's brain*. London: Routledge.

Gutteridge K (2007) Making a difference. *Midwives* 10(4): 173–175.

Hall J (2005) Midwifery basics: postnatal care – postnatal fertility control advice. *Practising Midwife* 8(5): 39–43.

Johnson R, Taylor W (2010) *Skills for Midwifery Practice*, 3rd edn. Edinburgh: Elsevier Churchill Livingstone.

Kettle C, Dowdswell T, Ismail KMK (2010) Absorbable suture materials for primary repair of episiotomy and second degree tears (review). *Cochrane Database of Systematic Reviews* **6**: CD000006.

Marchant S (2009a) Physiology and care in the puerperium. In: Fraser D, Cooper M (eds) *Myles Textbook for Midwives*, 15th edn. Edinburgh: Churchill Livingstone.

Marchant S (2009b) Physical problems and complications in the puerperium. In: Fraser D, Cooper M (eds) *Myles Textbook for Midwives*, 15th edn. Edinburgh: Churchill Livingstone.

McGowan I, Sinclair M, Owens M (2007) Maternal suicide: rates and trends. *Midwives* **10**(4): 167–169.

National Institute for Health and Clinical Excellence (NICE) (2006) *Routine Postnatal Care of Women and Their Babies*. Clinical Guideline No. 37. London: National Institute for Health and Clinical Excellence.

National Institute for Health and Clinical Excellence (NICE) (2007a) *Antenatal and Postnatal Mental Health*. Clinical Guideline No. 45. London: National Institute for Health and Clinical Excellence.

National Institute for Health and Clinical Excellence (NICE) (2007b) *Intrapartum Care: care of healthy women and their babies during childbirth*. Clinical Guideline No. 55. London: National Institute for Health and Clinical Excellence.

National Institute for Health and Clinical Excellence (NICE) (2010) *Neonatal Jaundice*. Clinical Guideline No. 98. London: National Institute for Health and Clinical Excellence.

National Institute for Health and Clinical Excellence (NICE) (2011) *Caesarean Section*. Clinical Guideline No. 132. London: National Institute for Health and Clinical Excellence.

Nursing and Midwifery Council (NMC) (2009) *Standards for Pre-Registration Midwifery Education*. London: Nursing and Midwifery Council.

Nursing and Midwifery Council (NMC) (2012) *Midwives' Rules and Standards*. London: Nursing and Midwifery Council.

Pollard M (2012*) Evidence-Based Care for Breastfeeding Mothers: a resource for midwives and allied healthcare professionals*. Oxford: Routledge.

Raynor MD, Oates MR (2009) Perinatal mental health. Part A, The psychological context of pregnancy and the puerperium. In: Fraser D, Cooper M (eds) *Myles Textbook for Midwives*, 15th edn. Edinburgh: Churchill Livingstone.

Royal College of Midwives (RCM) (2012) *Evidence Based Guidelines for Midwifery-Led Care in Labour: suturing the perineum*. London: Royal College of Midwives.

Royal College of Obstetricians and Gynaecologists (RCOG) (2007) *The Management Of Third- and Fourth-Degree Perineal Tears*. Green-top Guideline No. 29. London: Royal College of Obstetricians and Gynaecologists.

Royal College of Obstetricians and Gynaecologists (RCOG) (2009) *Reducing the Risk of Thrombosis and Embolism During Pregnancy and the Puerperium*. Green-top Guideline No. 37a. London: Royal College of Obstetricians and Gynaecologists.

Royal College of Psychiatrists (RCP) (2012a) *Mental Health in Pregnancy*. London: Royal College of Psychiatrists. Available at: www.rcpsych.ac.uk/expertadvice/problems/mentalhealthinpregnancy.aspx (accessed May 2013).

Royal College of Psychiatrists (RCP) (2012b) *Postnatal depression*. Available at: www.rcpsych.ac.uk/expertadvice/problems/postnatalmentalhealth/postnataldepression.aspx (accessed May 2013).

Steen M (2010) Care and consequences of perineal trauma. *British Journal of Midwifery* **18**(11): 358–362.

Steen M (2012) Risk, recognition and repair of perineal trauma. *British Journal of Midwifery* **20**(11): 768–722.

UK Newborn Screening Programme Centre (2012) *Guidelines for Newborn Blood Spot Sampling*. London: UK Newborn National Screening Committee.

UNICEF UK BFI (2010a) *Breastfeeding: a mother's journey*. Available at: www.unicef.org.uk/BabyFriendly/Health-Professionals/Care-Pathways/Breastfeeding/First-two-weeks/Baby-led-feeding/ (accessed May 2013).

UNICEF UK BFI (2010b) *Bottle Feeding: a mother's journey*. Available at: www.unicef.org.uk/BabyFriendly/Health-Professionals/Care-Pathways/Bottle_feeding/ (accessed May 2013).

UNICEF UK BFI (2010c) *Sore Nipples*. Available at: www.unicef.org.uk/BabyFriendly/Health-Professionals/Going-Baby-Friendly/FAQs/Breastfeeding-FAQ/Sore-nipples/ (accessed May 2013).

UNICEF UK BFI (2012) *Guide to the Baby Friendly Initiative Standards*. Available at: www.unicef.org.uk/BabyFriendly/Health-Professionals/New-Baby-Friendly-Standards/ (accessed May 2013).

UNICEF UK BFI/Department of Health (DH) (2012) *Guide to Bottle Feeding: how to prepare infant formula and sterilise feeding equipment to minimise the risks to your baby*. London: Department of Health.

Wooster E (2007) Supporting mental health. *Midwives* **10**(4): 170–172.

11

Medication and the Midwife
Cathy Hamilton

Aim

The aim of this chapter is to introduce the student midwife to her professional role and responsibilities in relation to the safe administration of medicine.

Learning outcomes

By the end of this chapter you will be able to:

1. demonstrate an understanding of definitions relating to medicines management
2. describe the legislation governing the supply and administration of medicines by a midwife (including midwives' exemptions, controlled drugs, general sale list medicines, prescription-only medications and patient group directions)
3. have an understanding of the principles governing the safe administration of medicines by a midwife
4. demonstrate an awareness of the implications of taking medicines for a pregnant and/or a breastfeeding woman
5. have an understanding of the routes by which medicines may be administered
6. know what to do in the case of a drug error and demonstrate awareness of your professional responsibilities in relation to the safe administration of medicines.

Introduction

The practice of midwifery is concerned with supporting women and their families through the normal, physiological process of childbirth. However, women may complain of discomfort or minor disorders associated with childbirth, they may become unwell during pregnancy or labour or they may have a

The Student's Guide to Becoming a Midwife, Second Edition. Edited by Ian Peate and Cathy Hamilton.
© 2014 John Wiley & Sons, Ltd. Published 2014 by John Wiley & Sons, Ltd.

pre-existing medical condition. In these cases, the midwife may be required to administer medicine to relieve the discomfort or to treat the condition. Headley et al. (2004) have reported that 92.4% of pregnant women in their research group had taken a medicinal product at least once during their pregnancies. At least a third of the women reported taking a pain-relieving medicine such as paracetamol, while 23% reported using an antacid to relieve symptoms of indigestion.

The use of medicinal products during pregnancy is such that it is important that midwives are competent to safely undertake all aspects of drug administration. This chapter aims to give an overview of issues relating to the use of medicines in the context of midwifery practice.

Legislation governing the administration of drugs

The Nursing and Midwifery Council (NMC) *Standards for Medicines Management* (NMC 2007) highlights the fact that the administration of medicines is an important aspect of the professional practice of all individuals registered with the Council. However, it is emphasised that it should not be viewed as a mechanical task which is performed exactly in accordance with the written prescription of a medical practitioner. This is where professional judgement and thought are important when each practitioner views the client as an individual, taking all aspects of her care into consideration (the holistic approach). This includes issues such as what other drugs the woman is taking, how they might interact with each other and what reactions she has had to a drug previously.

Rule 5 of the *Midwives' Rules and Standards* (NMC 2012) states that a practising midwife should only supply and administer those drugs for which she has received appropriate training. This includes being familiar with the dosage of the drug, any potential side-effects, restrictions to its use and method of administration.

The Medicines Act 1968

This legislation was introduced by the then Department of Health and Social Security following a review of legislation relating to medicines, prompted by the thalidomide tragedy of the early 1960s. During this time, many pregnant women took the drug thalidomide as treatment for morning sickness. It was not known at the time that this drug could have an adverse effect on the developing fetus as no testing on pregnant animals had been done prior to the drug being released to the public. This led to thousands of babies being born with severe and very distinctive limb deformities.

The Medicines Act 1968 brought together most of the previous laws relating to medicines and intro-duced other legal provisions for the control of medicines, including supply, possession and manufacture. It classifies medicinal drugs into three categories depending on the dangers they pose to the public and the risk of misuse:

1. Prescription-only medicines
2. Pharmacy-only medicines
3. General sale list medicines

Prescription-only medicines (POM)

These are medicines that can only be supplied and given to a client on the instruction of an appropriate practitioner (for example, a doctor or dentist). Since the Medicinal Products Prescription by Nurses Act 1992, health visitors and district nurses who have recorded their nurse prescribing qualification with the NMC are also able to prescribe certain medicines from the approved nurse prescribers list.

Pharmacy-only medicines (P)

Pharmacy-only medicine can only be bought from a registered pharmacy provided that the sale is supervised by the pharmacist, enabling the pharmacist to confirm with the client that it is safe for them to take the medicine. For example, the client will be asked if they are taking any other types of medicine which might interact or interfere with the requested medicine, or if they have any other condition, such as pregnancy, high blood pressure or cardiac problems, which might be affected by the medicine.

Some medicines may only be sold once the pharmacist is satisfied that certain circumstances have been fulfilled. For example, emergency contraception (also known as the 'morning-after pill') may only be sold to the person who actually requires the contraception and she must be over the age of 16 years.

General sale list medicines (GSL)

These do not need a prescription or the supervision of a pharmacist and can be obtained by members of the public from supermarkets or other retail outlets. Usually only a small pack size of the medicine may be sold in these stores. For example, the largest pack size of paracetamol that may be sold from a shop is 16 tablets whereas packs of 32 tablets may be sold from a pharmacy. Similarly, only low strengths of the medicine may be sold from a general store. For example, the highest strength of ibuprofen tablets that may be sold from a shop is 200 mg whereas tablets containing 400 mg may be sold from a pharmacy.

Some medicines may be reclassified from prescription only to pharmacy or from pharmacy to general sale list. This can happen once it is considered that the medicine is safe for most people to use. For example, aciclovir cream, which is used to treat cold sores, was initially available as prescription only. After a few years, it was reclassified to a pharmacy medicine, and recently it has been reclassified again to a general sale list medicine.

Midwives' exemptions and prescription-only medicines

Specific drugs, including those usually available only on prescription, may be supplied to midwives for use in their professional practice. In this case midwives are recognised as being exempt from certain restrictions on the sale or supply and administration of medicines under the Medicines Act 1968. Examples of drugs commonly used in midwifery practice include Syntometrine, which may be given during the third stage of labour to facilitate the delivery of the placenta, and pethidine, which may be administered as pain relief during labour. The midwife can administer both these drugs on her own responsibility without the need for a prescription.

A midwife may use these drugs only in her professional midwifery capacity. For example, she would not be permitted to administer the drug to a friend or family member unless she was caring for them during childbirth.

Preparations for use by midwives are shown in the list below. They are included in Schedule 5 (Parts 1 and 3) of the Prescription Only Medicines (Human Use) Order 1997 (often referred to as the 'POM' Order), the Medicines (Pharmacy and General Sale-Exemption) Order 1980 (SI 1980/1924) and the Medicines (Sale or Supply) (Miscellaneous Provisions) Regulations 1980 (SI 1980/1923).

In Part 1 of the POM Order (exemptions from restrictions on sale or supply), the midwife can supply the following medicines on her own initiative:

- Diclofenac
- Hydrocortizone acetate
- Miconazole
- Nystatin
- Phytomenadione

In Part 3 of the POM Order (exemptions from restrictions on administration), the midwife can administer the following medicines on her own initiative:

- Adrenaline
- Anti-D immunoglobulin
- Carboprost
- Cyclizine lactate
- Diamorphine
- Ergometrine maleate
- Gelofusine
- Hartmann's solution
- Hepatitis B vaccine
- Hepatitis immunoglobulin
- Lidocaine
- Lidocaine hydrochloride
- Morphine
- Naloxone hydrochloride (Narcan)
- Oxytocins (natural and synthetic)
- Pethidine hydrochloride
- Phytomenadione (vitamin K)
- Prochlorperazine
- Sodium chloride 0.9%

Whatever drugs a midwife uses in her practice, it is clearly stated in the *Midwives' Rules and Standards* (NMC 2012) that a midwife should not administer any drug unless she is familiar with its usage and has received appropriate training with regard to its use. This becomes particularly important now that the number of medicines included on the midwives' exemptions list has increased. There are implications for the continuous professional development and training needs of all midwives to ensure that they are updated on how to use and administer any particular drug.

Case study 11.1

Sharma is a first-year student midwife and is undertaking her first placement on the delivery suite. The woman she is caring for is in the first stage of labour and is requesting pethidine as a method of pain relief. Sharma asks Samantha, her mentor, if she should call the senior house officer to the ward to prescribe the drug. She is surprised when Samantha informs her that this is not necessary as pethidine is one of the drugs on the midwives' exemption list.

Samantha also explains to Sharma that as a student, while she can be involved in the checking and preparation of the pethidine with her, Sharma will not be permitted to actually administer the injection to the woman. The injection will need to be administered by a qualified midwife as it is a controlled drug.

Thankfully, though, as Samantha is a 'sign off mentor', Sharma will be still be able to practise administering other injections (such as Syntometrine) which are on the midwives' exemptions list under Samantha's direct supervision. This means that by the time she qualifies as a midwife in 3 years, she will feel competent to administer drugs by injection. Sharma is pleased to hear that she will get plenty of practice as giving injections is an area of midwifery practice she feels particularly anxious about!

Midwives' exemptions: the situation for students

The midwifery exemptions list was revised in 2010 (NMC 2010). This implemented changes in relation to the sale, supply and administration of medicine to allow midwives to supply and/or administer an updated range of POM. However, the change in legislation meant that student midwives were unable to achieve their competencies in the administration of medicines included on the exemptions list as the law permitted only qualified practitioners to do this and the responsibility could not be delegated to anyone else. There was some concern and confusion amongst students, educationalists and midwives about these issues. The NMC discussed the matter with the Medicine and Healthcare products Regulatory Authority (MHRA) to try to seek a solution to this dilemma which affected student midwives' ability to develop their competence in certain aspects of drug administration.

Another NMC circular in July 2011 (NMC 2011) led to further changes to midwives' exemptions, meaning that student midwives can now administer medicines contained on the exemptions list under the direct supervision of a 'sign off' mentor. This means that they have received specific mentor training and are qualified to assess ('sign off') students' competencies in practice. Direct supervision means that the midwife and student work alongside each other with the mentor actively watching the student undertake the preparation and administration of the drug.

However, while students may be involved in the preparation and checking of controlled drugs included on the midwives' exemptions list, under current legislation they are not able to actually administer them. This must still be done by a qualified midwife who cannot delegate this task.

Midwifery wisdom

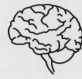

Students must never administer/supply medicinal products without direct supervision.

The *British National Formulary*

The *British National Formulary* (BNF) is a joint publication of the British Medical Association and the Royal Pharmaceutical Society of Great Britain. It is published twice a year under the authority of a Joint Formulary Committee which comprises representatives of the two professional bodies and of the UK health departments. The BNF aims to provide all healthcare professionals with sound, up-to-date information about the use of medicines. It includes key information on the selection, prescribing, dispensing and administration of medicines. Medicines generally prescribed in the UK are covered and those considered less suitable for prescribing are clearly identified. It is available in hard copy or electronically (www.bnf.org).

Administering medication

Principles

The midwife should ask herself the following questions before administering any medication to the women or babies in her care. These form the basic principles for the safe administration of medicines and are recommended by the NMC (NMC 2007).

- Are you familiar with the drug? For example, do you know how it works, the normal dosage, any potential side-effects or possible reason why it should not be given to this particular woman (contraindications)?
- Are you aware of the woman's plan of care and do you know that there is actually a need for her to receive the medication?
- Has all the relevant information about the medication been given to the woman and has she made an informed decision to have the drug?
- Have you confirmed the identity of the woman to ensure that the correct drug is given to the correct client? In maternity care, most women are conscious and are able to confirm who they are, but if the woman is unconscious, then her identity will need to be confirmed by checking the name and hospital number on her identity band.
- Does the woman have any known allergies?
- If appropriate, is the prescription chart clearly written and unambiguous?
- Does the prescription chart include the correct name of the drug, how it is to be administered (for example, orally or by injection into the muscle or vein), the amount to be given, how frequently it is to be given, when treatment started and the date when it should be completed?
- Has the medication reached its expiry date and is therefore unsuitable to use?

Checking of drugs

In order to reduce the number of drug errors, the NMC (2007) considers that it is unacceptable for a drug to be prepared before it is needed. An example of this in midwifery practice would be when a midwife draws up an injection of Syntometrine or Syntocinon into a syringe and leaves it by the bedside of the woman in labour ready for the third stage. If labour does not proceed as expected and there is a delay, then there is the potential for this drug to be given in error during rather than following labour. If an oxytocic drug such as Syntometrine is given during labour, this would lead to the potentially disastrous situation of the uterus undergoing a strong, sustained contraction with the fetus still inside.

With the same principle in mind, a midwife should not administer a drug which has been prepared by a colleague unless she was present while it was being prepared and is satisfied with the checking procedure (NMC 2007). An exception to this is when a woman already has an intravenous infusion in place which was prepared by a midwife and another midwife then takes over her care.

Controlled drugs

Certain POM are further classified as controlled drugs. Examples that a midwife might use in her professional practice are pethidine, diamorphine, morphine and pentazocine. In some cases, these medicines may be misused or sold illegally, so for this reason there are stricter legal controls on their supply – hence the term 'controlled drugs'.

There are controls on:

- who may prescribe these medicines
- how the prescription is written
- how much may be prescribed
- how the medicines are stored.

However, a registered midwife is able to administer certain controlled drugs on her own responsibility without a prescription from a medical practitioner under midwives' exemptions. Remember, a student

203

may be involved in the preparation and checking of a controlled drug with her midwife mentor but is not permitted to actual administer it to the client.

Misuse of Drugs Act 1971

This Act prevents the possession, supply and manufacture of medicinal and other products, except where this has been made legal by the Misuse of Drugs Regulations 1985. This was amended by the Misuse of Drugs Regulations 2001.

These regulations further divide the controlled drugs into five categories or schedules. The schedules are as follows:

- **Schedule 1**: drugs which may be used illegally and for social enjoyment such as drugs which stimulate hallucinations and a sense of euphoria. These drugs currently have no recognised medicinal uses. They include cannabis, coca leaf, LSD (lysergic acid diethylamide – 'acid') and mescaline. Only individuals with a Home Office licence may legally possess schedule 1 drugs for use in medical research.
- **Schedule 2**: drugs which may become addictive, for example, pethidine, diamorphine and morphine.
- **Schedule 3**: some barbiturates and pentazocine.
- **Schedule 4**: the benzodiazepine tranquillisers, for example, diazepam, nitrazepam and temazepam. Midwives may administer these drugs to help women sleep or relax during pregnancy or following childbirth.
- **Schedule 5**: medicines which may contain a small amount of a controlled drug, for example, certain pain-relieving drugs and cough mixtures.

Issues in the handling of controlled drugs

Supply

Community midwives or independent midwives may sometimes want to obtain a supply of a controlled drug such as pethidine for use at a homebirth. Legislation surrounding this is in accordance with the Prescription Only Medicine (Human Use) Order 1997. The midwife will need to obtain a Midwives Supply Order form from a supervisor of midwives (SOM). This order must be in writing, including the full name and occupation of the individual requesting the drug; it must state the purpose for which the drug is intended and include the total quantity of the drug to be obtained. As well as these details, it might be helpful for audit purposes for the midwife's NMC personal identification number (PIN) to be included as well as the contact details of the SOM and the name of the woman for whom the drug is to be administered.

The controlled drug is then supplied to the midwife by a pharmacist for use in her own professional practice only. In other words, it cannot be given to another midwife or healthcare practitioner to administer (NMC 2005a). The pharmacist should have a prior agreement with the midwife to supply the drug and should have a record of the midwife's signature.

On providing the drug, the name and amount of the drug supplied and name and address of the supplier should be recorded in the midwife's drugs book. This should also contain information about the dates the drug was given, the woman's name and the amount used.

The procedure as described above is intended for use by community-based midwives or independent midwives attending homebirths. Midwives working in NHS hospitals need to comply with local policies and procedures when administering controlled drugs, although it may be decided that they will follow the same procedures as community-based midwives (RCM 2010). In some NHS trusts, a standing order (see p.207) may be signed by a consultant obstetrician and the head of midwifery authorising the administration of controlled drugs by midwives based in the hospital.

For a homebirth, rather than the midwife obtaining a supply of controlled drugs, the woman may obtain a prescription for pethidine from her general practitioner. In this case, the drugs are owned by the woman and she becomes responsible for the destruction or return of any unwanted ampoules.

Storage of controlled drugs

Controlled drugs on schedules 1 and 2 must be kept in a locked cupboard within another non-moveable locked cupboard. Drugs on schedules 3, 4 and 5 do not need to be kept in the controlled drugs cupboard (i.e. double-locked), but should still be locked away.

Administration of a controlled drug

Two people, one of whom is a registered midwife or nurse, are required to check the drug, observe it being given and then sign the controlled drug register.

The recommended procedure is as follows:

- Confirm that the stock of the drug in the cupboard tallies with the drug register total.
- Record the woman's name, amount of drug to be given, date of administration and amount of stock remaining in the drug register.
- Check the name, amount and expiry date of the drug.
- Draw up the drug if being given by injection and take to the woman.
- Confirm her identity by checking her name band or asking her name and date of birth.
- Give the drug in the appropriate way and dispose of all equipment.
- Sign the drug register, including the time that the drug was actually administered.
- Record the name of drug, amount, route, time and date of administration in the appropriate documentation – for example, the prescription sheet and the woman's notes.

Destruction of unused controlled drugs

If a midwife has obtained a supply of controlled drugs which are no longer needed then she must destroy them, but only in the presence of an authorised person. This procedure is stipulated in the Misuse of Drugs Regulations 1985. An authorised person varies slightly throughout the UK but includes the following:

- A supervisor of midwives
- A regional pharmaceutical officer (England)
- A pharmaceutical officer of the Welsh Office
- A chief administrative pharmaceutical officer of the Health Boards (Scotland)
- An inspector appointed by the Department of Health and Social Services (Northern Ireland)
- Medical officers (England, Scotland, Wales)
- An inspector of the Royal Pharmaceutical Society of Great Britain
- A police officer
- An inspector of the Home Office drugs branch

A midwife is also permitted to take any unused controlled drugs back to the pharmacist who originally supplied them or to an appropriate medical officer but not to a supervisor of midwives.

If a woman has obtained her own prescription for pethidine, then by law these drugs are her property and she is responsible for destroying any which are not used. She should be advised to destroy the unused drugs, preferably with the midwife in attendance. Alternatively, they can be returned to the pharmacist but this must be done by the woman and not by the midwife acting on her behalf.

Activity 11.1

 Familiarise yourself with the procedures surrounding the supply, storage and administration of controlled drugs within your own maternity unit.

Patient group directions

Patient group directions (PGDs) are documents which make it legal for medicines to be given to groups of patients without individual prescriptions having to be written for each person (NMC 2007). They are useful for providing treatment for a clearly defined condition where there is a proven advantage for care without compromising the patient's safety. PGDs are drawn up locally by doctors, dentists, pharmacists and other healthcare professionals. They must be signed by a doctor and a pharmacist, both of whom should have been involved in developing the direction, and must be approved by the appropriate healthcare body.

If a medicine to be supplied or administered is on the midwives' exemption list, no PGD is needed. To date, none of the midwives' exemptions contained within the medicines legislation has been replaced by the PGD legislation and there is no legal need to change existing locally agreed policies into PGDs (NMC 2005b).

In midwifery practice, a PGD might be an appropriate option to consider if a group of women require on a regular basis a prescription-only drug which does not appear on the midwives' exemption list (NMC 2005b).

Unlicensed medicines

An unlicensed medicine is a medicine that has no marketing authorisation in place. This means that if an unlicensed medicine is given to a woman, the manufacturer may not have liability for any harm that may befall her as a result of taking the drug. It is the person who prescribes and dispenses that drug who assumes liability.

As a result of this, while doctors are free to prescribe drugs without an appropriate UK licence, they do so on their own responsibility and must accept full liability. However, the regulations state that a medicine can only be included in a PGD if it has a current UK marketing authorisation or a homeopathic certificate of registration (NMC 2005b). In addition, drugs usually have a UK product licence stating how they are to be used. Unlicensed medicines can be administered against a patient-specific direction but the patient's informed consent must be obtained so that it is clear that they are aware that they are taking an unlicensed product.

In certain exceptional circumstances, drugs with a marketing authorisation can be used outside the terms of their product licence (that means administered via a different route from that stated in the terms of the licence). In these cases, any PGD must clearly state that the drug is being used outside the terms of its licence with the reasons why this is necessary.

An example of this in midwifery practice is Syntocinon. This drug is on the midwives' exemption list and so does not legally need a PGD. It is usually administered via the intravenous route to increase uterine contractions during the first and second stages of labour.

However, it is not currently licensed in the UK for *intramuscular use* during the third stage of labour. Intramuscular Syntometrine is the oxytocic drug which has been used in the third stage of labour for the past 40 years (Rogers et al. 2011). The National Institute for Health Clinical Evidence (NICE) Intrapartumn Care guidelines, published in 2007, are based on the best available evidence and recommend the use of intramuscular Syntocinon rather than Syntometrine for the management of the active third stage of labour as it is considered more effective at preventing postpartum bleeding and also causes fewer side-effects (NICE 2007). Many maternity units are now changing practices to follow this recommendation (Rogers et al. 2011). In which case Syntocinon 10 iu could be considered for a PGD so that midwives are able to administer it intramuscularly without needing a prescription from a doctor.

Patient-specific directions

A patient-specific direction (PSD) can be used once a patient has been assessed by the prescriber, who then asks another healthcare professional to give a drug to the patient. A PSD is a form of prescription and can be for a single dose or a course of drugs to be given over several days. The PSD can be a written request in the medical notes or on the patient's drug chart (RCM 2010).

Standing orders or locally agreed policies

The use of standing orders for hospital-based midwives began in 1972. The Aitken Report (1958) had recommended that midwives working in hospitals be subject to the same regulations for the administration of medicines and controlled drugs as nurses. This suggestion was made in order to ensure safe and secure handling of medicines (RCM 2010), but it meant that all medicines given by a midwife would need to be prescribed by a doctor before they could be administered. This created many difficulties for midwives and led to unacceptable delays in treatment as women were forced to wait for their pain relief and oxytocic drugs to control bleeding during the third stage of labour.

In response, the (then) Department of Health and Social Security permitted doctors to authorise standing orders for the range of drugs used by midwives. Following this, the use of standing orders became widespread in maternity units (RCM 2010). The term 'standing order' may still be used in NHS trusts and may be used to refer to local guidelines for the administration of medicines. However, it should be noted that this term does not legally exist and there is no requirement in law to use standing orders for those medicines which midwives' exemptions legislation permits them to supply and administer anyway.

The NMC (2007) recommended that where midwives still use standing orders for medicines which are not covered by midwifery exemptions, processes are put in place to convert these to PGDs instead.

Activity 11.2

 Find out whether there are any standing orders and/or PGDs in your maternity unit. Which healthcare professionals have been involved in producing them? Are steps being taken to convert standing orders to PGDs as recommended by the NMC (2007)?

Teratogenic drugs

Any drug taken during pregnancy will cross the placenta and may affect the growth and development of the fetus. For this reason, any drug administered during pregnancy must offer benefits to the woman which outweigh the risk to the baby. Drugs which may have a potentially adverse effect on the fetus resulting in malformation or death are called teratogens. This is more of an issue during the early part of pregnancy when the baby's organs are developing. Much of the fetal development occurs before the woman even knows that she is pregnant. Thalidomide has already been mentioned, but there are many others. Women with known medical conditions such as epilepsy and depression have difficult decisions to make.

For example, women taking the antidepressant paroxetine have been warned to avoid taking it in the early part of pregnancy due to the association of heart defects in babies born to women who have taken the drug (MHRA 2013).

Drugs and breastfeeding

If a breastfeeding woman takes any drug, then there is a potential risk that the substance may enter the baby's bloodstream via the breastmilk and possibly cause an adverse reaction. For example, the antidepressant amfebutamone has been shown to cause seizures in babies (Chaudron & Schoenecker 2004). As highlighted in the previous section, the risk of taking any drug needs to be weighed against the benefit to the mother.

The age of the baby is an important factor in deciding what the risk of an adverse reaction is. For example, a premature baby whose kidneys and liver are not fully mature may not be able to detoxify the drug effectively and toxic levels may accumulate in the baby's body and cause an adverse reaction. On the other hand, an older baby who is being weaned onto solid food will be taking less breastmilk and as a consequence will not be exposed to such high levels of the ingested drug.

If the woman is given a drug by injection which is destroyed in the gut (for example, insulin and heparin), this will not pass into the baby's circulation and so is safe to take while breastfeeding.

Certain drugs affect lactation by reducing milk production. For example, oral contraceptives containing oestrogen (the combined pill) have this effect.

Routes of administration

Midwives should be competent to administer medication by a variety of routes.

Oral

Medication taken by mouth (orally) will be absorbed via the gastrointestinal tract. In order for a woman or baby to take a drug orally, they must be willing to take the medication, alert and capable of swallowing (Johnson & Taylor 2010). As oral medications can be affected by other constituents in the stomach, it is important that the manufacturer's instructions are followed and the drug taken as directed – for example, before, during or after eating.

Oral medications can be available in several different preparations:

- *Tablets*: usually should be swallowed whole. If scored, they can be cut in half using a tablet cutter. Some tablets are coated with an outer layer to protect the stomach lining or to make them easier to swallow. If they are bitten and chewed, this effect is lost.
- *Capsules*: these should also be swallowed whole and not chewed.

- *Granules and powders*: these should be dissolved thoroughly (usually in water) before being given. Certain drugs such as paracetamol are available in soluble form for women who have difficulty swallowing tablets.
- *Elixir*: certain drugs are also available in liquid form. The midwife should ensure that she shakes the bottle several times before measuring out the required amount to ensure thorough mixing of the drug. If giving a drug in liquid form to a baby, then the required amount should be drawn up into a sterile syringe and inserted into the baby's mouth, usually towards the cheek (Johnson & Taylor 2010). Some hospitals now use special oral syringes in order to administer liquid medication to babies. These look very similar to ordinary syringes but with the markings appearing in blue rather than black. They also come with a hub, which prevents any of the medication leaking out of the sides.
- *Lozenges*: these should be sucked rather than swallowed. They are usually used to treat conditions in the mouth such as a fungal infection.
- *Sublingual medication*: these are absorbed under the tongue.

Injection

Drugs are given by injection if they cannot be absorbed or are absorbed too slowly when given orally. Drugs given by injection are given parenterally – that is, they are taken into the body in a manner other than through the digestive tract, by intravenous or intramuscular injection.

Intramuscular (IM) injection

The drug is given straight into a muscle. The midwife needs to have a good knowledge of anatomy when choosing the best site to give an IM injection to make sure that she avoids nerves, bone and blood vessels.

Popular sites for an IM injection include the deltoid muscle (upper, outer part of the arm), the quadriceps muscle (upper, outer part of the leg) and the gluteus maximus muscle (the upper, outer quarter of the buttock).

Subcutaneous (SC) injection

This injection is given into the area beneath the skin containing connective tissue and fat. As these tissues have a reduced blood supply, absorption is slower. Examples of drugs given by SC injection are insulin and heparin.

Intradermal injection

This injection is given just below the skin and is often used to administer local anaesthetic (lidocaine) prior to repair of the perineum following childbirth.

Intravenous (IV) injection

Drugs given straight into the bloodstream via a vein work very quickly. This is advantageous if a quick effect is needed but not so good if the woman reacts badly to the drug or has an allergic reaction to it. Drugs can be given intravenously as a bolus or IV 'push' injection, as an intermittent infusion (via a drip) or via a syringe driver (equipment which pushes a measured dose into the vein over a set period of time). Sometimes, women can control the amount of drug given via the syringe driver at the push of a button. This is known as patient-controlled analgesia (PCA) and is used in some maternity units so that women can control their postoperative pain relief following a caesarean section.

The midwife must be fully trained and informed in all aspects of IV drug administration. In some areas it is considered an extended role of the midwife and extra training is required following initial registration as a midwife. Regular updating may also be required in order to maintain competence (Johnson & Taylor 2010). However, all midwives are able to give IV ergometrine maleate for the treatment of postpartum haemorrhage (severe bleeding following childbirth) in an emergency. This is in accordance with Rule 5 of the *Midwives' Rules and Standards* (NMC 2012), which states that only in an emergency situation can a midwife provide care which she has not been trained to give.

Complementary and alternative therapies

Complementary and alternative medicine can be defined as any type of healthcare which does not form part of the traditional, mainstream medical approach (Tiran 2011). Women are increasingly turning to natural remedies (homeopathy, aromatherapy and acupuncture amongst others) to help them cope with the discomforts associated with pregnancy, childbirth and the postnatal period as they are reluctant to use pharmacological preparations which may have adverse side-effects for themselves or the baby (Tiran 2011).

A midwife who wishes to use alternative therapies during the course of her midwifery practice must have successfully completed the required training and have been judged competent in its use (NMC 2012).

Midwives who are not fully qualified complementary therapists can use aspects of the treatment as long as they have received training in its correct usage (Tiran 2011). For example, there are a few essential oils specifically recommended for labour which a midwife may use without being a fully qualified aromatherapist as long as she has received the appropriate training. Essential oils such as clary sage, lavender and jasmine can be massaged into the abdomen, used as a room spray or put into a warm bath (Tiran 2011).

However, it is very important that midwives who wish to use such treatments are fully versed in their correct usage to avoid potential problems and incomplete advice. For example, it has been found that some midwives give insufficient information to women about the use of raspberry leaf tea during labour to enhance the contractions and others are unable to explain how cabbage leaves work to reduce breast engorgement (Tiran 2011).

If a woman wants to use natural remedies during childbirth and the midwife believes that the substances chosen might be detrimental to the woman or her baby or interfere with traditional treatment which has already been given, then the midwife must discuss this with the woman. In accordance with the NMC *Code* (2008), however, the midwife must respect the rights of the woman to make her own decisions in relation to her care. All the midwife can do in these circumstances is to ensure as far as she can that the woman's decisions are informed.

Drug errors

Case study 11.2

Alice is a newly qualified midwife working on a postnatal ward. She has just realised that by mistake she has given an antibiotic to one of the women in her care instead of the pain relief the woman had requested. The woman seems fine and is unaware of the error.

For a split second Alice wonders about not saying anything as she is sure that no harm will be caused to the woman by this error. However, she also remembers her NMC *Code* and *Midwives' Rules* which clearly state that as a professional, she must act in the woman's best interests.

Tearfully Alice reports her error to the ward manager. The manager calls the doctor to inform her of the drug error and she agrees to attend the ward to examine the woman concerned. Meanwhile, the manager accompanies Alice as she explains to the woman that a mistake has been made.

The woman listens to Alice but is not overly concerned. She has had antibiotics many times and has never had a reaction. She is more anxious that she receives her pain relief as she still has severe after-pains. She is breastfeeding but is reassured that the single dose of antibiotic she has received should not adversely affect her baby and there is no need to stop feeding. She is warned, though, that occasionally breastfed babies whose mothers take antibiotics might experience loose stools.

The doctor arrives and also speaks to the mother. The ward manager and Alice make entries in the mother's medical records to show that an incident has occurred. An incident form is also completed. Alice then contacts the supervisor of midwives (SOM) on call that day and talks the incident through with her. The SOM agrees that the best course of action has been taken. She recommends to Alice that she meets her named SOM to reflect on the incident and to discuss strategies that may prevent a future mistake for Alice and all other midwives working on the ward. As this is Alice's first drug error and as she reported her mistake straight away, no further action is taken.

Alice is very shaken by the incident and in future is meticulous about checking all medicines with another practitioner as she knows this is best practice. She is a good role model for student midwives too as she undertakes the checking procedure so methodically. She also makes sure she discusses with the women in her care what medication they are going to receive so that they can work in partnership with her to prevent future drug errors.

In the event that the wrong drug or wrong dosage of drug is given to a woman or baby, it is essential that this is reported to the senior midwifery staff and a doctor as soon as it has been recognised so that appropriate action can be taken to rectify the situation and hopefully cause less harm to the woman. For example, in the scenario cited above, the woman might be allergic to the antibiotic administered, in which case she may require urgent treatment.

Following an audit of the administration of postoperative pain relief and heparin in a maternity unit, Birch & Culshaw (2003) suggested that drug errors in obstetrics are a common and hidden phenomenon and that multiprofessional working is needed to ensure that safe working practices are put in place to reduce the numbers of errors.

In the event of any kind of drug error occurring, a careful local investigation is required to look in detail at what occurred and why. Often drug errors are due to deficiencies in process, such as commonly mistaken drugs being stored together or midwives undertaking a particularly heavy workload at any particular time.

A multidisciplinary approach is recommended so that teams of healthcare professionals, including midwives, doctors and pharmacists, can work together to ensure that potential improvements in the administration of medicines are fully discussed and disseminated within the team (NMC 2012).

Conclusion

This chapter has demonstrated how important it is for midwives to have sound knowledge of legislation related to medicines, the various routes of administration and the checking procedures. A multidisciplinary approach between midwives, doctors and pharmacists is recommended to ensure that safe and effective policies are put in place in terms of the prescribing, dispensing and administration of drugs. The role of the midwife also involves ensuring that women in her care are aware of risks and benefits associated with taking medicines during pregnancy and labour so that they can make informed choices about their treatment. If there is any doubt about the safety or suitability of a medicine, then the midwife should refer to another healthcare professional such as a pharmacist, who will have more detailed expert knowledge about the potential effect of the particular medicine.

Fundamental to the issue is the midwife following the *Midwives' Rules and Standards* (NMC 2012), which clearly state that she shall only use those medicines in her practice for which she has received appropriate training and is familiar with the dosage and method of administration.

The fact that the midwife is able to supply and administer a number of medicines on her own responsibility, through the use of midwives' exemptions, highlights her unique role as an autonomous practitioner able to provide a first-class, woman-centred service.

Quiz

Please answer 'true' or 'false' to the following questions to test your knowledge.

1. A student midwife can administer pethidine under the direct supervision of a qualified midwife.
2. The term' standing orders' is not a legal definition.
3. A prescription chart is required before any drug is administered.
4. Two midwives should always check a drug before it is administered to a client.
5. *Standards for Medicines Management* (2007) is the latest NMC document relating to the administration of drugs.
6. Midwives' exemptions are drugs which can only be administered by a midwife.
7. 'Direct supervision' of a student midwife implies that a student and her mentor check a drug together and then the student goes onto the ward to give the drug to the client.
8. A midwife should always countersign the prescription chart and/or medical records when a student midwife has administered a drug.
9. A woman does not need to be informed if a drug is given to her in error.
10. A subcutaneous (SC) injection is given straight into the muscle.

References

Aitkin Report, Standing Advisory Committee, Joint Sub-committee Ministry of Health (1958) *Control of Dangerous Drugs and Poisons in Hospitals*. London: HMSO.

Birch L, Culshaw A (2003) Drug error in maternity care: a multi-professional issue. *British Journal of Midwifery* **11**(3): 173–178.

British National Forumulary (BNF) (2004) *British National Formulary Extra: News 6. BNF response to new study on medication use during pregnancy*. London: British Medical Association and the Royal Pharmaceutical Society.

Chaudron LH, Schoenecker CJ (2004) Bupropion and breast feeding: a case of a possible infant seizure (letter). *Journal of Clinical Psychiatry* **65**(6): 881–882.

Headley J, Northstone K, Simmons H, Golding L (2004) Medication use during pregnancy: data from the Avon longitudinal study of parents and children. *European Journal of Clinical Pharmacology* **60**: 355–361.

Johnson R, Taylor W (2010) *Skills for Midwifery Practice*, 3rd edn. Edinburgh: Churchill Livingstone.

Medicinal Products Prescription by Nurses Act (1992) London: HMSO.

Medicines Act (1968) London: HMSO.

Medicines and Healthcare products Regulatory Agency (MHRA) (2013) *Update on Risks of Birth Defects in Babies Born to Mothers Taking Paroxetine*. www.mhra.gov.uk/home/groups/pl-p/documents/websiteresources/con2022700.pdf (accessed May 2013).

Misuse of Drugs Act (1971) London: HMSO.

National Institute for Health and Clinical Excellence (NICE) (2007) *Intrapartum.*
Care: care of healthy women and their babies during childbirth. Clinical Guideline No. 55. London: National Institute for Health and Clinical Excellence.

Nursing and Midwifery Council (NMC) (2005a) *Midwives Supply Orders.* Circular 25/2005. London: Nursing and Midwifery Council.

Nursing and Midwifery Council (NMC) (2005b) *Medicines Legislation: what it means for midwives.* Available at: www.nmcuk.org/Documents/Circulars/2005circulars/NMC%20circular%2001_2005.pdf (accessed May 2013).

Nursing and Midwifery Council (NMC) (2007) *Standards for Medicine Management.* Available at: www.nmc-uk.org/Documents/NMC-Publications/NMC-Standards-for-medicines-management.pdf (accessed May 2013).

Nursing and Midwifery Council (NMC) (2008) *The Code: standards, conduct, performance and ethics for nurse and midwives.* London: Nursing and Midwifery Council.

Nursing and Midwifery Council (NMC) (2010) *Changes to Midwives Exemptions.* NMC Circular 06/2010. Available at: www.nmc-uk.org/Documents/Circulars/2010circulars/NMCcircular06_2010.pdf (accessed May 2013).

Nursing and Midwifery Council (NMC) (2011) *Changes to Midwives' Exemptions.* NMC Circular 07/2011. Available at: www.nmcuk.org/Documents/Circulars/2011Circulars/nmcCircular07-2011-Midwives-Exemptions.pdf (accessed May 2013).

Nursing and Midwifery Council (NMC) (2012) *Midwives' Rules and Standards.* London: Nursing and Midwifery Council.

Prescriptions Only Medicines (Human Use) Order 1997 (IS 1997/1830 Schedule 5) London: HMSO.

Rogers C, Villar R, Pischal P, Yearley C (2011) Effects of syntocinon use in active management of the third stage of labour. *British Journal of Midwifery* **19**: 371–378.

Royal College of Midwives (RCM) (2010) *Midwife and Medicine Legislation A6: an information paper.* London: Royal College of Midwives.

Tiran D (2011) Complementary therapies in maternity care: responsibilities of midwives. In: Macdonald S, Magill-Cuerden J (eds) *Mayes Midwifery,* 14th edn. London: BaillièreTindall.

12

The Midwife and Public Health
Carmel Bagness and Patricia Lindsay

Aim

To provide an overview of the midwife's role within the national public health agenda, and to relate this to wider global public health concerns.

Learning outcomes

By the end of this chapter you will be able to:

1. state what public health is
2. describe the public health role of the midwife in the UK
3. list some influences on the health of populations
4. discuss at least six public health issues of concern to midwives
5. describe the Millennium Development Goals.

Introduction

Pregnancy is a natural phenomenon and is very much influenced by the wider social context in which the mother, baby and family live. Midwives are uniquely placed to influence the health and well-being of women during their childbearing experience and as such, all midwives have a role in understanding the importance of preventing illness and disease, whilst promoting health and well-being by providing high-quality evidence-based care. Women and babies should be as well, if not fitter and healthier, after pregnancy and birth as they were before.

Although geopolitically, the UK is regarded as a single entity, healthcare systems and management vary across the four countries, and where possible the authors have made such distinctions.

Public health has been defined as being 'about helping people to stay healthy and avoid getting ill' (DH 2012a). This includes specific areas such as nutrition, recreational substance use (licit and illicit), sexual

The Student's Guide to Becoming a Midwife, Second Edition. Edited by Ian Peate and Cathy Hamilton.
© 2014 John Wiley & Sons, Ltd. Published 2014 by John Wiley & Sons, Ltd.

health, pregnancy, immunisation and children's health. The main concerns of public health are twofold: the health of populations and the health of individuals or groups within a population. Population health needs are embraced within overarching measures such as food and water safety, road safety and the provision of free at point of care health services. These are applied to the whole population, with standards often enshrined in legislation, and monitored through non-departmental public bodies such as the Environment Agency or the Care Quality Commission (CQC) in England.

Much public health activity in the UK is derived from government, and the drivers are both political and economic, as the burden of disease is costly to a nation in which the state subsidises health and social care. A new structure, Public Health England, introduced in April 2013, has the remit to protect public health by delivering on the objectives of the Public Health Outcomes Framework (DH 2011a, 2012b). The Health & Social Care Act 2012 is the legislation responsible for this; at national level, Public Health England will be the executive agency responsible for delivering the wider agenda, whilst at local level, the move of public health services into local authorities is planned to create a multiprofessional approach to delivering local strategies to support better healthcare for the population.

Epidemiology is a further useful concept for the midwife to understand. The World Health Organization (WHO 2012a) defines it as 'the study of the distribution and determinants of health-related states or events'. It focuses on understanding health risks and the spread of disease within and beyond specific populations. The Health Protection Agency (HPA), an independent body, undertakes health surveillance on behalf of the government in England, and its main concern is communicable diseases, where the HPA gathers data on the incidence of a range of infections such as gastrointestinal, healthcare-associated (including methicillin-resistant *Staphylococcus aureus*, MRSA) and blood-borne diseases such as HIV. The HPA monitors the incidence of vaccine-preventable infections such as measles and whooping cough. It also gathers data on environmental problems such as chemical hazards and poisons. The HPA has now become part of Public Health England.

In England, under the Health Protection (Notification) Regulations 2010, some diseases such as tuberculosis (TB) and measles have to be notified to local authority proper officers (HPA 2012a). Public Health Wales, Health Protection Scotland and Health & Social Care Northern Ireland have very similar arrangements for notifying diseases which present a particular risk. This information is used to alert authorities to the risk of disease outbreaks which threaten public health and may demand a rapid response, and to monitor trends in communicable diseases. The list changes from time to time; for example, from 2010 ophthalmia neonatorum is no longer a notifiable disease (HPA 2012a).

Midwifery wisdom

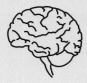

The midwife should regularly update her knowledge about notifiable diseases and their status in order to protect her patients and the public.

New initiatives are introduced as evidence becomes available. For example, an increase in whooping cough (1230 cases reported up to August 2012 in England and Wales, which included nine deaths, compared to only 910 cases during the whole of 2011 (HPA 2012b) prompted the DH (DH 2012c) to initiate a short-term immunisation programme to reduce the spread of whooping cough, commencing in October 2012. This is administered during the third trimester of pregnancy to boost the short-term immunity passed on by pregnant women to protect their newborn, who normally cannot be vaccinated until they are 2 months old.

The health of the population is influenced by personal/lifestyle choices and by environmental factors, such as living conditions, type (or absence) of work, diet and exposure to toxins. Midwives working in the

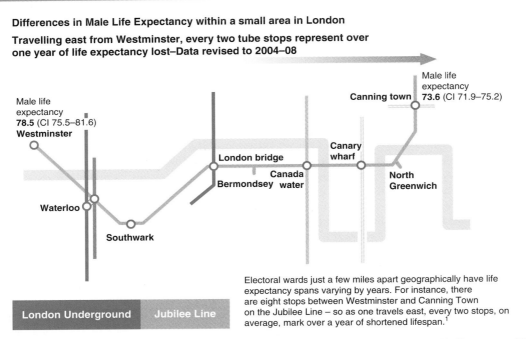

Differences in Male Life Expectancy within a small area in London

Travelling east from Westminster, every two tube stops represent over one year of life expectancy lost–Data revised to 2004–08

Male life expectancy **73.6** (CI 71.9–75.2)

Canning town

Male life expectancy **78.5** (CI 75.5–81.6)
Westminster

Canary wharf

London bridge

Canada water

Bermondsey

North Greenwich

Waterloo

Southwark

London Underground   Jubilee Line

Electoral wards just a few miles apart geographically have life expectancy spans varying by years. For instance, there are eight stops between Westminster and Canning Town on the Jubilee Line – so as one travels east, every two stops, on average, mark over a year of shortened lifespan.[1]

[1]Source: Analysis by London Health Observatory of ONS and GLA data for 2004–08. Diagram produced by Department of Health

Figure 12.1   The Jubilee Line of health inequality.
Source: London Health Observatory (2010), reproduced with permission.

community are aware of inequalities in health and sometimes find that there are areas of affluence, with better health outcomes, close to areas of deprivation.

The London Health Observatory has produced a vivid image illustrating this, where the measure is life expectancy (Figure 12.1). Although the map refers to males, female life expectancy follows a similar trend, with a range of 84.2–80.6 years, travelling east along the same line between the same 'stations' as the male (Ball & Tewdwr-Jones 2012). Health outcomes in urban areas are strongly determined by social and economic inequality, the assertion here being that travelling east from the more affluent areas sees a reduction in the health and well-being of the population. This pattern is not peculiar to London and the same trends may be observed across the UK, with life expectancy generally lower in urban and deprived areas (Kyte & Wells 2010).

Midwifery wisdom

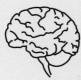

It is important for the midwife to understand how healthcare is structured locally, so having an understanding of the local authority and healthcare systems will be of benefit. This can begin by asking your midwife mentor and visiting websites that outline the systems such as your borough council or county council in England, and searching for Health and Social Care pages. In Scotland, look at National Health Service (NHS) in Scotland and local health boards, for Northern Ireland this will be the Health and Social Care in Northern Ireland (or HSC) and in Wales, NHS Wales will direct you to some useful websites.

Mortality and morbidity

Maternal and neonatal mortality and morbidity are part of the measurement used to assess how well (or not) a health service is performing. Maternal mortality can be defined as the number of deaths during pregnancy or within 42 days after the end of pregnancy, regardless of the gestation. It is usually expressed as the number of deaths per 100,000 maternities. Maternal deaths are classed as direct, that is, resulting directly from complications arising during the pregnancy, labour or puerperium. Examples are deaths from haemorrhage or pre-eclampsia. Indirect deaths result from a pre-existing disorder which has been made worse by the pregnancy, for example cardiac disease. Late deaths are those which occur more than 42 days (but less than 1 year) after the end of the pregnancy, due to direct or indirect causes, and coincidental deaths are deaths from causes not related to pregnancy or birth, but where death happened to occur during the childbearing period (CMACE 2011). Perinatal mortality includes all stillbirths and deaths within the first week of life, per 1000 registered births (Sidebotham & Walsh 2011). Neonatal mortality refers to babies who were born alive but died within 28 days of birth. Infant mortality is the number of deaths occurring within the first year of life. The infant mortality rate in 2010 was 4.2 deaths per 1000 live births, the lowest ever recorded for England and Wales (ONS, 2012). The report also noted that infant mortality rates were high among babies of mothers aged under 20 years and over 40 years. The infant mortality rate in Scotland in 2010 was 3.7 per 1000 births (Scottish Government 2012).

Morbidity refers to injury or illness resulting from pregnancy or birth (House of Commons 2009). In the UK, the overall number of maternal deaths has fallen over the last 3 years (CMACE 2011). However, this period also saw a rise in the number of women dying from infection, particularly community-acquired infections involving β-haemolytic streptococcus Lancefield group A (CMACE 2011).

Midwifery wisdom

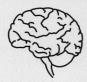

The death of a mother is always a tragedy, and the midwife needs to understand how this can happen and more importantly, how it can be prevented or at least the risks reduced. To read more about the details of maternal mortality across the UK, the detailed publication *Saving Mothers' Lives: reviewing maternal deaths to make motherhood safer: 2006–2008* is available online at http://onlinelibrary.wiley.com/doi/10.1111/j.1471-0528.2010.02847.x/abstract

Public health and provision for maternity services

The provision for maternity services should include high-quality midwifery services, which have a well-educated workforce, who understand the principles of the public health agenda and how it can impact on the health and well-being of individual women and their families. Midwives in the UK have been an all-graduate profession since 2008, with clearly defined standards for that education set by the Nursing and Midwifery Council (NMC 2009). In the UK, midwifery is regulated by the NMC which sets standards for high-quality care developed to safeguard the health and well-being of the public. This includes a focus on all aspects of public health relating to pregnancy and childbearing women, including sexual and reproductive health services. The engagement of midwives needs to be collaborative in nature, working across the health and social care sectors, as well as being able to provide continuity of care for the family throughout pregnancy, birth and beyond.

Public health focuses on enabling everyone to take responsibility for their own health, preventing disease and supporting the whole population towards understanding the benefits of a healthy lifestyle. The role of the midwife in this key process acknowledges that midwives see women at a critical period in their lives, at a time when they are focusing on their own health and that of the unborn child. This provides a window of opportunity to educate and inform on the benefits of a healthy life style, at a time when the broader public health goals and aspirations can be integrated into existing midwifery practice.

In 2010, an independent report by Sir Michael Marmot reviewed the heath inequalities across England and concluded that inequalities in heath were derived from social inequalities (Marmot 2010). The report suggested that health outcomes could be significantly improved by fairer distribution of health and social life opportunities, particularly for women and children. One of the key focuses on this was giving every child the best start in life.

From a midwifery perspective, this called on midwives to focus more on the public health elements of their role. In 2010, the *Midwifery 2020* report, a four-country Chief Nursing Officer-commissioned report looking at the direction of midwifery services and roles across the UK for the next decade, devoted an entire section to the public health role of the midwife. The vision of the Public Health workstream of the report was that midwifery could contribute to a lifetime impact on health: 'a healthier society right from the start, beginning with excellent midwifery care' (DH 2010, p3).

Midwifery wisdom

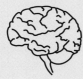

It is worth considering your personal views on public health, and how that might impact on advice you give to women. Have you thought about how your views might influence the conversations you have with pregnant women?

The report described two distinct roles for midwives: all midwives have a role in prevention of ill health and promotion of better lifestyles, whilst some midwives may specialise in the detailed area of public health, including having a strategic role both locally and nationally. The report acknowledged that in order to achieve improved population health, the following components were essential:

- midwives as first point of professional contact
- knowledgeable, confident and skilled midwives
- compassionate and emotionally literate midwives
- equality and diversity aware midwives
- respect for midwifery expertise within teams.

Midwives, working collaboratively across the local community, can identify resources and other health and social care professionals who can effectively contribute to a care pathway that is both individualised and holistic, with outcomes focused on a healthier life for mother, baby and family. Midwives, in their unique role, have opportunities to enhance health and well-being through focused parent education and effective antenatal, labour and postnatal care. Many maternity units have midwives who are specialists in smoking cessation, identifying and managing violence against women, reproductive health and family planning. These people will act as a resource for all midwives, as well as being the main contributor to the local public health agenda for both individual women (their families) and the wider population.

The planning of midwifery care and the contribution of midwifery expertise to the development of local health strategies are a key component of enhancing local health outcomes. Continuing professional development means that midwives need to constantly maintain and enhance the skills and knowledge required to engage with local government on public health briefings, as well as understanding local population challenges and needs. Successful commissioning of maternity services is also critical in ensuring that the right service is provided for the right population in a timely and productive manner, whilst being cost-effective. Being aware of local trends, national statistics and strategies around infectious diseases, obesity, smoking, alcohol and drug misuse is essential knowledge for the practising midwife in implementing effective care. An example would be the midwife engaging with organisations such as the National Institute for Health and Clinical Excellence (NICE) which has launched public health briefings for local government, to help local management of major health issues in communities across the UK (NICE 2012).

Midwifery wisdom

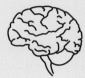

All midwives must keep their knowledge up to date to meet the requirements of the regulator, the NMC, through a process of post-registration education and practice (PREP) (NMC 2011), and also to maintain professional competence. Make a note to check the internet sites of bodies such as NICE and the DH regularly. Sign up for alerts, newsletters or updates where possible; for example with the Royal College of Midwives, the Royal College of Nursing, the *Health Service Journal*, MIDIRS or the NHS Institute for Innovation and Improvement.

Specific public health issues of importance to midwifery

The role of the midwife has included public health issues from the earliest days of the profession. Initially these were confined to the reduction of maternal mortality, the management of transmissible disease, such as TB or syphilis, in childbearing women and the promotion of safe infant feeding practices (Berkeley 1922, Clendening 1942, Loudon 1992, Truby King 1945). This remit has expanded to cover many more areas, some of which are mentioned below.

It may seem that in some cases, much of the midwife's work is attempting to achieve a satisfactory outcome from an unsatisfactory situation, for example, where a woman enters pregnancy in relatively poor health because of diet or lifestyle. However, it is better to prevent or ameliorate the causes of poor health rather than manage the consequences later on (RCN 2012). This is why supporting women to eat healthily and to breastfeed is so important, as this gives the infant a good foundation for better health in later childhood. It is also important that midwives remember that some health practices have different interpretations in other cultures. For example, bed sharing with a newborn infant is part of normal childrearing practice in many cultures around the world, although not necessarily in the UK. Similarly, female genital mutilation (FGM) (female genital cutting/female circumcision) is practised in some cultures but is illegal in the UK.

Some areas of public health are very clearly the responsibility of the midwife. These are usually issues which impinge on the health and well-being of either the mother or the fetus, or both, and which can influence health outcomes. Some of these are briefly discussed here.

Infant feeding

Infant feeding is a key public health concern because the way a baby is fed in the early weeks and months of life influences future health. Breastmilk is a unique biologically active fluid which not only contains all the nutrients the newborn requires but provides some protection against infection, including gastrointestinal infections. There is some evidence that breastfeeding is associated with a lower risk of sudden infant death syndrome and diabetes and hypertension in later life (Martin et al. 2005, Owen et al. 2006, Vennemann et al. 2009). There are benefits to maternal health too and women who breastfeed are less likely to develop breast cancer and certain types of ovarian cancer (Jordan et al. 2010, Stuebe et al. 2009). If the mother is unable to breastfeed, or does not wish to, modern infant formula milks are a safe substitute providing that the equipment is clean and sterilised and the formula used according to the manufacturers' instructions.

It should be remembered that feeding a baby is about more than just putting milk into its stomach. Whichever method is chosen, it should be a pleasurable experience for both mother and child, and one which promotes appropriate infant growth and development and reinforces a loving, nurturing relationship.

Domestic abuse

A definition of domestic abuse or violence is: 'Any incident of threatening behaviour, violence or abuse (psychological, physical, sexual, financial or emotional) between adults who are or have been intimate partners or family members, regardless of gender or sexuality' (Home Office 2012). The definition also encompasses forced marriage, female genital mutilation and 'honour'-related violence. The Government has extended the definition to include girls of 16 and 17 years of age. While men can be victims, most are women and 5% of women a year experience one or more assaults (Home Office 2010). The issue is of concern to midwives because the violent behaviour may start, or become worse, in pregnancy. This imperils the health, and sometimes the life, of both the woman and the fetus. Existing children living in a violent home are at risk of abuse. Exposure to violence is also psychologically damaging to a child.

At the first antenatal appointment (the 'booking' appointment), midwives should ask (discreetly) if the woman is suffering, or is at risk of, domestic violence. If she is, then the woman is offered support and advice and measures may be taken to protect the child when it is born. Social workers and the police may become involved, depending on the situation. If the woman says that there is no violence, midwives must still be alert to warning signs. These include frequent attendance at the doctor's surgery with genital or urinary infections, unexplained bruising, especially over the abdomen or breasts, frequent hospital admissions during pregnancy and overbearing or controlling behaviour on the part of the partner. Any discussion with the woman about domestic violence should not take place in the presence of the partner and must be recorded in the hospital (not the hand-held) notes, including care planning and actions taken.

Midwifery wisdom

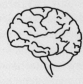

Midwives must remember that questions around domestic abuse must be asked in a sensitive and respectful manner. The topic should be raised at booking and again later in the pregnancy as many women do not reveal abuse the first time they are asked. Also the violent behaviour may begin for the first time after the booking appointment. A useful way to commence a conversation may be by asking if the woman feels safe at home.

Obesity

The Department of Health estimates that 23% of adults in England are obese and note the health risks that this presents to individuals, such as type 2 diabetes (DH 2011b). The risks of obesity in pregnancy and childbirth are considerable. These include higher rates of pre-eclampsia, miscarriage, fetal anomaly, haemorrhage and wound infection. Obese women are more likely to require a caesarean section (CMACE/RCOG 2010). In the latest enquiry into maternal deaths, 47% of the women who died from direct causes were overweight or obese (Lewis 2011). Midwifery responsibilities include giving information and advice, close monitoring during pregnancy and a moving and handling assessment in the third trimester. Midwives make referral to specialists as appropriate, for example dieticians, obstetricians and anaesthetists, as this is considered to be a high-risk pregnancy. Thromboprophylaxis during labour and in the early postnatal period will be required.

Smoking, drugs and alcohol

Tobacco, alcohol and street drugs are used by many people. In England, surveys found that 6.8% of adults had used cannabis during the survey period 2010–2011, 21% of adults were smokers (with 12.7% of mothers still smoking at the time of delivery) and 4% of women reported no change in their drinking habits during pregnancy(NHS Information Centre 2011, 2012a–c). There are concerns about all of these, as they have negative consequences for health and may be addictive. This is particularly true for pregnant women, as the toxins, including nicotine and carbon monoxide, cross the placenta.

Cigarette smoking is associated with cancer, respiratory and cardiac disease in adults. During pregnancy, its impact on placental development and function can produce fetal growth restriction. The effects continue after birth, and neonatal growth and cell function may be impaired (Serobyan et al. 2005).

Heavy use of alcohol affects fertility and is associated with an increased risk of miscarriage and stillbirth (RCM 2010). Fetal alcohol spectrum disorder may result from continuing to drink during pregnancy and this affects the physical and intellectual development of the child. Unfortunately, there is no safe level of intake and many women prefer not to drink alcohol when pregnant and thus avoid the risk. The Department of Health estimates that one in 100 babies is born with some degree of alcohol-related brain damage. A booklet and a film have been produced to inform the public and support midwives in reducing the number of affected babies (DH 2012d).

The use of illegal drugs in pregnancy exposes the mother and fetus to the harmful effects of the substance, some of which cause lasting damage. Depending on the route used to take the drug, women may find themselves exposed to the risk of infections. The woman's diet may suffer as she may be unable to afford good-quality food and if prostitution is her means of funding her drug habit, the risk of sexually transmitted infections and violence is considerable.

Female genital mutilation

This describes any activity which alters the female genitalia for non-medical reasons. The WHO recognises four types of mutilation (WHO 2012b). The damage ranges from removal of the clitoral prepuce to infibulation, which involves narrowing of the vaginal orifice, and apposition of the labia, with or without clitoral excision. The procedure is usually carried out in childhood, and certainly before the girl reaches adulthood. Since the Female Genital Mutilation Act of 2003, it is illegal in the UK. There are no health benefits and detrimental effects may include gynaecological and urinary problems, obstructed labour, severe genital tract damage in labour and fetal compromise. Midwives caring for women who have undergone such procedures should develop a plan of care with the woman, which can include referral to a gynaecologist for review. Reversal of the infibulated state is usually carried out in the second trimester of the pregnancy. The midwife and the health visitor should be aware that, if the infant is female, the parents may wish the procedure to be carried out on the child. This is illegal in the UK and it is possible that safeguarding procedures may be required to protect the child from harm.

Midwifery wisdom

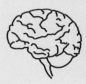

Female genital mutilation is a very challenging issue and you may not have come in contact with it before, so it is vital that you have an understanding of this practice. The Forward website is a useful resource to begin with: www.forwarduk.org.uk/key-issues/fgm

Sexual and reproductive health

Part of the public health work of the midwife encompasses sexual health and reproductive health. This includes fertility and contraception. Midwives may be involved in preconception care and advice, to optimise health before pregnancy and, hopefully, improve outcomes. This advice should include diet, smoking and alcohol intake which might affect fertility and fetal health. Women with medical conditions such as diabetes mellitus or cardiac disease should be counselled before pregnancy and in collaboration with the medical specialists caring for the woman (DH 2004).

Sexually transmitted infections (STIs) may affect fertility, the most common being chlamydia, for which there is a national screening programme for people under 25 in England. Currently, this is the only country in the UK which has a formal national screening programme. STIs also affect fetal and maternal health and all pregnant women are offered screening for syphilis and HIV, which are two of the most serious, with long-lasting consequences. With prompt recognition and careful management, these infections need not necessarily lead to poor outcomes. The midwife should not make judgements about who might, or might not, need screening. For example, lesbian couples may also need advice and counselling. Women with a history of sexual abuse may find the intrusive nature of some elements of midwifery care, such as vaginal examination, unacceptable and midwives must be sensitive to this and adapt care to the woman's needs.

Midwifery wisdom

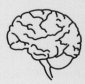

If vaginal examination is not acceptable to the woman, it is possible, in many cases, to assess labour progress by close observation of other signs. These include the woman's speech and behaviour, looking for the purple line in the buttock cleft, descent of the uterine fundus with fetal descent and watching for prominence of the rhombus of Michaelis in the sacral area (also known as the quadrilateral of Michaelis) which is a kite-shaped area that includes the three lower lumbar vertebrae.

In the postnatal period midwives will advise women about contraception. Fertility may return surprisingly quickly, especially if the woman is not breastfeeding, and most would prefer not to become pregnant immediately after the birth. Most women will resume sexual intercourse within 6 weeks of the birth. The return of ovulation is uncommon before 6 weeks, even in women who choose to formula feed, but some may have begun ovulating by then (Jackson & Glasier 2011). Midwives should remember that breastfeeding is not entirely reliable in delaying ovulation and all women should be advised about the need for contraception before resuming intercourse following birth.

Sudden infant death syndrome

Sudden infant death syndrome (SIDS), also known as sudden unexpected death in infancy (SUDI) or cot death, is 'the sudden unexpected death of any infant or young child which is unexpected by history and where a thorough post-mortem examination fails to demonstrate an adequate cause of death' (Beckwith 1970). Most babies who die are less than 1 year old and over 72% are less than 4 months; 34% of deaths occur during the winter months and it is slightly more common in boys (FSID 2012). While no cause of death can be confirmed, there are a number of factors which appear to increase the risk for a baby. These include maternal smoking, a teenage mother, preterm birth, low birthweight, formula feeding and baby care practices such as laying the infant on its stomach to sleep. Bed sharing (co-sleeping) is known to increase the risk of SIDS if the mother is a smoker, has taken drugs or alcohol, or is very tired (Blair et al. 2009). UNICEF has produced advice leaflets for parents and professionals (UNICEF 2011), identifying that the safest place for a baby to sleep is in a cot beside the parents' bed.

A sudden infant death is always referred to the coroner as the death is unexplained, and a police officer is likely to visit the home, which can add to the distress of the parents. In 2010 the SIDS rate for England and Wales was 0.35 per 1000 live births (ONS 2012), continuing the trend towards falling rates since 1988. SIDS is one of the few public health 'good news' stories as significant progress has been made towards reducing the number of families affected by this distressing situation. Research is ongoing to try to reduce the rate further. The Foundation for the Study of Infant Deaths has introduced the CONI (Care of the Next Infant) Scheme which aims to support parents and professionals during a subsequent pregnancy.

Global policy perspectives

The global policy perspective on public health and maternity care focuses around an ambitious project adopted by the United Nations (UN) in September 2000. The UN Millennium Declaration committed to a new global partnership to reduce extreme poverty and set out a series of time-bound targets with a deadline of 2015. The eight Millennium Development Goals (MGDs), as they became known, ranged from halving extreme poverty to halting the spread of HIV/AIDS and providing universal primary education for all children. In order to achieve this, they concentrated on reducing maternal and neonatal/infant mortality, as well as promoting gender equality and empowering women to have more control over their reproduction and life choices. Table 12.1 provides an overview of the goals and targets.

In September 2010, the UN launched the Every Woman Every Child (UN 2010) campaign which aims to save the lives of 16 million women and children by 2015. It focused world attention on the need to enhance economic support, strengthen national policy and improve local service provision for the most vulnerable women and children. This global strategy identified four key gains:

- It reduces poverty.
- It stimulates economic productivity and growth.
- It is cost-effective.
- It helps women and children realise their fundamental human rights.

Table 12.1   Overview of Millennium Development Goals (data from UN 2000)

	Millennium Development Goals	Targets
1	ERADICATE EXTREME POVERTY and HUNGER	1. Halve, between 1990 and 2015, the proportion of people whose income is less than $1 a day 2. Achieve full and productive employment and decent work for all, including women and young people 3. Halve, between 1990 and 2015, the proportion of people who suffer from hunger
2	ACHIEVE UNIVERSAL PRIMARY EDUCATION	1. Ensure that, by 2015, children everywhere, boys and girls alike, will be able to complete a full course of primary schooling
3	PROMOTE GENDER EQUALITY AND EMPOWER WOMEN	1. Eliminate gender disparity in primary and secondary education, preferably by 2005, and in all levels of education, no later than 2015
4	REDUCE CHILD MORTALITY	1. Reduce by two-thirds, between 1990 and 2015, the mortality rate of children under five
5	IMPROVE MATERNAL HEALTH	1. Reduce by three-quarters, between 1990 and 2015, the maternal mortality ratio 2. Achieve, by 2015, universal access to reproductive health
6	COMBAT HIV/AIDS, MALARIA AND OTHER DISEASES	1. Halt and begin to reverse, by 2015, the spread of HIV/AIDS 2. Achieve, by 2010, universal access to treatment for HIV/AIDS for all those who need it 3. Halt and begin to reverse, by 2015, the incidence of malaria and other major diseases
7	ENSURE ENVIRONMENTAL SUSTAINABILITY	1. Integrate the principles of sustainable development into country policies and programmes and reverse the loss of environmental resources 2. Reduce biodiversity loss, achieving, by 2010, a significant reduction in the rate of loss 3. Halve, by 2015, the proportion of the population without sustainable access to safe drinking water and basic sanitation 4. Achieve, by 2020, a significant improvement in the lives of at least 100 million slum dwellers
8	DEVELOP A GLOBAL PARTNERSHIP FOR DEVELOPMENT	1. Develop further an open, rule-based, predictable, non-discriminatory trading and financial system 2. Address the special needs of least developed countries, landlocked countries and small island developing states 3. Deal comprehensively with developing countries' debt 4. In co-operation with pharmaceutical companies, provide access to affordable, essential drugs in developing countries 5. In co-operation with the private sector, make available benefits of new technologies, especially information and communication technologies

In 2012 the UN published its 2012 annual report updating progress on the MGDs. Some encouraging news was reported that child survival rates were improving and although decreases in maternal mortality were far from their 2015 target, significant improvements in health were being seen in some areas. One of the real challenges has been the lack of reliable and accurate data on maternal mortality. In 2010, the WHO reported on global trends in maternal mortality and suggested that 'An estimated 358,000 maternal deaths occurred worldwide in 2008, a 34% decline from the levels of 1990. Despite this decline, developing countries continued to account for 99% (355 000) of the deaths'. Compare this with the UK, which in 2011 was 11.39 deaths per 100,000 maternities compared to 13.95 per 100,000 maternities for the previous triennium, 2003–5 (Lewis 2011).

It is often suggested that getting pregnant can be one of the most dangerous activities a woman can undergo in some countries. The role the midwife can play in the UK and globally has been shown to make a positive difference to the health and well-being of women. The recent Birth Place in England research study (NPEU 2011) demonstrated that overall birthing in England is safe, but it relies on high-quality evidence-based care and an understanding of how services should be managed according to the potential risk status of the mother when pregnant and throughout her birth experience.

Globally, one of the key health professionals contributing to these improvements is the midwife, who can administer interventions to prevent and manage life-threatening complications such as heavy bleeding or refer the woman to a higher level of care when needed. Midwives are also in a prime position to develop a relationship with the woman, using that contact to educate and inform on the benefits of improving their lifestyle, or enabling them to seek appropriate help where their choices may be limited by poverty, violence and/or discrimination. This role is not confined to countries that are less well developed but includes UK midwives, who can utilise the evidence available to enhance care. In developing regions of the world, the proportion of deliveries attended by skilled health personnel rose from 55% in 1990 to 65% in 2010. However, gender inequality and discrimination against children and women persist, in particular in relation to access to healthcare and education, work and economic resources, and participation in government decision making, which continues to undermine efforts to achieve the MGDs (UN 2012).

The International Confederation of Midwives (ICM) works with midwives globally to secure and enhance women's right and access to midwifery care before, during and after childbirth. In June 2011, the ICM launched a key report (UNFPA 2011) which for the first time provided statistical analysis of the challenges facing some of the poorest countries across the globe. The vision of the movement behind the report is summed up thus:

> *The drive for safer motherhood continues to gain strength as more women worldwide achieve access to midwifery care. Our vision is for a world where every woman has access to a midwife's care for herself and her baby.*

(UNFPA 2011)

Midwifery wisdom

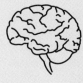 A key midwifery skill is about listening to women, so if you want to find out more about midwifery abroad, you should take the opportunity to ask women you meet about healthcare and specifically midwifery in their country of origin. You could also look at the ICM website, which provides further information and useful links to understanding midwifery across the globe. This in turn will help you understand why some women do not understand the healthcare systems and processes in the UK.

Conclusion

In 1948, the WHO defined health as 'A complete state of physical, mental and social well-being and not simply the absence of disease or infirmity' (WHO 1948). This view has moved forward and now focuses on the positive aspects of health rather than just the absence of disease, and midwives in partnership with their obstetric colleagues and related healthcare professionals have a key role in improving the health and well-being of all women and families they come in contact with.

While great strides have been made in improving the health of the maternity population, there remain some areas of concern. An example here would be the rising level of obesity in the community. Tackling this is likely to prove difficult. In times of relative financial hardship, food expenditure for families is often affected. A healthy diet may be perceived to be expensive, and cheaper, less healthy foods may be more affordable for some women. There is also scope to consider the current approach to public health measures for the childbearing population. Many of these, it could be argued, could be seen as paternalistic and based on a medical rather than a social model of health. They may also be viewed as being politically driven and therefore may not always be tailored to the needs of those they profess to serve.

Whatever the motivation behind the strategy, the role the midwife can play cannot be overemphasised. Midwives are ideally placed to encourage women to consider their health at a critical time in their lives, where targeted interventions such as reducing obesity, smoking cessation programmes and other screening programmes can be mobilised to, at the least, deliver safe effective public health measures and at best provide the tools to enhance family health.

Midwives in their personal well-being as well as their professional lives have a platform available to them to enhance the health and well-being of the local population. Midwives are also encouraged to be more politically active and engage in the wider debates about how, on a national level, better health can be promoted and enhanced.

Quiz

1. How would you describe the role of the midwife in public health to a friend who asks you?
2. Make a list of some reasons why deprivation affects health and life expectancy.
3. Find your local guidelines for domestic violence in pregnancy. What contacts do they give for local refuges? If there is no contact, find out if there is one in the area you will be practising.
4. Find out about screening for STIs in your area. What chlamydia screening programme is in place?
5. Make a list of some influences on the health of populations across the UK.
6. What are the five most common causes of maternal mortality in the UK?
7. Identify five risks that women who are considered obese are exposed to when they become pregnant.
8. Reflect on the answers you have given so far, and consider now how you would respectfully ask women questions to find out more about their lifestyle choices.
9. Describe the Millennium Development Goals that most affect the role of the midwife.
10. Which of the following statements best describes why the midwife has an important role to play in public health?
    (a) Midwives are the first point of professional contact and are ideally suited to have positive relationships and impacts on women's health.
    (b) Midwives make great role models for promoting a healthier lifestyle and life choices.
    (c) Midwives are part of the multiprofessional healthcare team whose primary objective is to improve the health of individuals and the local population.
    (d) Midwives have a professional duty to treat all women with respect and dignity, whilst encouraging them to change their lifestyles towards healthier living for themselves and their family.

References

Ball S, Tewdwr-Jones M (2012) *The UCL London 2062 Project: an interdisciplinary perspective of London today and a London of tomorrow*. London: University College London. Available at: www.ucl.ac.uk/london-2062/documents/2062-19July-2011.pdf (accessed May 2013).

Beckwith J (1970) Discussion of terminology and definition of the sudden infant death syndrome. In: Bergman A, Beckwith J, Ray C (eds) *Sudden Infant Death Syndrome: proceedings of the Second International Conference on the Causes of Sudden Death in Infants*. Seattle: University of Washington Press, pp14–22.

Berkley C (1922) *A Handbook of Midwifery*. London: Cassell.

Blair P, Sidebotham P, Evason-Coombe C, Edmonds M, Heckstall-Smith E, Fleming P (2009) Hazardous cosleeping environments and risk factors amenable to change: case-control study of SIDS in south west England. *British Medical Journal* **339**: b3666.

Clendening L (1942) *The Dover Source Book of Medical History*. New York: Dover Publications.

Centre for Maternal and Child Enquiries (CMACE) (2011) *Saving Mothers' Lives: reviewing maternal deaths to make motherhood safer – 2006–08. The Eighth Report of the Confidential Enquiries into Maternal Deaths in the United Kingdom. British Journal of Obstetrics and Gynaecology* **118**(Suppl. 1): 1–203.

Centre for Maternal and Child Enquiries/Royal College of Obstetricians and Gynaecologists (CMACE/RCOG) (2010) *Management of Women with Obesity in Pregnancy*. Centre for Maternal and Child Enquiries and Royal College of Obstetricians and Gynaecologists. Available at: www.rcog.org.uk/files/rcog-corp/CMACERCOGJoint GuidelineManagementWomenObesityPregnancya.pdf (accessed May 2013).

Department of Health (DH) (2004) *Standard 11, National Service Framework for Children, Young People and Maternity*. London: Department of Health. Available at: http://webarchive.nationalarchives.gov.uk/20130107105354/http://www.dh.gov.uk/prod_consum_dh/groups/dh_digitalassets/@dh/@en/documents/digitalasset/dh_4090523.pdf (accessed May 2013).

Department of Health (DH) (2010) *Midwifery 2020: delivering expectations*. London: Department of Health.

Department of Health (DH) (2011a) *Public Health England's Operating Model*. Available at: www.dh.gov.uk/prod_consum_dh/groups/dh_digitalassets/documents/digitalasset/dh_131892.pdf, (accessed May 2013).

Department of Health (DH) (2011b) *Healthy Lives, Healthy People: a call to action on obesity in England*. Available at: www.dh.gov.uk/en/Publicationsandstatistics/Publications/PublicationsPolicyAndGuidance/DH_130401 (accessed May 2013).

Department of Health (DH) (2012a) *Public Health, Adult Social Care and the NHS*. Available at: www.dh.gov.uk/health/category/policy-areas/public-health/ (accessed May 2013).

Department of Health (DH) (2012b) *Structure of Public Health England*. London: Department of Health. Available at: http://healthandcare.dh.gov.uk/phe-structure/ (accessed May 2013).

Department of Health (DH) (2012c) Pregnant women to be offered whooping cough vaccination. Available at: www.dh.gov.uk/health/2012/09/whooping-cough/ (accessed May 2013).

Department of Health (DH) (2012d) *Children, Families and Maternity e-Bulletin*. Available at: https://www.gov.uk/government/uploads/system/uploads/attachment_data/file/127029/Children-Families-and-Maternity-bulletin-October-2012.pdf.pdf (accessed May 2013).

Foundation for the Study of Infant Deaths (FSID) (2012) *Cot Death Facts and Figures*. London: Foundation for the Study of Infant Deaths. Available at: http://fsid.org.uk/document.doc?id=97 (accessed May 2013).

Health Protection Agency (HPA) (2012a) *List of Notifiable Diseases*. Available at: www.hpa.org.uk/Topics/InfectiousDiseases/InfectionsAZ/NotificationsOfInfectiousDiseases/ListOfNotifiableDiseases/ (accessed May 2013).

Health Protection Agency (2012b) HPA welcomes introduction of whooping cough vaccination for pregnant women as outbreak continues. Available at: www.hpa.org.uk/webw/HPAweb&HPAwebStandard/HPAweb_C/1317136 292634 (accessed May 2013).

Home Office (2010) *Crime in England and Wales 2009/2010*. Available at: http://webarchive.nationalarchives.gov.uk/20110218135832/http://rds.homeoffice.gov.uk/rds/pdfs10/hosb1210.pdf (accessed May 2013).

Home Office (2012) *Domestic Violence*. Available at: www.gov.uk/government/news/new-definition-of-domestic-violence-and-abuse-to-include-16-and-17-year-olds (accessed May 2013).

227

House of Commons (2009) *Better Off Dead? A report on maternal morbidity from the UK All-Party Parliamentary Group on population, development and reproductive health*. London: Portcullis House. Available at: www.appg-popdevrh.org.uk/Publications/Maternal%20Morbidity%20Hearings/Maternal%20Morbidity%20Report%20-%20FINAL%20single%20page.pdf, (accessed May 2013).

Jackson E., Glasier A (2011) Return of ovulation and menses in postpartum non-lactating women: a systematic review. *Obstetrics and Gynecology* **117**(3): 677–662.

Jordan S, Siskind V, Green A, Whiteman D, Webb P (2010) Breastfeeding and risk of epithelial ovarian cancer. *Cancer Causes and Control* **21**(1):109–116.

Kyte L, Wells C (2010) Variations in life expectancy between rural and urban areas of England, 2001–07. *Health Statistics Quarterly* **Summer**: **46**.

Lewis G. (2011) *Saving Mothers' Lives: Reviewing maternal deaths to make motherhood safer—2006–08 The Eighth Report of the Confidential Enquiries into Maternal Deaths in the United Kingdom BJOG* 118 (Suppl. 1), 1–203.

London Health Observatory (2010) *Jubilee Line of Health Inequality 2004–2008*. Analysis by London Health Observatory of ONS and GLA data for 2004–2008. Available at: www.lho.org.uk/viewResource.aspx?id=15463 (accessed May 2013).

Loudon I (1992) The transformation of maternal mortality. *British Medical Journal* **305**(1926): 1557–1560.

Marmot M (2010) *Marmot Review: fair society, healthy lives*. London: UCL Institute of Health Equality. Available at: www.instituteofhealthequity.org/ (accessed May 2013).

Martin R, Gunnell D, Davey Smith G (2005) Breastfeeding in infancy and blood pressure in later life: systematic review and meta-analysis. *American Journal of Epidemiology* **161**(1): 15–26.

National Quality Board (2012) *Quality in the New Health System – maintaining and improving quality from April 2013*. London: Department of Health. Available at: www.gov.uk/government/uploads/system/uploads/attachment_data/file/126950/Quality-in-the-new-system-maintaining-and-improving-quality-from-April-2013-FINAL-2.pdf.pdf (accessed May 2013).

NHS Information Centre (2011) *Statistics on Drug Misuse: England 2011*. Available at: https://catalogue.ic.nhs.uk/publications/public-health/drug-misuse/drug-misu-eng-2011/drug-misu-eng-2011-rep.pdf (accessed May 2013).

NHS Information Centre (2012a) *Statistics on Smoking: England*. Available at: https://catalogue.ic.nhs.uk/publications/public-health/smoking/smok-eng-2011/smok-eng-2011-rep.pdf (accessed May 2013).

NHS Information Centre (2012b) *Statistics on Women's Smoking Status at Time of Delivery: England, Quarter 1, 2012/13*. Available at: https://catalogue.ic.nhs.uk/publications/public-health/smoking/stat-wome-smok-time-deli-eng-q1-12-13/stat-wome-smok-time-dele-eng-q1-12-13-rep.pdf (accessed May 2013).

NHS Information Centre (2012c) *Statistics on Alcohol: England*. Available at: https://catalogue.ic.nhs.uk/publications/public-health/alcohol/alco-eng-2012/alco-eng-2012-rep.pdf (accessed May 2013).

National Institute of Health and Clinical Excellence (NICE) (2012) *About Public Health*. Available at: www.nice.org.uk/aboutnice/whatwedo/aboutpublichealthguidance/about_public_health_guidance.jsp (accessed May 2013).

Nursing and Midwifery Council (NMC) (2009) *Standards for Pre-Registration Midwifery Education*. London: Nursing and Midwifery Council. Available at: www.nmc-uk.org/Educators/Standards-for-education/Standards-for-pre-registration-midwifery-education/ (accessed May 2013).

Nursing and Midwifery Council (NMC) (2011) *The PREP Handbook: post-registration education and practice*. London: Nursing and Midwifery Council. Available at: www.nmc-uk.org/Publications/Standards/ (accessed May 2013).

National Perinatal Epidemiology Unit (NPEU) (2011) *The Birthplace in England Research Programme*. Available at: www.npeu.ox.ac.uk/birthplace/results (accessed May 2013).

Office for National Statistics (ONS) (2012) *Unexplained Deaths in Infancy – England and Wales 2010*. London: Office for National Statistics. Available at: www.ons.gov.uk/ons/dcp171778_276544.pdf (accessed May 2013).

Owen C, Martin R, Whincup P, Davey Smith G, Cook D (2006) Does breastfeeding influence risk of type 2 diabetes in later life? A quantitative analysis of published evidence. *American Journal of Clinical Nutrition* **84**(5): 1043–1054.

Royal College of Midwives (RCM) (2010) *Alcohol and Pregnancy: guidance paper*. London: Royal College of Midwives. Available at: www.rcm.org.uk/EasySiteWeb/getresource.axd?AssetID=112535 (accessed May 2013).

Royal College of Nursing (RCN) (2012) *Going Upstream: nursing's contribution to public health*. London: Royal College of Nursing. Available at: www.rcn.org.uk/__data/assets/pdf_file/0007/433699/004203.pdf (accessed May 2013).

Scottish Government (2012) *Infant Mortality Statistics*. Available at: www.scotland.gov.uk/News/Releases/2012/01/infantmortality31012012 (accessed May 2013).

Serobyan N, Orlovskaya I, Kozlov V, Khaldoyanidi SK (2005) Exposure to nicotine during gestation interferes with the colonization of fetal bone marrow by hematopoietic stem/progenitor cells. *Stem Cells and Development* **14**(1): 81–91.

Sidebotham M, Walsh T (2011) Epidemiology. In: Macdonald S, Magill-Cuerden J (eds) *Mayes' Midwifery*. London: Baillière Tindall.

Stuebe A, Willett W, Michels K (2009) Lactation and incidence of premenopausal breast cancer: a longitudinal study. *Archives of Internal Medicine* **169**(15): 1364–1371.

Truby King F (1945) *Feeding and Care of Baby*. London: Whitcombe and Tombs.

United Nations (UN) (2000) *The Millennium Development Goals*. Available at: www.un.org/millenniumgoals/ (accessed May 2013).

United Nations (UN) (2010) *Global Strategy for Women's and Children's Health*. Available at: http://www.who.int/pmnch/activities/jointactionplan/en/ and www.everywomaneverychild.org (accessed May 2013).

United Nations (UN) (2012) *The Millennium Development Goals Report 2012*. Available at: www.un.org/en/development/desa/publications/mdg-report-2012.html (accessed May 2013).

United Nations Population Fund (UNFPA) (2011) *State of the World's Midwifery 2011: delivering health, saving lives*. Available at: www.internationalmidwives.org and www.unfpa.org/sowmy/home.html (accessed May 2013).

UNICEF (2011) *Caring for Your Baby at Night*. www.unicef.org.uk/BabyFriendly/Resources/Resources-for-parents/Caring-for-your-baby-at-night/ (accessed May 2013).

Vennemann M, Bajanowski T, Brinkmann B, et al. for the GeSID Study Group (2009) Does breastfeeding reduce the risk of sudden infant death syndrome? *Pediatrics* **123**(3): e406–e410.

World Health Organization (WHO) (1948) *Definition of Health*. Available at: www.who.int/about/definition/en/print.html (accessed May 2013).

World Health Organization (WHO) (2010) *Trends in Maternal Mortality: 1990 to 2008*. Available at: whqlibdoc.who.int/publications/2010/9789241500265_eng.pdf (accessed May 2013).

World Health Organization (WHO) (2012a) *Epidemiology*. Available at: www.who.int/topics/epidemiology/en/ (accessed May 2013).

World Health Organization (WHO) (2012b) *Classification of Female Genital Mutilation*. Available at: www.who.int/reproductivehealth/topics/fgm/overview/en/index.html and www.who.int/topics/female_genital_mutilation/en/ (accessed May 2013).

Regulating the Midwifery Profession

Carole Yearley and Emma Dawson-Goodey

Aim

The midwife is a registered practitioner and is accountable to the Nursing and Midwifery Council (NMC). This chapter looks at the structure and function of the NMC. It also looks at how the NMC strives towards the protection of the public whilst upholding the reputation of the profession.

Learning outcomes

By the end of this chapter you will be able to:

1. demonstrate an understanding of the background to midwifery regulation
2. describe the structure of the NMC
3. discuss in broad terms the relevant articles of the Nursing and Midwifery Order 2001
4. identify and discuss the functions of the NMC which include standards of education, maintenance of a register, post-registration education and practice (PREP), standards and fitness to practise
5. discuss the responsibilities of the midwife in order to practise safely.

Introduction

The public expects midwifery practice to be of a competent standard and midwives have a high level of respect. Society has become better informed and expectations are rising. The midwife–client relationship is perhaps unique; it is based on trust and deals with our most valuable possession, health and the

The Student's Guide to Becoming a Midwife, Second Edition. Edited by Ian Peate and Cathy Hamilton.
© 2014 John Wiley & Sons, Ltd. Published 2014 by John Wiley & Sons, Ltd.

health of our baby. When the woman's expectations are not met or when an error is made, this relationship is damaged. The result of this may be detrimental to health or even cause death. The cost to each person is therefore exceedingly high. The professional must then be closely examined and held accountable. Women need to feel that midwives have achieved an appropriate level of education and are professionally competent.

Self-regulation

Regulation of the midwifery profession was first defined in 1902 when the British government passed the Midwives Act. The need to prepare and educate midwives for their role had been finally endorsed by the government, which acknowledged the relationship between educated midwives and better outcomes for women and babies during childbirth. The title 'midwife' became protected by law and along with this established the principle that only trained practitioners (midwives or doctors) could attend women during childbirth. The professionalisation of midwives became established through a self-regulating approach, giving the profession wide-ranging powers and autonomy over its direction and protocols for care. This was essentially a contract between the state and the profession.

Subsequent amendments over a significant period of time led to the creation of the NMC by 2002. The NMC is an example of state-licensed self-regulation, i.e. the rules and principles established by institutions are given support from the state by legislation. This approach provides the NMC with a high degree of authority.

The structure of the council is set out under the Nursing and Midwifery Order 2001 (Statutory Instruments 2002/253). The NMC is currently composed of four statutory committees:

1. Investigating Committee (IC)
2. Conduct and Competence Committee (CCC)
3. Health Committee (HC)
4. Midwifery Committee.

The IC, CCC and HC are concerned with fitness to practise allegations.

The Department of Health (DH 2007) published a report which sets out the government's strategy for reforming and modernising the system of healthcare regulation. In line with the recommendations in the White Paper *Trust, Assurance and Safety: the regulation of health professionals in the 21st century* (DH 2007), the composition of the Council has changed to a smaller, more board-like structure to include lay persons and, most importantly, registrant members do not form a majority. The White Paper suggests that 'the existence of professional majorities undermines councils' independence and their perceived independence' (1.10, p25). The NMC now has 12 lay and registrant members appointed by the Privy Council, including one member from each of the four UK countries.

The core function of the NMC is to establish standards of education, training, conduct and perfor-mance for nursing and midwifery and to ensure those standards are maintained, thereby safeguarding the health and well-being of the public. These functions are fundamental in the key tasks of the Nursing and Midwifery Order 2001 (Statutory Instruments 2002/253), which include the following:

- Part III Registration, whose purpose is to maintain a register of nurses and midwives eligible to practise in the UK. It is therefore illegal to practise as a midwife or nurse in the UK without being on the register.
- Part IV Education and Training, whose responsibility is to establish standards of education and training for both pre-registration and post-registration nursing and midwifery in order to register and remain on the register. Part IV also includes the validation of courses in approved universities.

231

- Part V Fitness to Practise considers allegations against nurses and midwives.
- Part VIII Midwifery Committee establishes the rules for midwifery standards and provides guidance for local supervisors of midwives.

Midwifery wisdom

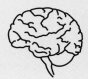

To stay on the NMC register, you have to renew your registration every 3 years. You also pay an annual fee at the end of the first and second year of the registration period.

More than a century on from the Midwives Act 1902, protection of the public remains at the heart of self-regulation and the NMC. As did the previous regulatory authority the United Kingdom Central Council for Nurses, Midwives and Health Visitors (1983–2002), the NMC has had to embrace the fundamental tenets of these two different professions yet has maintained the specialist and specific interests and concerns relating to midwifery practice through establishing the Midwifery Committee. This professionally appointed, yet statutorily required group leads and affirms the direction and implications of legislation for the midwifery profession, both collaboratively with and/or independently of the regulation proposed for nurses. Concurrently, the NMC addresses political debates which challenge the impacts and consequences of being a self-regulating organisation. This appraisal comes especially in light of past events (DH 2004, Kennedy 2001, Redfern 2001, Smith 2004) which have undermined the public's confidence generally in a range of health professions' ability to police their own practitioners. The core functions of the NMC can be found in Figure 13.1.

Figure 13.2 is a representation of how the NMC structures serve to regulate midwives. Understanding these will enable practitioners to utilise the boundaries set by the NMC to enable them to reach their full potential as midwives. Rules are not intended to restrict professionals but to empower them, so they can feel confident of their professional remit and sphere of practice. Midwives who feel empowered, in turn, empower women in their decision making and together they create a strong allegiance for achieving excellence in practice.

Standards and guidelines

In order to safeguard the health and well-being of the public, the NMC also publishes standards of practice and guidance. The fundamental standard of practice for both nurses and midwives is currently *The Code: standards of conduct, performance and ethics for nurses and midwives* (NMC 2008). In addition, midwives must practise in accordance with the NMC *Midwives' Rules* (2012a). *The Code* aims to improve accountability and personal responsibility through a number of statements which reflect a wide set of principles, including 'consent and confidentiality', 'working as a team', 'use the best available evidence' and 'record keeping'. *The Code* also encompasses principles relating to the way care is delivered, the basis for ethics – for example 'act with integrity'. It further identifies a positive duty to respect equality and diversity.

Adhering to these standards allows nurses and midwives to use their professional judgement and to justify their actions. Nurses and midwives do have a professional duty to practise accordingly and if a nurse/midwife fails to adhere to the standards then this can be referred to a fitness to practise hearing.

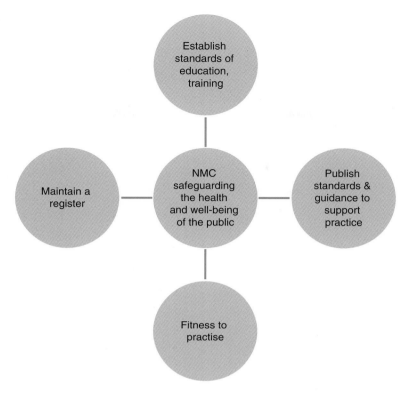

Figure 13.1   The core functions of the NMC.

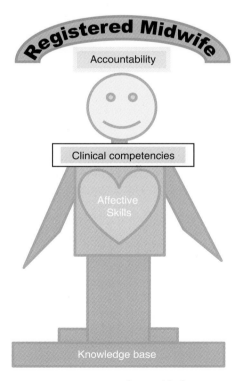

Figure 13.2   How the NMC structures serve to regulate midwives.

Activity 13.1

To help you to familiarise yourself with *The Code* (NMC 2008) and the *Midwives' Rules*, read the following scenarios and reflect on how the standards may be used to support the midwife or have been breached by her. Scenario 1 should help you identify where you feel the standards can support the midwife. Scenario 2 should help you to identify where you feel the midwife is in breach of those standards. Scenario 3 illustrates how the rules can support midwives in practice; Scenario 4 illustrates a situation where it appears that the rules have been contravened.

Scenario 1

Abby, a midwife, has been told by the doctor on the labour ward to rupture the membranes of a low-risk labouring woman. The doctor says that she always likes the membranes ruptured in labour. There is no clinical indication to perform this and the client also does not wish to have this done.

Scenario 2

Mary is a midwife working in a very busy antenatal clinic. She is booking a woman who speaks very little English. There is no-one there to translate. Mary gesticulates that she needs to take blood from her and proceeds to take blood for screening purposes. Later that day, the woman's husband phones the clinic and is very upset that this procedure was done without full explanation to his wife about the tests.

Scenario 3

Gita is a community midwife who has booked Sarah, pregnant with her second baby. Sarah's first baby was born by caesarean section for a breech presentation. Sarah tells Gita that she would like to have this baby at home using a birthing pool. Which rule(s) specifically relate to this situation and how can Gita use them to ensure that her practice meets the rule(s) and standard(s)?

Scenario 4

Liz, a midwife, has been on sick leave with back pain for some weeks. Her pregnant friend, Jo, calls her late one night and asks Liz to come to her home as Jo is in labour. Liz goes to the house as she thinks that the birth is imminent and takes her community midwifery bag and home birth equipment. When she arrives, Jo's labour is progressing and she asks Liz to stay with her for the birth. The baby is born 1 hour later and Liz attends the delivery. Mother and baby are well. Which rule(s) specifically relate to this situation and which, in your opinion, have been breached?

The suggested answers appear at the end of the chapter.

The Nursing and Midwifery Council *Midwives' Rules*

In addition to standard setting, under the Nursing and Midwifery Order 2001 (Statutory Instruments 2002/253), referred to as the Order, the NMC is also required to set the rules by which registered midwives must abide in addition to those relating to local supervising authorities and how they must discharge the function of supervision of midwives. The rules detail the requirements for midwives and their practice. The revised *Midwives' Rules and Standards* (NMC 2012a) came into effect on 1st January 2013 and replace the previous rules. Under each rule, standards for the exercise by for the exercise by the local supervising authorities of their supervisory role provides further detail for the expected standard. With regard to the rules included under the section 'Obligations and scope of practice', guidance on the midwife standard is included which sets out the behaviour that would be reasonably expected of a midwife. For midwives, the *Midwives' Rules* (NMC 2012a) and *The Code* (NMC 2008) are the fundamental 'tools of the trade'; they are the tenets of daily practice and should be used by midwives to self-assess the quality of their practice and are also used to judge others' practice standards.

The NMC has also produced guidance publications which provide further information in relation to the standards documents – for example, *Standards for Medicines Management* (NMC 2010) and *Record Keeping* (NMC 2009a). These publications provide nurses, midwives and students with a series of principles to support their practice. The standards and guidance are all available to view on the NMC website: www.nmc-uk.org/Publications.

The consequences of breaching *The Code* and the *Midwives' Rules* may be serious for mothers, babies and midwives. The following section will focus on the role of the NMC and its fitness to practise procedures which deal with these breaches.

Fitness to practise

There are two legal documents that preside over the NMC fitness to practise (FtP) procedures. First, the Nursing and Midwifery Order 2001 (Statutory Instruments 2002/253) (called the Order) Part V makes provisions for fitness to practise which establish and review the standards of conduct, performance and ethics expected of registrants. The Council's function is to consider allegations which fall within article 22 (1) that may impair fitness to practise by reasons of misconduct, lack of competence, conviction or caution in the UK, ill health, entry on register has been fraudulently procured/incorrect or at the NMC's own initiation. The second document is the Nursing and Midwifery (Fitness to Practise) Rules Order of Council 2004 SI2004/1761 (called the fitness to practise rules) and subsequent Nursing and Midwifery (Fitness to Practise) (Amendment) Rules Order of Council 2007, which provide the procedural rules for hearings. The NMC's definition of fitness to practise is 'suitability to be on the register without any restrictions' (NMC 2011a).

The NMC has three statutory practice committees that deal with fitness to practise allegations:

1. Investigating Committee (IC)
2. Conduct and Competence Committee (CCC)
3. Health Committee (HC).

Hearings and meetings are held before a panel of the relevant committee. IC hearings and meetings are held in private. CCC hearings are nearly always heard in public, demonstrating the NMC's public accountability. However, this may depend upon the nature of the allegations, whether there is any public interest in dealing with them at a hearing and finally if it relates to the health of the registrant.

Midwifery wisdom

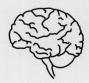
If you are ever asked to write a factual account as a student concerning care issues or allegations of misconduct, you should always speak with your midwifery lecturer or a supervisor of midwives who can offer professional support and guidance.

The White Paper *Trust, Assurance and Safety: the regulation of health professionals in the 21st century* (DH 2007 4.33, p66) states that 'the independence and impartiality of those who pass judgement on health professions in fitness to practise proceedings is central and professional confidence in their findings and the sanctions that they impose'. With this in mind, the NMC can demonstrate its independent approach to fitness to practise proceedings as NMC Council members are not allowed to sit on any of the fitness to practise panels. In addition, practice panel members who are appointed to the IC are unable to sit on the CCC and vice versa.

Each IC, CCC and HC panel must include a minimum of three members, one of whom must be from the same health professional field and is registered on the same part of the NMC register as the person concerned. Therefore if the person concerned is a midwife and the allegation relates to midwifery practice, one of the panel members must be a midwife. The panel must also include at least one lay member. The panels have a chair who may be a registered or lay person. It is envisaged that having lay members appointed will give the public greater confidence in the outcomes of fitness to practise hearings. Legal assessors must also be present: they are not panel members involved in the decision making but are present to clarify and advise on the various points of law. CCC hearings are held in public, but HC hearings are held in private to maintain registrants' confidentiality regarding their personal health matters.

The hearings are typically held at NMC offices throughout the UK. CCC hearings may be observed by the public and registrants. Encouraging midwives and student midwives to attend a hearing can give them a unique opportunity to further improve their understanding of the functions of the NMC fitness to practise procedures. The purpose of the visit is not to scare or promote anxiety but rather as a form of experiential learning.

Activity 13.2

If you would like to observe a hearing, access the NMC website www.nmc-uk.org, view the FtP pages and follow the instructions on 'attending a hearing as an observer'. Reservations may be made on line.

In order to increase your understanding of the nature of allegations and the outcomes, access the NMC website to read the outcomes of completed CCC hearings or click on this link: www.nmc-uk.org/Hearings/Hearings-and-outcomes/.

Allegations are heard through adjudication at hearings or meetings. The NMC describes 'adjudication' as 'the process of deciding whether an allegation is proved and, if so, what action or sanction to take' (NMC 2011b). Ultimately hearings/meeting must have the public interest and protection of the public as their primary focus. In addition, the interests of the registrant must also be balanced into the equation. It is important that the panels strive to uphold proper standards of conduct and maintain public confidence in the profession, i.e. its reputation. They must also provide fairness between the parties.

The reader may assume that many nurses/midwives are referred to the NMC and that many of those referred are ultimately 'struck off'. However, this is not the case. It is important to note that according to the NMC Annual Report 2011–2012 (NMC 2011c), there are over 671,000 nurses and midwives registered with the NMC in the UK and of those, approximately 0.6% are referred and less than 0.1% are given a sanction.

Activity 13.3

Make a list of what you consider are misdemeanours which may result in a referral to the NMC. Consider who can make a referral to the NMC.

The NMC Annual Report 2011–2012 (NMC 2011c) identifies that the highest percentages of referrals were made by the employer, followed by a member of the public, service user or patient and then the police. The Report identifies the types of allegations relating to misconduct, including, amongst others, patient neglect, maladministration of drugs, record keeping, dishonesty, abuse of patients/ colleagues (physical, sexual, verbal, inappropriate relationship), pornography, racism and sleeping on duty. Allegations relating to lack of competence include, amongst others, patient care, lack of knowledge, skill and judgement. Examples of criminal allegations may include alcohol/drugs misuse, theft, child pornography and murder.

Integral to the principles of justice is the necessity to separate investigation, prosecution and adjudication. In relation to hearings, essentially the order of proceedings is governed by the Nursing and Midwifery (Fitness to Practise) (Amendment) Rules Order of Council 2007. Fitness to practise proceedings are civil, not criminal proceedings. Allegations are first considered by the screening team which includes NMC officers. Their purpose in the main is to identify the nature of the allegation, establish whether the allegation falls within article 22(1) of the Nursing and Midwifery Order 2001 and to establish whether the allegation is in the form required by the NMC. It may be necessary for the team to undertake further enquiries to establish whether the allegations fall within the remit of the NMC. Having reviewed the case, the screening team will either close the case or refer to a practice committee under article 22(5). Generally cases are referred for further consideration to the IC. However, some cases are not relevant; for example, a member of the public who writes to the NMC to complain that her neighbour, who is a registered midwife, has a noisy dog.

The IC will review the evidence and may seek further information from NMC staff or legal firms acting on their behalf. The registrant is sent notice of the procedures and is duly informed at each stage of the process. Cases relating to a registrant's state of health may also require health reports. The panel will consider written representation from the registrant. Having gathered all the necessary information, an IC panel will convene and, after deliberation, conclude one of the following in respect of whether there is a case to answer in relation to an allegation of impaired fitness to practise in accordance with the Nursing and Midwifery Order 2001 article 26:

- No case to answer
- Case to answer in respect of an allegation of impaired fitness to practise – refer to CCC
- Case to answer in respect of an allegation of impaired fitness to practise relating to a health issue – refer to HC
- Refer to separate IC to consider allegations of fraudulent or incorrect entry on the register

The order of proceedings for CCC and HC is generally as follows. The panel is asked to consider whether the facts relating to the allegation are found proven. Since 2008 the panel uses the civil

237

standard of proof, namely the balance of probabilities, i.e. is more likely to be true than not (Nursing and Midwifery (Fitness to Practise) (Amendment) Rules Order of Council 2007). Following the fact finding stage, the panel must then consider whether the facts found proved amount to misconduct. The NMC (2011d) defines misconduct as 'Behaviour which falls short of what can reasonably be expected of a nurse or midwife'. If misconduct is found, the panel must next consider whether the registrant's fitness to practise is currently impaired (i.e. to remain on the register without any restrictions at the time of the hearing/meeting). It is often at this stage that the panel refers to the NMC standards, namely *The Code* (NMC 2008) and *Midwives' Rules and Standards* (NMC 2012a), to consider whether any have been breached and to what extent. The legal assessor presents to the panel any relevant case law which has set a precedent. This is applied during the panel's determination. Where a nurse or midwife has made an appeal against the outcome of a hearing to the High Court, the judgement can be used as a precedent for other hearings. In addition, appeals made through other professional regulatory bodies such as the General Medical Council and the Health Professional Council may also be cited. The relevant case may then be cited in the panel's determination.

The panel is invited to consider any mitigation the registrant may present. This might for example include personal or family circumstances that affected their practice. The panel may also be invited to take into consideration any favourable references or testimonials produced on the registrant's behalf in response to their current practice. During the impairment stage, the panel members are required to use their professional judgement rather than any specific legal standard of proof when considering the evidence.

At the final stage, if the panel finds that the registrant's fitness to practise is currently impaired then it may apply sanctions. If sanctions are being considered, the panel should refer to the NMC (2012b) *Indicative Sanctions Guidance to Panels*, 'to provide consistency and transparency in decision making'. The panel must have in mind the protection of the public, the public interest and the registrant's own interests. The sanctions available to the CCC and HC are set out in article 29(5) of the Nursing and Midwifery Order 2001 and are as follows:

- No case to answer
- Caution on records up to 5 years
- Impose conditions of practice for up to 3 years
- Suspend for up to 1 year then may extend
- Strike off (however, a panel cannot initially strike off immediately if impairment is as result of lack of competence or ill health unless the registrant has been suspended for 2 years)

Full details of the NMC *Indicative Sanctions Guidance* are available via the NMC website: www.nmc-uk.org/Documents/PanelSupportGroup/Green%20Guidance%20Documents/1785245%20ISG.PDF.

Article 31 rule 8 of the Nursing and Midwifery Order 2001 gives powers to the IC, CCC and HC to restrict the registrant's practice using Interim Orders (IO) whilst allegations are investigated or when the hearing has been concluded. Interim Orders may be in the form of suspension from practice or restrictions to practice. Following HC and CCC hearings, the registrant has up to 28 days to appeal so sanctions may not be enforced until the appeal period is over. Therefore if the CCC panel has made a striking-off order, a suspension order or a conditions of practice order, the panel may wish to invoke an IO. The panel must be satisfied that the following 'test' applies in order to invoke an IO: to protect the public or in the public interest (this includes maintaining confidence in the profession), or in the interests of the person concerned (NMC 2013). If the panel is satisfied that the IO meets one or more of these categories then an IO may be applied.

Figure 13.3 provides an overview of the NMC's fitness to practise procedures.

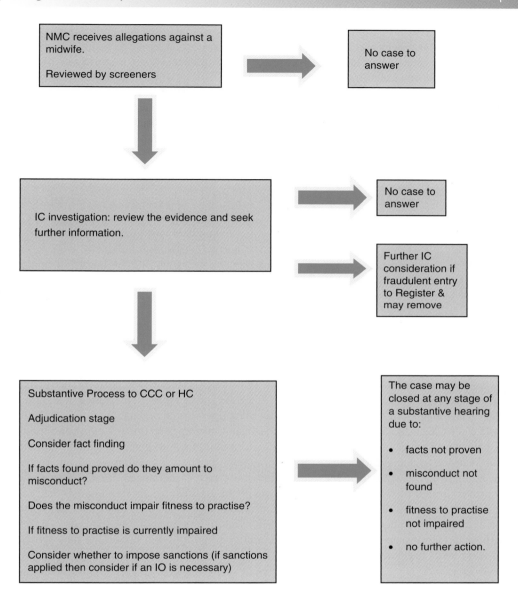

Figure 13.3   NMC fitness to practise procedures.

Who regulates the regulators?

Before 1st December 2012, the independent regulators for the NMC were known as the Council for Healthcare Regulatory Excellence (CHRE). The CHRE was established under the NHS Reform and Health Care Professions Act 2002. Its role was to ensure that regulatory bodies functioned to promote the interests of patients and the public. It included members from each of the regulatory bodies and oversaw the following regulatory bodies: General Medical Council, General Dental Council, Nursing and Midwifery Council, General Optical Council, General Osteopathic Council, Royal Pharmaceutical Society of GB,

Pharmaceutical Society of Northern Ireland and Health Professional Council. It endeavoured to promote best practice and consistency across the professions. Furthermore, it aimed to establish best principles for good professional self-regulation. The CHRE also had statutory powers to intervene in the conduct of the regulatory body if the public interest is not served.

Following completed NMC hearings, all cases were reviewed by the CHRE. Having read and considered individual cases, the CHRE had the power to refer cases of 'undue leniency' to the High Court under the provisions of section 29(4)(b) of the NHS Reform and Health Professions Act 2002. An example of this process can be found in the Council for Healthcare Regulatory Excellence v (1) Nursing and Midwifery Council (2) Grant [2011] EWHC 927 (Admin).

Activity 13.4

To read the judgment in full, use your browser and type in: CHRE v NMC and P Grant [2011] EWHC 927 (Admin). Click on the link [PDF] Judgment-CHRE.

Having read the Grant case via this link which details the facts and findings by Cox J, use the *Indicative Sanctions Guidance* (NMC 2012b) to consider what sanction you would apply. To read the final decision and reasons regarding the Grant case, access the following link:

www.nmc-uk.org/Documents/FTPOutcomes/2011/October2011/Reasons%20GRANT%20CCCSH %20%2020111010.pdf.

Recently the CHRE was commissioned to undertake a strategic review of NMC performance (CHRE 2012). In both its interim and final report, in January 2012, significant issues were identified in all areas within the NMC. Wide-ranging criticisms were made concerning operational management, people and culture issues, and the NMC's regulatory functions, with particular reference to underfunding and the management of cases. As part of its review, the CHRE has formulated a number of recommendations and a timescale in order to achieve the necessary improvements. There has been significant restructuring with new appointments within the NMC in order to initiate such vast changes. The CHRE anticipates that these improvements should be visible within 2 years (CHRE 2012).

From 1st December 2012 under the Health and Social Care Act 2012, the CHRE has legally been renamed as the Professional Standards Authority for Health and Social Care (PSA). Its responsibilities include those previously performed by the CHRE and in addition it will undertake new functions, for example social work regulation.

The Nursing and Midwifery Council and pre-registration midwifery education

The European Union Directive Recognition of Professional Qualifications 2005/36/EC Article 40 (Statutory Instrument 2005/3354, Statutory Instrument 2007/3101) defines midwifery and recognises the unique professional qualification that a midwife holds. This permits midwives, on successful completion of an approved midwifery training programme, to be admitted onto the midwifery part of the register and to be eligible to practise midwifery in the UK. It also allows midwives who qualified within 27 member countries of the EU to have the automatic right to join the NMC register and to practise midwifery in the UK. Article 5(1)] gives authority to the NMC to set the standards for education and training to qualify as a midwife.

Whilst the professional demands on midwives have evolved significantly since the turn of the century and the Midwives Act of 1902, the key tenets of setting standards for safe and effective midwifery practice at the point of registration remain paramount. In order for the key tenets to be met, the NMC sets the standards of midwifery education so that midwives are competent and capable of fully embracing the role of a midwife at the point of entry onto the register.

Activity 13.5

 Anyone can access the NMC register to search for a nurse or midwife by their PIN number and/or name. Practitioners holding effective registration on specific part(s) of the register can be identified which means they are eligible to practise in the UK. If you are a qualified midwife, use the link to search for your own or another midwife's practitioner details on the Search the Register page on the NMC website. www.nmc-uk.org/SearchRegisterResults?pid=o

241

The structure and content of midwifery education programmes

Figure 13.2 illustrates that a sound knowledge base is the cornerstone for safe and effective practice. It is necessary to enable midwives to practise within their 'scope of practice' rule 5 (NMC 2012a, p13) to ensure professional competence. The NMC has detailed the fundamental principles that must be encompassed within every midwifery education programme, against which student midwives must be able to demonstrate their competence:

- Provision of women-centred care
- Ethical and legal obligations
- Respect for individuals and communities
- Quality and excellence
- The changing nature and context of midwifery practice
- Lifelong learning
- Evidence-based practice

Specific to each principle above are certain competencies which students must achieve. These competencies are assessed through a variety of clinical and theoretical assessments to show that the required standard in each has been reached. These are identified under four domains: effective midwifery practice, professional and ethical practice, developing the midwife and others, and achieving quality care through evaluation and research. Against each domain relevant essential skill clusters (ESCs) are listed (NMC 2009b). Set progression points (i.e. at the end of each year) enable students' progress to be formally reviewed; a 12-week period built into programmes ensures that any outstanding assessments have been achieved before students are permitted to progress to the next level of study.

Whilst the NMC sets the education standards, it does not provide the training. This is devolved to universities. Universities wishing to provide a programme of midwifery education must attain NMC approval. This is to ensure that they meet the standards specified by the regulator. Although scope exists to develop innovative midwifery programmes, the NMC must be satisfied that these programmes meet all the requirements before issuing approval. This is done through a formal validation quality assurance process. Following initial approval, midwifery programmes must be reapproved by the NMC at regular intervals to ensure they remain current. The *Standards for Pre-Registration Midwifery Education* (NMC 2009b) set out the benchmarks expected by the NMC in terms of structure and content of all UK midwifery training programmes.

Activity 13.6

Use the *Standards for Pre-Registration Midwifery Education* (NMC 2009b) to consider the following aspects:

1. Make a list of the types of assessments that students may undertake during a midwifery programme.
2. Why are assessments undertaken at university and in practice?
3. Who is qualified to assess the student?

Assuring quality

The lead midwife for education (LME) holds a key statutory role in the quality assurance process. She is a practising midwife who holds a recorded midwifery teaching qualification and is responsible for professional leadership of midwifery in each university. Each approved institute of education (AEI) providing a midwifery education programme must have appointed a LME who 'forms an essential part of the quality assurance process and … must demonstrate to the NMC that the standards leading to either registration or a recording on the midwives' part of the register are being maintained' (NMC 2009b, p7). The LME therefore is the conduit of the NMC to ensure that the quality of midwifery education is maintained according to the standards. In addition to the NMC, LMEs must also work in close collaborative partnerships with other key groups to provide strategic direction on programme development and delivery and to ensure that appropriate numbers of students are trained to meet the demands of local maternity services. Most importantly, LMEs must ensure that education programmes meet the needs of women who use the maternity services (see Figure 13.4 which illustrates the interface of the LME with other groups).

Assuring quality relates not only to the quality of the education programmes but also to the quality of a student's character. In accordance with rule 6(1)(a)(ii) of the registration rules, under the Order (Statutory Instruments 2002/253), on successful completion of a student's training, the LME must sign the supporting declaration of good health and good character which is forwarded to the NMC to permit the student to be entered on to the NMC register. This is signed at the discretion of the LME and is a measure by which the NMC can be assured that at the point of entry, the student complies with the expectations set out in *The Code* (NMC 2008), a vital standard for ensuring public protection. Therefore, a student may have achieved success in all the theory and practice components of their educational programme but should evidence identify that she may not be of sufficient good health and/or good character, the LME has the right to refuse to sign the declaration. This is to ensure that students are able to provide safe and effective care for mothers and babies. Students need to be regularly reminded that, like qualified midwives, their conduct and professional behaviour both in and out of work may affect the profession they aspire to join. The NMC provides guidance on the professional conduct expected of nursing and midwifery students in order for them to be fit to practise (NMC 2011e).

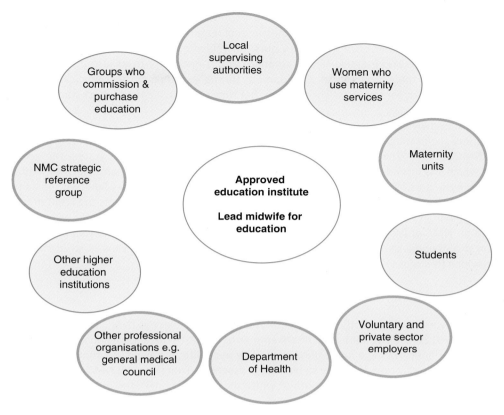

Figure 13.4 Interfacing with others.

Activity 13.7

In a group with the support of a supervisor of midwives, identify how you would define 'good health' and 'good character'.

- What sorts of behaviours might result in a student not being considered as meeting the standards expected of a midwife?
- In relation to a student's behaviour, why is this relevant outside work?

Following your discussion, summarise the key points and then refer to the *Guidance on Professional Conduct for Nursing and Midwifery Students* (NMC Nursing and Midwifery Council, NMC, 2011e) to checkyouranswers:www.nmc-uk.org/Documents/NMC-Publications/NMC-Guidance-on-professional-conduct.pdf.

Post-Registration Education and Practice (PREP) standards

Registration with the NMC is essential to enable newly qualified nurses and midwives to practise. Remaining on the NMC register is not automatic. The NMC requires that registrants renew their registration every 3 years, by means of a signed Notification of Practice (NOP) form and payment of the registration fee, paid each year and thereafter as a retention fee. On signing the NOP form, registrants are making a declaration that they have met the ongoing requirements to remain on part or parts of the register, depending on their profession, as a nurse or midwife. This is referred to as the NMC Post-Registration Education and Practice (PREP) standard and is necessary to ensure that nurses and midwives continue with their professional development throughout their professional careers in order to remain up to date with contemporary practice so that they can provide the highest standard of patient/client care.

In addition, midwives are also required to submit an annual Intention to Practise (ITP) form to their named supervisor of midwives (SOM) in accordance with current rule 3 (NMC Nursing and Midwifery Council, NMC, 2012a). The ITP form is a signed declaration by the midwife, stating the geographical region in which she intends to practise and also that she has met with her named SOM for supervisory review within the past 12 months. This is signed by the named SOM as verification that the named SOM is satisfied that the information about the midwife is correct and that she meets the NMC requirements regarding eligibility to practise. Failure to meet these will mean that the practitioner will be required to undertake an NMC approved return to nursing or midwifery course. A SOM is well placed to provide advice on professional development to midwives and the supervisory review is an ideal confidential forum in which to discuss these issues.

The PREP requirements

In this section we will explore the PREP requirements in more detail (NMC Nursing and Midwifery Council, NMC, 2011f) and use some practice examples to illustrate the application of PREP standards for individual practitioners. Being a nurse and/or midwife necessitates having the knowledge and skills for the role; thus the application of theory to practice is essential. Therefore the NMC PREP standards have two components, practice and theory, both of which must be demonstrated in order to remain eligible to practise as a nurse or midwife.

- *The PREP (Practice) Standard*: 'You must have worked in some capacity by virtue of your nursing or midwifery qualification during the previous 3 years for a minimum of 450 hours, or have successfully undertaken an approved return to practice course within the last 3 years' (NMC Nursing and Midwifery Council, NMC, 2011f, p4).
- *The PREP (Continuing Professional Development) Standard*: 'You must have undertaken and recorded your continuing professional development (CPD) over the 3 years prior to the renewal of your registration' (NMC Nursing and Midwifery Council, NMC, 2011f, p4).

The practice standard of 450 hours relates to the separate registration as a nurse or midwife. Therefore, if you are dual registered and wish to continue to practise as a nurse and midwife then the practice hours must be recorded separately for each professional part of the register. *The PREP Handbook* summarises the required practice standard (NMC Nursing and Midwifery Council, NMC, 2011f, p5).

The PREP (Continuing Professional Development) Standard requires that registrants have undertaken at least 35 hours of learning activity relevant to their practice during the 3 years prior to renewal of their registration. This can be formal learning such as a course, module or study. It can be informal and include activities such as a literature review on a particular topic area, reading and reflecting on an article, local policy or a professional discussion related to clinical practice. Whilst there is no official format, *The PREP Handbook* provides a helpful template to record your learning (NMC Nursing and Midwifery Council, NMC, 2011f, p9). The use of reflective models in recording PREP learning activities, such as outlined in Johns (1996) and Boud et al. (1985), is helpful as the stages of the reflective cycle can help practitioners return to a situation, and identify and document key thoughts and feelings about the incident.

Midwifery wisdom

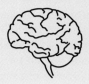

As soon as you commence your midwifery education and throughout your programme of study, you are strongly advised to keep a reflective diary, but please remember to ensure that the rules of confidentiality are maintained.

Activity 13.8

Eligibility to practise

With reference to *The PREP Handbook* (NMC Nursing and Midwifery Council, NMC, 2011f), consider the practitioner's situation and identify what she must do to remain eligible to practise and how she would provide assurance to the NMC that the standards are being achieved.

Rosa is employed as a practice nurse working in a GP clinic but she is also a registered midwife and would like to retain both qualifications. Her primary remit at work covers health promotion, sexual health and diabetes. She runs a diabetes clinic to which pregnant diabetic women are referred.

In terms of meeting her PREP requirements as a nurse and a midwife, what does she need to consider and to demonstrate in order to remain eligible to practise?

Eligibility to practise responses

As Rosa wishes to retain dual registration as a nurse and a midwife, she needs to record separately her nursing and midwifery practice hours in the 3 preceding years of submitting her NOP form. She is required to record 450 practice hours specifically relating to her nursing activities and 450 hours specific to midwifery practice. She cannot record the same practice hours twice, for example, the care she provides to pregnant women in the GP diabetic clinic, although some activities may relate to both her nursing and midwifery registration. As Rosa wishes to retain her midwifery qualification, she must submit her ITP to her named SOM each year in accordance to rule 3 (NMC Nursing and Midwifery Council, NMC, 2012a). She must also meet with her named SOM for her supervisory review. Rosa may wish to consider increasing her midwifery practice hours to ensure she meets the midwifery practice standards; this may include applying for an annualised midwifery contract or working as a bank midwife. In addition, Rosa will need to undertake 35 practice hours of CPD activities that are relevant to her nursing and midwifery practice to ensure she remains up to date.

The future of PREP: moving towards revalidation

The current arrangements for achieving PREP have been well established since the inception of the NMC PREP standards in 2004, following the shift from the UKCC triennial refresher courses for midwives. The present system relies on various strategies as previously discussed to assure the NMC that individuals are meeting the requirements. However, Council acknowledges that these current methods could be strengthened to ensure greater consistency in providing assurance that all practitioners are achieving the standards (NMC Nursing and Midwifery Council, NMC, 2012c).

This process is under review; the NMC argues that revalidation will ensure the continuing fitness to practise of nurses and midwives after initial NMC registration (NMC Nursing and Midwifery Council, NMC, 2012c). It is likely that revalidation processes in the future will include some of the steps currently in place such as self-declaration and audit. These are in addition to other measures and systems applied by employers, nurses and midwives which support maintenance of fitness to practise beyond the point of initial registration, one such example being appraisal. Midwifery is a useful model to explore for revalidation as it includes supervision of midwives. It is anticipated that by 2014, revalidation will be introduced as the means by which an effective, evidence-based and affordable system will provide ongoing, robust assurance to the NMC that nurses and midwives are fit to practise.

Conclusion

The Nursing and Midwifery Council is the professional body which regulates nurses and midwives in the United Kingdom. Its ultimate aim is to protect and maintain the safety of the public. This chapter has outlined the four statutory functions of the NMC which govern the regulation of nurses and midwives. Activities have been included to encourage readers to consider how codes, rules, standards and guidance apply to practice dilemmas and professional situations which midwives and nurses encounter on a regular basis. It is anticipated that readers will have a deeper understanding and embrace the regulatory framework as a means to support practice and women's choices. The importance of public protection as the key tenet of the NMC is emphasised and the consequences of breaching the regulations are discussed, illustrated with examples drawn from real life.

The NMC is regulated by the PSA. In order to practise safely and competently, midwives need to work within the NMC standards and guidance. The NMC fitness to practise procedures aim to reassure the public that there is an impartial process for investigating allegations, thereby promoting public confidence in its self-regulatory function. The NMC endeavours to provide a system which is efficient in protecting the public and maintaining public confidence in the profession. However, whilst there are challenges ahead for the NMC, protection of the public has to remain at the heart of professional regulation.

Activity 13.9

Suggested responses to scenarios 1–4

Scenario 1
Following the doctor's request, Abby should consider whether there is any evidence to support the procedure. If the request is based on anecdotal evidence or just personal preference then Abby could refer to *The Code*: 'Provide a high standard of practice and care at all times' (NMC Nursing and Midwifery Council, NMC, 2008, p6). *The Code* identifies that 'care must be based on best available evidence'. In addition, the client herself does not want to have this procedure so the client has not given her consent (p3).

Scenario 2
On this occasion it appears that Mary tried to explain the procedure by gesticulating. However, if a client does not speak English it is very difficult to be sure that she understands and that the

requirements for a valid consent are met (NMC Nursing and Midwifery Council, NMC, 2008, p3). In addition, *The Code* identifies that 'arrangements to meet people's language and communication needs' should be made (p3), so it would be appropriate to find a suitable interpreter in this situation.

Scenario 3
Rule 5 of the *Midwives' Rules and Standards* provides helpful advice and guidance. Gita must ensure that Sarah's needs are the primary focus of her practice and should 'work in partnership with the woman and her family' (NMC Nursing and Midwifery Council, NMC, 2012a, p15). Should Sarah decide to birth at home, Gita must respect this decision and support her wishes by continuing to provide the highest standards of midwifery care. In planning this, Gita may need professional support and guidance from a SOM. The SOM may help Gita to identify and address any learning needs she may have to ensure that she recognises any deviations that arise and acts appropriately.

Scenario 4
In this situation Liz is currently on sick leave from work and has therefore been assessed as not being fit enough to work. As such, Liz is in breach of rule 5 (NMC Nursing and Midwifery Council, NMC, 2012a). Whilst it may have been her intention to provide support to Jo as a friend during labour, on arrival Liz had adequate time to contact the on-call midwife to attend the delivery. Had she done this, Liz still could have remained with Jo as a friend but without providing midwifery care. In making the decision to take her community bag and home birth equipment to Jo's home, Liz demonstrated that it was more likely than not that she intended to provide midwifery care. In accordance with rule 9, 'Supervision and reporting' (NMC Nursing and Midwifery Council, NMC, 2012a, p26), 24 hours access to a SOM would have been available, so Liz should have contacted the SOM as a source of professional advice and guidance to enable her to practise within her statutory framework.

References

Boud D, Keogh R, Walker D (1985) *Reflection: turning experience into learning*. London: Kogan Page.

Council for Healthcare Regulatory Excellence (CHRE) v (1) Nursing and Midwifery Council (2) Grant [2011] EWHC 927 (Admin). Available at: www.chre.org.uk/_img/pics/library/110414_Grant_Judgment.pdf (accessed May 2013).

Council for Healthcare Regulatory Excellence (CHRE) (2012) *Performance Review Report 2011–2012*. Available at: http://tinyurl.com/cshudys (accessed May 2013).

Department of Health (DH) (2004) Independent Investigation into How the NHS Handled Allegations about the Conduct of Clifford Ayling. London: Department of Health.

Department of Health (DH) (2007) *Trust, Assurance and Safety: the regulation of health professionals in the 21st century (White Paper)*. Available at: www.official-documents.gov.uk/document/cm70/7013/7013.pdf (accessed May 2013).

European Union Directive Recognition of Professional Qualifications 2005/36/EC Article 40 (Statutory Instrument 2005/3354, Statutory Instrument 2007/3101).

Health and Social Care Act 2012 (Consequential Amendments – the Professional Standards Authority for Health and Social Care) Order 2012. http://legislation.data.gov.uk/uksi/2012/2672/made/data.htm?wrap=true (accessed May 2013).

Johns C (1996) Visualizing and realizing caring in practice through guided reflection. *Journal of Advanced Nursing* **24**: 1135–43.

Kennedy I (2001) *Learning from Bristol: The Report of the Public Enquiry into Children's Heart Surgery at The Bristol Royal Infirmary 1984–1995*. London: HMSO.

National Health Service Reform and Health Professions Act (2002) www.legislation.gov.uk/ukpga/2002/17/contents (accessed May 2013).

Nursing and Midwifery Council (2004) (Fitness to Practise) Rules Order of Council Statutory Instrument 2004 No. 1761. London: Nursing and Midwifery Council.

Nursing and Midwifery Council (Fitness to Practise) (Amendment) Rules Order of Council 2007. London: Nursing and Midwifery Council.

Nursing and Midwifery Council (NMC) (2008) *The Code: standards of conduct, performance and ethics for nurses and midwives*. Available at: www.nmc-uk.org/Documents/Standards/The-code-A4-20100406.pdf (accessed May 2013).

Nursing and Midwifery Council (NMC) (2009a) *Record Keeping: guidance for nurses and midwives*. Available at: www.nmc-uk.org/Documents/NMC-Publications/NMC-Record-Keeping-Guidance.pdf (accessed May 2013).

Nursing and Midwifery Council (NMC) (2009b) *Standards for Pre-Registration Midwifery Education*. London: Nursing and Midwifery Council.

Nursing and Midwifery Council (NMC) (2010) *Standards for Medicines Management*. Available at: www.nmc-uk.org/Documents/NMC-Publications/NMC-Standards-for-medicines-management.pdf (accessed May 2013).

Nursing and Midwifery Council (NMC) (2011a) *What is Fitness to Practise?* Available at: www.nmc-uk.org/Hearings/What-is-fitness-to-practise (accessed May 2013).

Nursing and Midwifery Council (NMC) (2011b) *How the Process Works*. Available at: www.nmc-uk.org/Hearings/How-the-process-works (accessed May 2013).

Nursing and Midwifery Council (NMC) (2011c) *Nursing and Midwifery Council Annual Fitness to Practise Report 2010–2011*. London: Nursing and Midwifery Council.

Nursing and Midwifery Council (NMC) (2011d) *Misconduct*. Available at: www.nmc-uk.org/Employers-and-managers/Fitness-to-practise/Misconduct (accessed May 2013).

Nursing and Midwifery Council (NMC) (2011e) *Guidance on Professional Conduct for Nursing and Midwifery Students*. London: Nursing and Midwifery Council.

Nursing and Midwifery Council (NMC) (2011f) *The PREP Handbook*. Available at: www.nmc-uk.org/Documents/Standards/NMC_Prep-handbook_2011.pdf (accessed May 2013).

Nursing and Midwifery Council (NMC) (2012a) *Midwives' Rules and Standards*. Available at: www.nmc-uk.org/Documents/NMC-Publications/Midwives%20Rules%20and%20Standards%202012.pdf (accessed May 2013).

Nursing and Midwifery Council (NMC) (2012b) *Indicative Sanctions Guidance to Panels*. Available at: www.nmc-uk.org/Documents/PanelSupportGroup/Green%20Guidance%20Documents/1785245%20ISG.PDF (accessed May 2013).

Nursing and Midwifery Council (NMC) (2012c) *The NMC and Revalidation*. London: Nursing and Midwifery Council.

Nursing and Midwifery Council (NMC) (2013) *Guidance to Panels Considering Whether to Make an Interim Order*. Available at: www.nmc-uk.org/Documents/PanelSupportGroup/Green%20Guidance%20Documents/Guidance%20to%20panels%20considering%20whether%20to%20make%20an%20IO.PDF (accessed June 2013).

RedfernM (2001) *The Royal Liverpool Children's Inquiry*. London: House of Commons.

Smith J (2004) *Shipman Inquiry Fifth Report: safeguarding patients: lessons from the past – proposals for the future*. London: HMSO.

Statutory Instruments 2002/253 The Nursing and Midwifery Order 2001 No. 253. Available at: www.legislation.gov.uk/uksi/2002/253/made/data.pdf (accessed May 2013).

14

The Impact of Cultural Issues on the Practice of Midwifery

Celia Wildeman

Aim

The aim of this chapter is to explore contemporary issues that influence midwifery practice in the context of culture-sensitive care so that midwives can address the emerging challenges in the best interests of their clients.

Learning outcomes

By the end of the chapter you will be able to:

1. define culture and differentiate between culture, race and ethnicity
2. critically analyse and debate contemporary issues that arise in the context of culturally sensitive midwifery care
3. evaluate personal/professional practice and consider how to construct a workable philosophy of client care that will make a difference to the provision and delivery of high-class and culturally sensitive care
4. discuss the importance of the role and function of an interprofessional team approach to midwifery care and how this can create a climate of tolerance and change
5. reflect on and critically examine the impact of power dynamics on the interprofessional team and clients.

The Student's Guide to Becoming a Midwife, Second Edition. Edited by Ian Peate and Cathy Hamilton.
© 2014 John Wiley & Sons, Ltd. Published 2014 by John Wiley & Sons, Ltd.

Introduction

Literature and research have consistently highlighted the extent of the motivation or non-motivation of midwives to engage with the concept of culture and even to embrace people from the diverse cultural mix who entrust their lives to them (Rowe & Garcia 2005). Houghton (2008) holds the view that caring for a woman who speaks little or no English and often has complex care needs is a common occurrence for many midwives in the UK today.

Indeed, the essential nature of midwives working in a culturally sensitive manner has long had a steady footing in midwifery circles (Bowler 2008, English National Board 2001). A moder midwife lives and works in a complex multiracial and multicultural society, one in which she is perceived as a role model, friend, confidante and advocate (Hunt 2003). It is therefore vital that she is able to think, feel and act inside and outside the societal box to enhance midwifery care for those of her clients who are considered already to be at a disadvantage in society.

Some midwives may shy away from political issues that have a direct impact on the care of the client. Two such political issues are poverty and health inequalities. (Smith et al. 2005). Thinking outside the box would require the midwife to move away from what would be considered safe territory (Wickham 2007). She would need to network with agencies and personnel who would not normally be considered part of the healthcare team. Agencies such as the Citizens Advice Bureau (CAB) have resources and expertise potentially useful to the clients to whom this chapter intends to give a voice. The National Institute for Health and Clinical Excellence (NICE) (2008) provides up-to-date and evidence-based literature and guidance to healthcare professionals and women. It emphasises to women that 'your care and the information you are given about it should take account of any religious, ethnic or cultural needs you may have'. Indeed, the significance of the client and health professional being aware of the role of advocacy in enhancing quality care was stated (NICE 2008).

Case study 14.1

 Helen Begum was born in Birmingham though her parents are from Pakistan. She speaks fluent English but because of her cultural beliefs and practices, she is having problems conforming to what are considered the norms of antenatal care.
How would you define culture?

There is no one definition of culture and it is important not to be constrained by any one definition; howeverm it is useful to have ideas around the concept of culture. This may offer the student of midwifery and midwives guiding tools that can enhance understanding of the diverse needs and expectations of people, such as Helen, who may be similar and different from themselves.

It may also facilitate a mindset in which they are receptive to change in the way they perceive clients who do not visibly conform to the norms of society, for example, travellers, refugees and asylum seekers (Wiseman 2011). Risk to health increases because of different health-seeking behaviours of different cultural groups (Bridle 2012, Wiseman, 2011;). The Nursing and Midwifery Council (NMC) requires midwives to act as advocates for those in their care, helping them to access relevant health and social care, information and support (NMC 2008).

These norms of society are not usually transparent particularly to people who may have limited language skills and also low or infrequent exposure to people and/or experiences from the dominant culture. They do, however, have equality rights and in some cases protection from discrimination (Griffith 2010).

There is no one 'lens' through which to construct a definition of culture (Hoffman 2007). This is because the midwife is often unconscious of her thinking, feelings and actions that may be influencing her decision making and attitudes to a particular client. Burr (2003) warns against the tendency to believe that knowledge and assumptions that guide us in our dealings with other people are 'truths'. She is of the opinion that 'our current accepted ways of understanding the world is a product not of objective observation of the world, but of the social processes and interactions in which people are constantly engaged with each other'. This view is supported by Reynolds & Manfusa (2005), who argued that a significant number of midwives do not believe that cultural issues are relevant or significantly important. Their lack of awareness and familiarity of interaction with people from diverse cultural backgrounds prevent them gaining deeper understanding of the cultural aspects of midwifery care. Reynolds & Manfusa therefore suggest that midwives give greater priority to getting to know about the client's cultural beliefs and expectations so as to meet their individual needs and preferences. Sudworth et al. (2012) endorse this view. They highlighted the significance of trust in the midwife–woman relationship and asserted that 'communication is the key to effective delivery of care and in understanding cultural barriers which may impinge on the quality of care' (Sudworth et al. 2012, Thompson 2003).

For the purposes of this chapter, various definitions will be suggested to facilitate the student's autonomy in determining a personal working definition of culture; this free choice is in keeping with the philosophy that underpins the contents and tone of the text. The expectation is that midwives and student midwives will feel personally committed to working in a culturally sensitive way with their clients rather than just doing it because it is a professional obligation. Development of cultural competence is vital to a high standard of midwifery care.

Schott & Henley (2007) expressed the view that culture is a set of norms, values, assumptions and perceptions (both explicit and implicit) and social conventions which enable members of a group, community or nation to function cohesively. Schott & Henley are of the opinion that 'culture vitally affects every aspect of our daily life, how we live, think, behave and how we view and analyse the world'.

Burnham & Harris (2002) argue for the usefulness of understanding the difference between three inter-related concepts, namely, race, ethnicity and culture. They define race as 'a personal biological inheritance'. Clearly a person's race is immediately apparent and assumptions, stereotypes and equally dangerous judgements can be readily made which are believed to be truths (Burr 2003). Culture is defined (Burnham & Harris 2002) as 'the social network within which conversations about race and ethnicity evolve' and ethnicity is the 'way a person thinks about the biological inheritance'. They imply that the meaning of ethnicity and culture is constantly emerging and changing; they are not static concepts but dynamic. This suggests that as the practitioner familiarises herself with the client's cultural norms and expectations, she will be more willing to become transparent about prejudices, ideas and practices so that her ideas and biases may become more open and available for refreshment and reconstruction (Burnham & Harris 2002, Sudworth et al. 2012).

Helman (2007) defines culture as a 'set of guidelines that individuals inherit as members of a particular society, and that tell them how to view the world, how to experience it emotionally and how to behave in it in relation to other people, to supernatural forces or gods and to the natural environment'. Norms and rules are usually obscure and only come to light when they are broken. Midwives are in a privileged position in which they have the necessary education and training (NICE 2010) accept difference in their clients' knowledge and behaviour without judging them harshly.

There are many similarities in the authors' definitions of culture in that they have personal, familiar and societal connotations. However, Helman (2007) highlights the significance of an individual's belief system around the kind of person she is or can become, personal responsibility or even duty to transmit these beliefs across generations by the 'use of symbols, language, art and ritual'. It is apparent that the client's cultural lens through which she perceives and understands her world is extremely important to her and will be fiercely protected from perceived threat by anyone, including the midwife, who may seem likely to do harm.

Case study 14.2

 Amy is 16 years old. She is a single young woman who has limited social support. She is at the antenatal clinic for a routine check up at 28 weeks' gestation. Your practice mentor has asked you to do the antenatal examination. This includes questioning Amy about her well-being. On enquiring about her nutritional state, you discover that she is not eating regularly and sufficiently. She is worried about finance and identifies this as the main reason why she is neglecting her nutitional intake.

How would you go about finding a solution to this problem?

When responding to Case study 14.2, it is important that Amy is treated with respect and concern, which includes not falling into a parent/child mode of conversation (Walsh 2005). The student is in a powerful position because Amy, like most women, wants the best for her baby and is therefore receptive to advice even when it is not given in a sensitive manner. It would be helpful to show genuine curiosity about the reasons why she felt that she could not afford nutritious food. Once you have gathered the relevant information, it is important to consult your practice mentor so that a possible solution can be found. This might be to:

- arrange for the community or teenage pregnancy midwife to visit Amy at home. This might enable her to feel supported and the midwife to assess her social situation and needs
- refer her to the dietician so that her nutritional needs can be determined and she can increase her motivation to meet the dietary requirements necessary to sustain a healthy pregnancy
- provide her with information about the CAB so that she can enquire about her eligibility for social benefits
- think further outside the box and make an appointment to see her Member of Parliament to discuss pregnancy-related issues in the context of poverty and inequalities.

Having considered Case study 14.2, the midwifery student should be in a position to consolidate a working definition of culture. This may facilitate a mindset that supports a personal and professional position where she treats her clients as individuals irrespective of their cultural or other differences.

The morality of working in a cultural context

Hart et al. (2003) highlight the 'positive ways in which health professionals work, often in stressful and under-resourced contexts', to achieve health benefits for disadvantaged groups of clients. However, though they acknowledge this positive approach, they stress that this is not universal. They highlight the consistent nature of evidence of how interactions between health professionals, healthcare institutions and service users result in clients feeling oppressed and humiliated rather than cared for, particularly in the case of disadvantaged service users. These are issues also revealed by he Centre for Maternal and Child Enquiries (CEMACE 2011) and (Esegbona-Adeigbe 2011). It is important that practitioners feel good about the way they work with their clients. However, it is also necessary for midwives to be willing to reflect on and face the challenges and criticisms about any shortfall in care provision and/or delivery that negatively impacts on clients who already suffer disadvantages in the society in which they live (Ahmad & Bradby 2009).

Carter (2001) asserts that by having a 'greater understanding of ourselves through developed self-awareness we are more likely to have increased self-respect, which in turn leads to a greater respect of others'. It appears that the practitioner's sense of self, who she is, how she arrived at this awareness and the social and professional context in which she operates provides a rich source of information that will inform her moral and ethical position.

The NMC (2008) supports an ethico-legal position of equity for all the midwife's clients/patients. It states that:

> all registered nurses, midwives and specialist community public health nurses are person-ally accountable for their practice and that they should in the exercise of their duty:
>
> - respect the patient/client as an individual
> - obtain consent before you give any treatment and care
> - protect confidential information
> - co-operate with others in the team
> - maintain your professional knowledge and competence
> - be trustworthy
> - act to identify and minimise risk to patients and clients.

Case study 14.3

Jane has arrived on the delivery suite and is in established labour. She is a single white woman with no supportive birth partner. She is extremely scared and appears not to be coping well with the pain.

You are the student midwife allocated to care for Jane. After the initial history taking and measuring of vital signs, you inform your practice mentor of your findings and discuss the plan of care. Jane did not complete her birth plan. She has, however, stated that she does not want any male professionals involved in her care.

What are the ethical issues?

The student midwife may be aware that she has a duty to care for Jane in as non-judgemental a way as possible. Ethically, she needs to take the time to interact with Jane and find out what are her needs and expectations. In this case, there were no visible clues about why Jane decided not to accept care from male professionals. She had the usually considered British name of Jane, and spoke English articulately.

An exploratory approach based on Jane's right to choose would have discovered that she was of a Muslim faith that she did not disclose at her booking assessment as she felt that this information would be perceived negatively. It is also useful to consider that, in the past, Jane may have experienced violence, sexual abuse or inappropriate treatment that would cause her to be distrustful of men. She was extremely afraid of being judged by health professionals and did not want to jeopardise her care and that of her baby.

In this case it would be good practice for the midwife to keep an open mind, listen actively, be supportive and empathic. The midwife would also be acting as an advocate by informing the multiprofessional team on a need-to-know basis and documenting Jane's wishes to ensure that quality care can be continued and a record is maintained.

The NMC (2008) in the *Code of Professional Conduct* also states that registrants must 'recognise and respect the role of patients and clients as partners in their care and the contribution they can make to it'. It continues that the practitioner should identify the client's preferences regarding care and respect these within the limits of professional practice, existing legislation, resources and goals of the therapeutic relationship. These ethical ideals are well supported by the Equality Act (2006) which will be discussed later in the chapter.

Indeed, you are personally accountable for ensuring that you promote and protect the interests and dignity of patients and clients, irrespective of gender, age, race, ability, sexuality, economic status, lifestyle, culture and religions or political beliefs. In the case discussed in Case study 14.3, Jane clearly needed the support of a non-judgemental, culturally sensitive midwife who could see beyond her decision not to have male professionals involved in her care. The potential for upholding difference and therefore inducing conflict would then be avoided and a more positive alliance ensured. Jane's right to 'autonomous' (NMC 2008) decision making in this instance would meet with the NMCs approval and the Equality Act which 'aims to ensure that people are treated fairly and equally' and 'enjoy the privileges of fairness and respect irrespective of who or where ever they are' (Commission for Equality and Human Rights 2006).

Similar ethical/moral positions are expressed by various authors. For example, Quinn & Harding (2001) endorse the government's view that 'NHS care has to be shaped around the convenience and concerns of patients'. To achieve this goal, it is considered that 'patients must have more say in their own treatment and more influence over the way the NHS works' (DH 2004a).

Clearly, the morality of midwifery care is complex. In professional practice, the practitioner's ethical position can conflict with her beliefs around how she would like to conduct herself as a midwife and the image she portrays. Ethical decisions are not straightforward.

Case study 14.4

Chloe has stated in her birth plan that she wishes for a natural birth. This means that she does not want technology as a means to monitor progress of the baby.

She is admitted to the antenatal ward as her blood pressure is elevated, there is protein in her urine and oedema of her face and sacral area. It is normal professional practice as part of the assessment of her care to carry out a cardiotocograph. Chloe has refused to give her consent to have fetal monitoring.

How would you deal with this situation?

In response to the previous case study, there are several approaches that could be considered. You may try to persuade Chloe to think more widely about her options, after showing her that you are receptive and sensitive to her decision by acknowledging positively that she made this decision in the best interests of herself and her baby. However, her circumstances have changed in that she and her baby are at increased risk of obstetric complications that could affect their well-being. Her blood pressure is elevated, there is proteinuria and non-dependent oedema. All three signs are suggestive of pre-eclampsia, an obstetric complication of pregnancy that increases the chances of a poor outcome for the client and her baby. It is important to document Jane's wishes and concerns and refer the case to a midwife or your mentor for further action.

The ethical dilemma in this case is enormous. The right of Chloe to be autonomous and make her own decisions creates tensions with the professional duty of the midwife to 'act to identify and minimise risk to patients and clients' (NMC 2008). Indeed, to exercise her accountability and responsibility the midwife must provide 'safe and competent' care (NMC 2008).

Midwifery practice in a culturally sensitive climate of care

Today midwives work in a climate of change, one in which collaboration and partnerships need to be forged to ensure delivery of good standards of care. Fletcher (2001) expressed the view that the midwife should build on existing partnerships (e.g. obstetricians, paediatricians) and develop new ones, for example, with the private and voluntary sectors, that will enable midwives to respond positively to the challenges of 'the new NHS'.

One of the biggest challenges for the midwife of today is her ability to understand and act upon the diverse needs and expectations of a multicultural clientele. Helman (2007) observes that the tendency to generalise is ever present. For example, blanket policies and procedures are put in place to meet the needs of clients of all cultures irrespective of the relevance to them as individuals. Breastfeeding policies, for example, sometimes create immense stress and unhappiness for many clients and their families who are expected to accept rules and customs that are alien to them. The potential for conflict is ever present, one of the reasons being that people, including healthcare professionals, make assumptions that they believe to be truth. Helman (2007) therefore asserts that one should differentiate between 'the rules of a culture, which govern how one should think and behave, and how people actually behave in real life'. This guideline is worthy of note in particular because generalisations can be dangerous, for they often lead to the development of stereotypes and then to cultural misunderstandings, prejudices and discrimination (Helman 2007). The midwife's professional practice must therefore be grounded in best available evidence and guided by her employer's policies and procedures.

Activity 14.1

Read the equal opportunities policy associated with your current placement. It might be useful to organise a study group including peers and colleagues and share the content and your findings.

Following this, invite your mentor(s) to a discussion group and reflect on what is required from you by your employer.

What are the possible implications for your developing midwifery practice?

Some of the following might have emerged:

- The employer's expectations of the practitioner's interactions with clients.
- The legal framework that governs the practice of midwives in the context of equal opportunities, fairness and justice.
- The sanctions that are in place to monitor, control and discipline practitioners who do not achieve the legal and/or professional standard.
- Your own and others' theoretical and personal codes of ethics for delivery of client care.

The values you hold personally and professionally will influence your treatment of clients irrespective of the culture. Fry (2002) states that 'a value is a worthwhile standard or quality of a person or social group'. She reminds practitioners that 'cultural values are the accepted and dominant standards of a particular cultural group'. Indeed, these values function in conjunction with belief systems to give 'meaning and worth to the existence and experiences of the group'. The midwife therefore in daily practice

255

needs to be aware that 'every culture has values and beliefs about health and illness and about what is morally acceptable behaviour in the provision of health promoting care to people' (Fry 2002). Some cultures, for example the British, 'place a high premium on the sovereignty of the individual and the rights of the individual to make choices about their lives' (Fry 2002). Others, for example, people of traditional Greek and Italian origin and many traditional groups founded in South Asia, place a high value on the family, collective and communal decision making and the 'over-riding obligation of individual family members to place the interest of their family above their own' (Fry 2002).

Clearly, these descriptions of some cultural ways of being are not absolute. There are bound to be subcultures within these that may not necessarily comply with the majority of their cultural group. This highlights the need for clarity by the midwife in her dealings with cultural group members. It is important for her to be aware that sameness is not synonymous with those who appear to be from the same or similar cultural groups. Racial (and indeed cultural) stereotyping in midwifery has been shown to negatively influence the care of women, for example Asian women (Kirkham et al. 2002, Rowe & Garcia 2005). Informed choice and decision making by midwifery clients can be influenced significantly by the predisposition to place clients in the straitjacket of stereotyping.

The Confidential Enquiry into Maternal and Child Health (CEMACE 2011), in providing its findings and recommendations for midwifery practice, highlights some of the following risk factors for maternal deaths:

- social disadvantage
- poor communities
- minority ethnic groups
- late booking and poor attendance
- domestic violence.

All of these are of key relevance to the culturally diverse groups that midwives interact with on a daily basis. This heightened awareness, with compounding evidence to support it, has the potential to persuade midwives to take the lead in pushing for change. This is necessary to improve the lives of their clients by facilitating acceptance rather than exclusion and indeed to reduce maternal and perinatal mortality and morbidity (CEMACE 2011).

Skinner (2001) has warned of the difficulties that midwives will face if they are unable to cultivate a culture of change. The significant ingredient, according to Skinner (2001), is empowerment, autonomy and increasing confidence that the care they give to their clients is relevant to their needs and preferences. The issue of self-belief needs to be added to this assertion. Midwives are the lead professional in over 70% of maternity cases, and the challenge of change is an exciting venture for some (Skinner 2001). The opposing view is that traditional beliefs and attitudes to care inevitably will be affected and lead to dissonance and possible outright fear. However, midwives need to be prepared to lead the campaign for change in the best interests of their disadvantaged clients.

The CEMACE (2011) and Raven et al. (2007) emphasise the important role of midwives in ensuring that local maternity services reach and maintain contact with all pregnant women. This, they suggest, could be achieved through various basic yet essential processes, for example advocating for professional interpreters for women who do not speak English and the 'strengthening or development of a robust and effective communication system'. The important value of statutory midwifery supervision (CEMACE 2011; LSA 2012) in providing impetus for change in the form of the midwife developing and utilising skills of advocacy, antidiscriminatory and antioppressive practices clearly is relevant to midwifery care in the 21st century and beyond. Midwifery practice must be clothed in high principles and values that put clients at the centre of all that is done by the midwife. As the CEMACE (2011) points out, many midwives carry out their work in the context of deprivation and poverty and with women having difficulty accessing services. At the same time, 'the midwife may often be the only professional who is able to build an element of trust with the woman' (CEMACE 2011).

How the midwife organises and delivers her practice will influence the quality of the maternity experience that the client receives as well as the midwife's satisfaction in her work. The midwife must be aware that 'where the services are not meeting the medical or cultural needs of women, midwives act as advocates to ensure that appropriate services are delivered, interpreting services are available and cross-organisational communication is of the highest standard' (CEMACE 2011). That is the stuff that midwifery practice should be made of and maybe the power dynamic will then change to one of equity rather than midwife domination, as can appear presently to be the case.

The power dynamics of midwifery practice

The *Code of Professional Conduct* expects registered practitioners, including the midwife, to 'recognise and respect the role of patients and clients as partners in their care and the contribution they can make to it' (NMC 2008). Indeed, the practitioner is accountable for ensuring that she 'promotes and protects the interests and dignity of patients and clients, irrespective of gender, age, race, ability, sexuality, economic status, lifestyle, culture and religion or political beliefs'. According to the meaning of the above guidance, the midwife is accountable to her clients to ensure that they receive as good a quality of care, however they define it, as received by anyone from the dominant culture. Kitzinger (2000) asserts that 'birth is women's business, takes place in women's space and is choreographed by women'. Though Kitzinger (2000) made her comments in the birth context, they are also relevant to any situation in which midwives interact with their clients.

Burr (2003) believes that power can be thought of as the 'extent of a person's access to sought after resources, such as money, leisure time, rewarding jobs and the extent to which they have the capacity to have some effect on their world'. The ability to influence your environment can only become a reality through empowerment brought about as a result of being treated equally. The White Paper *Fairness for All* (DH 2004b) suggests that 'unjust treatment can make a person feel isolated, scared and misunderstood'. This is a situation that midwives can prevent through proactivity and insightfulness.

Midwives have resources available to them (knowledge and skills) and this puts them in a powerful position; clients want and need these available resources, particularly those who are disadvantaged because of cultural differences. They are positioned within minority groups rather than the dominant cultural group which inevitably means that they constantly jostle for scarce resources, human and material. Midwives therefore should not be complacent but humble and appreciative of their powerful position. They can use this to influence policy and change and to empower rather than exclude clients who already suffer the effects of substandard care (CEMACE 2011). Burr (2003) supports the notion that 'knowledge increases a person's power'. She asserts Foucault's (1976) idea that 'knowledge is power over others, the power to define others'.

To change the dynamics of unequal power positions between the midwife and her culturally disadvantaged clients, midwives need to be committed to instigating and delivering care that is antidiscriminatory and antioppressive, so as to meet the individual needs of clients and their families and to comply with legal requirements (Griffith 2010). 'Individuals have no control over the cultural background in which they are born' (Millen 2002). Thompson (2009) asserts that professionals should 'value diversity' and that 'developing antidiscriminatory practice is an essential part of good practice'. However, he acknowledges that issues to do with this aspect of care are a 'minefield of difficulties at both a theoretical and practical level' (Thompson 2009).

Information giving and receiving are time intensive in the role and responsibilities of the midwife. In the current climate, where clients and midwives alike perceive her as extremely busy, the midwife needs

257

always to be aware that the power of communicating at all levels and in all contexts is axiomatic to her very survival.

Activity 14.2

The student of midwifery may find the cultural awareness quiz at the end of this chapter useful and interesting. It will enable her to develop curiosity about her clients. Interest in clients (Henderson 2005) enhances familiarity and this in turn breaks down cultural barriers (Reynolds & Manfusa 2005).

Focusing on individual difference, familiarity around cultural groups and the willingness to orientate to the needs and expectations of these client groups will stand the student of midwifery in good stead. Axten (2003) is of the opinion that 'feeling secure means being in control and that placing ourselves in positions where we can control others increases our sense of security'. Midwives need to disown any false sense of security and instead embrace the challenge of really getting to know and understand the diverse client groups that entrust their care to them. Facing cultural issues provides a midwife with the opportunity to reduce the widening gap that exists between the dominant and minority cultures (DH 2005). This is indeed a position of humility and privilege.

Conclusion

The CEMACE report (CEMACE 2011) notes that the 'midwife may often be the only professional who is able to build an element of trust with the woman'. This puts her in a privileged and powerful position.

Midwives have an opportunity to make a difference to the lives of clients who may already experience disadvantage from all quarters. Indeed, it is consistently stated and noted that 'midwives are perfectly placed as advocates for the safe delivery of maternity care' (CEMACE 2011). The challenge is and always will be – are midwives prepared to stand up and be counted to ensure that their clients are central to their work?

Professional directives and guidance include the *Midwives' Rules and Standards* (NMC 2012), *Code of Professional Conduct* (NMC 2008) and most recently the Equality Act (2006). The Act provides for the establishment of the Commission for Equality and Human Rights (CEHR). This new framework is part of the government's wider programme of reform to challenge discrimination and inequality and to promote equality and diversity. The CEHR must also take on responsibility for the promotion of human rights. Midwives essentially must keep themselves up to date with these changes so as to work always in an culturally intelligent and sensitive manner. This should enable them to truly advocate for and empower their clients.

Cultural awareness quiz

Please complete the quiz. It should take about 1 hour. It can be completed individually or as a group. It might be useful to arrange a study room at your university's learning and resources centre or invite your mentor(s) on your practice site to complete the quiz with you.

1. When is Ramadan and what must Muslims *not* do during this period?
2. Why do Spanish people have two surnames?
3. Why does the Christian festival of Easter move dates each year?
4. What group is defined by the 5 Ks and what are they?
5. What is Halal meat?
6. What is the origin of Halloween?
7. What religion is practised by most Indians?
8. What religion is practised by most Pakistanis?
9. What is the official language of India?
10. What are the main religions of Afro-Caribbean people ?
11. What is the official language of Pakistan?
12. From which West Indian Island do most Afro-Caribbean people in the UK come?
13. Who is/was St Christopher?
14. What is a Bar Mitzvah?
15. What is Rastafarianism?
16. What information about Rastafarianism would enhance medical and midwifery care?
17. How many times each day do Muslims have to pray and what do they have to do beforehand?
18. What is Nirvana?
19. Where do most Buddhist international students come from?
20. What food is acceptable to most religions?
21. What is the ethnic origin of a person with a white British father and a black Trinidadian mother?

References

Ahmad W, Bradby H (eds) (2009) *Ethnicity, Health and Health Care: understanding diversity, tackling disadvantage*. Oxford: Blackwell Publishing Ltd.

Axten S (2003) Power: how it is used and sometimes abused. *British Medical Journal* **11**(11): 681–684.

Bowler I (2008) They're not the same as us: midwives' stereotypes of South Asian descent maternity patients. *Sociology, Health and Illness* **15**(2): 157–178.

Bridle L (2012) Asylum seekers and refugees accessing maternity care – literature review and discussion. *MIDRS Midwifery Digest* **22** (1): 7–12.

Burnham J, Harris Q (2002) *Emerging Ethnicity: a tale of three cultures*. In Dwivedi K, Varma V (eds) *Meeting the Needs of Ethnic Minority Children: a handbook for professionals*. London: Jessica Kingsley.

Burr V (2003) *An Introduction to Social Constructionism*. London: Routledge.

Carter D (2001) Developing self-awareness. In: *Midwives in Action*. London: English National Board, pp 10–18.

Commission for Equality and Human Rights (2006) *The Equality Act*. London: Commission for Equality and Human Rights.

Confidential Enquiry into Maternal and Child Enquiries (CEMACE) (2011) *Why Mothers Die*. London: Confidential Enquiry into Maternal and Child Enquiries.

Department of Health (DH) (2004a) *The NHS Plan: a plan for investment, a plan for reform*. London: Department of Health.

Department of Health (DH) (2004b) *Fairness for All: a new Commission for Equality and Human Rights*. London: Department of Health.

Department of Health (DH) (2005) *Tackling Health Inequalities: status report on the programme for action*. London: Department of Health.

English National Board (2001) *Midwives in Action*. London: English National Board.

Esegbona-Adeigbe S (2011) Acquiring cultural competence in caring for black African women. *British Journal of Midwifery* **19**(8): 486–489.

Fletcher S (2001) Partnership working. In: *Midwives in Action*. London: English National Board, pp 28–33.

Foucault M (1976) *The Will to Knowledge*. Paris: Gallimard.

Fry FT (2002) *Ethics in Nursing Practice: a guide to ethical decision-making*, 2nd edn. Oxford: Blackwell Publishing Ltd.

Griffith R (2010) The Equality Act. *British Journal of Midwifery* **18**(11): 732–733.

Hart A, Lockley R, Henwood F, Pankhurst F, Hall V, Sommerville F (2003) *Researching Professional Education, Addressing Inequalities in Health: new directions in midwifery education and practice*. London: Nursing and Midwifery Council.

Helman C (2007) *Culture, Health and Illness*, 5th edn. London: Arnold.

Henderson C (2005) Midwives can help reduce inequalities. *British Journal of Midwifery* **13**(9): 681–684.

Hoffman L (2007) The art of witness – a bright new edge. In: Anderson H, Gehart D (eds) *Collaborative Therapy: relationships and conversations that make a difference*. New York: Taylor and Francis, pp63–79.

Houghton G (2008) Women seeking asylum: are communication needs being met? *British Journal of Midwifery* **16**(3): 142.

Hunt S (2003) Tackling disadvantage in maternity care. In: *Midwives in Action: a resource*. London: Nursing and Midwifery Council.

Kirkham M, Stapleton H, Curtis P, Thomas G (2002) Stereotyping as a professional defence mechanism. *British Journal of Midwifery* **10**(9): 549–552.

Kitzinger S (2000) Some cultural perspectives of birth. *British Journal of Midwifery* **8**(12): 746–750.

Local Supervising Authority (LSA) (2012) *Annual Report to the Nursing and Midwifery Council*. London: Local Supervising Authority.

Millen R (2002) *Anti-Discriminatory Practice: a guide for workers in child care and education*, 2nd edn. London: Continuum.

National Institute for Health and Clinical Excellence (NICE) (2008) *Routine Antenatal Care for Healthy Pregnant Women*. Clinical Guideline No. 62. London: National Institute for Health and Clinical Excellence.

National Institute for Health and Clinical Excellence (NICE) (2010) *Pregnancy and Complex Social Factors – a model for service provision for pregnant women with complex social factors*. Clinical Guideline No. 110. London: National Institute for Health and Clinical Excellence.

Nursing and Midwifery Council (NMC) (2008) *The Code: standards of conduct, performance and ethics for nurses and midwives*. London: Nursing and Midwifery Council.

Nursing and Midwifery Council (NMC) (2012) *Midwives' Rules and Standards*. London: Nursing and Midwifery Council.

Quinn P, Harding C (2001) Involving clients and responding to women's needs. *Midwives in Action* **2**(4): 34–40.

Raven JH, Chen Q, Tolhurst R, Garner P (2007) Traditional beliefs and practices in the postpartum period in Fujian Province, China: a qualitative study. *MIDRS Midwifery Digest* **17**(4): 560–569.

Reynolds F, Manfusa S (2005) Views on cultural barriers to caring for South Asian women. *British Journal of Midwifery* **13**(4): 236–242.

Rowe R, Garcia J (2005) Ethnic minorities access to antenatal screening. *British Journal of Midwifery* **13**(2): 101–104.

Schott J, Henley A (2007) *Culture, Religion and Childbearing in a Multi-racial Society*. Oxford: Butterworth-Heinemann.

Skinner G (2001) Developing the culture. In: *Midwives in Action*. London: English National Board, pp 41–48.

Smith C, Constantine P, Redmayne T (2005) Midwives can help to reduce inequalities. *British Medical Journal* **13**(9): 540–542.

Sudworth F, Williams A, Heron-Marx S (2012) Maternity services in a multi-cultural Britain: using Q methology to explore the views of first and second generation women of Pakistani origin. *MIDRS Midwifery Digest* **22**(1): 52–62.

Thompson N (2003) *Communication and Language: a handbook of theory and practice*. London: Palgrave Macmillan.

Thompson N (2009) *People Skills*, 2nd edn. London: Palgrave Macmillan.

Walsh D (2005) Professional power and maternity care: the many faces of paternalism. *British Journal of Midwifery* **13**(11): 70.

Wickham S (2007) A decade of polarity. *Practising Midwife* **10**(3): 44–45.

Wiseman O (2011) Undocumented migrants and maternity care. *British Journal of Midwifery* **19**(1): 38–42.

15

Legislation and the Midwife
Cathy Hamilton

Aim

To introduce the student midwife to the practice of midwifery within a contemporary legal framework.

Learning outcomes

By the end of this chapter you will be able to:

1. demonstrate a basic understanding of key legal terms and ethical principles in order to carry out midwifery practice within the law
2. understand the difference between criminal and civil law
3. develop an awareness of legal issues of particular relevance to midwifery practice
4. understand of some of the complex issues relating to obtaining consent for treatment and examination
5. demonstrate an awareness of where to go to access further advice and guidance in relation to these complex issues
6. show an awareness of some of the most relevant Acts of Parliament which might influence your midwifery practice.

What is the law?

Law can be defined as a rule of conduct or procedure established by custom, agreement or authority. It is the mechanism by which society regulates the order and control of people who live in it. The legal system itself is enforced by a political body (Jones & Jenkins 2004). The law produces rules by which all members

The Student's Guide to Becoming a Midwife, Second Edition. Edited by Ian Peate and Cathy Hamilton.
© 2014 John Wiley & Sons, Ltd. Published 2014 by John Wiley & Sons, Ltd.

of society are expected to abide. There are rules to deal with conflict, punish unacceptable behaviour and protect society's members from harm (Jones & Jenkins 2004). If someone is accused of 'breaking the law', the accuser should be able to cite the source of the law to which reference is being made (Dimond 2006). If the statement is accurate, then the appropriate Act of Parliament or a previous decided case can be cited. Without the law, there would be anarchy, fear and confusion (Jones & Jenkins 2004).

The law is classified as criminal or civil. A criminal offence is said to have been committed when the accused takes part in a forbidden activity. As a result, he or she will face criminal proceedings in a court of law (Dimond 2011). In this case, the prosecution must prove 'beyond reasonable doubt' the guilt of the accused. In the Crown Court, if the accused pleads 'not guilty', the case is put before a jury of 12 randomly selected members of the public, who will determine among themselves the defendant's guilt or innocence.

Civil law relates to the rights of private citizens or institutions. Civil proceedings take place between individuals with a view to obtaining compensation or a remedy, such as an injunction preventing contact between two individuals (Dimond 2011). The standard of proof in civil courts is based on the 'balance of probabilities'. This means that it must be demonstrated that it is 'more probable than not' that the accused is guilty of misconduct.

There are three main sources of English law: statutory law, common law and European law.

Statutory law

A statute is a formal written rule of a country or state. Statutes are Acts of Parliament and as such are the most important source of law. An Act creates a new law or changes an existing one. An Act is a Bill approved by both the House of Commons and the House of Lords and formally approved by the reigning monarch (given royal assent). Once implemented, an Act becomes law and applies to the whole of the UK or to specifically defined countries within the UK. In contrast to an Act, a Bill is a proposal to produce a new law or amend an existing one that is presented for debate before Parliament.

In order to be passed, an Act of Parliament needs to proceed through a number of stages for consideration and debate. When the government is considering introducing new legislation, it has various ways to proceed. It can bring the issue straight to Parliament or it can consult the public first. A Green Paper is a government consultative document, which is circulated in order to obtain the views of the general public, civil servants and ministers – in fact, any interested parties who may add to the debate. Following this, a White Paper is issued, which sets out in everyday language the government's intentions in relation to implementation of the proposed law.

Examples of Green and White Papers relevant to midwives are *Our Healthier Nation* (DH 1998), a Green Paper which formed a background to the White Paper *Saving Lives: Our Healthier Nation* (DH 1999), which was presented to Parliament the following year.

More recently, the latest government presented its long term strategy for improving public health in the White Paper entitled *Healthy Lives, Healthy People: our strategy for public health in England* (DH 2010).

Activity 15.1

 Visit the Department of Health website (www.dh.gov.uk) to access these Green and White Papers. Search the website to see what other consultations of relevance to midwifery are currently being undertaken. Consider contributing to these.

Statutory Instruments (SIs) are a form of legislation which allows the provisions of an Act of Parliament to be brought into force or altered without Parliament having to pass a new Act. They are also known as secondary, delegated or subordinate legislation (House of Commons 2007).

An example of how this system works is the Nursing and Midwifery Order 2001 (SI 2002 No. 253). In 2002 the Nursing and Midwifery Council (NMC) replaced the United Kingdom Central Council for Nursing, Midwifery and Health Visiting (UKCC) following this Order. The SI is complicated but comes from section 60 of the Health Act 1999, which allows secondary legislation to amend primary legislation in the regulation of healthcare professions. The Order repealed the Nurses, Midwives and Health Visitors Act 1997 and placed all the relevant regulations in the Order. The NMC was then enabled to produce a new *Code of Professional Conduct* (NMC 2002) (Jones & Jenkins 2004).

Secondary legislation has the same legal power as primary legislation provided the content remains within the authority of the original Act (Jones & Jenkins 2004).

Common law or case law

This type of law is determined by the decisions of judges in relation to particular cases. The decisions of the courts create precedents which cannot be over-ridden by a court lower down in the hierarchy. For example, a judge in a County Court may not go against a decision made in a similar case in a High Court; the Court of Appeal may not go against decisions made in the House of Lords. However, a judge may decide that the case being heard is different from previous ones which allows the judge to reach a different decision as long as the different feature is clearly highlighted in the judge's summing up. See Figure 15.1 for an overview of the hierarchy of the court system.

Decisions are recorded in All England Law Reports (All ER) or Weekly Law Reports (WLR) so that everyone associated with the law can have easy access to them.

An example of a case which has great relevance in healthcare is *Bolam v Friern Hospital Management* [1957] 1 WLR 582. The reference informs the reader that it was reported in 1957 in the first volume of Weekly Law Reports on page 582. This case is also reported in All England Law Reports as *Bolam v Friern Hospital Management* [1957] 2 All ER 118.

This particular case concerned a man who had been given electroconvulsive therapy without a muscle relaxant or anaesthetic and suffered a fractured jaw as a result. He claimed that his doctor had been negligent in his care. However, the judge, Mr Justice McNair, ruled that a doctor is not guilty of negligence if a responsible body of medical opinion considers that he has acted properly even if not all members of the medical profession share this view. This landmark case put peer judgement at the centre of assessing clinical care and led to the instigation of the so-called Bolam test.

European law

Since Britain joined the European Community (EC) in 1973 and following the signing of the Maastricht Treaty in 1992, which led to the formation of the European Union (EU), it is obliged as a member state to ensure that EU directives and regulations are enforced in the UK. All UK law must also fit within the framework of EU legislation and appeals can be made to the European Court of Justice.

A regulation is binding on all member states from the time it is developed without the need for the states to pass any enabling laws. A directive, however, is binding only in terms of the outcomes which must be achieved and not how they are brought about. In these cases the member states themselves may decide what laws are required in order to fulfil the directive.

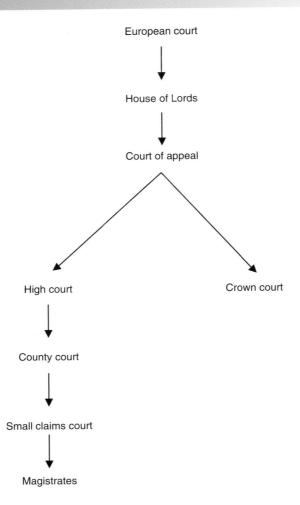

Figure 15.1   The hierarchy of the court system.

An example of a directive relevant to midwifery is the inclusion in the *Midwives' Rules and Standards* of the Midwives Directive 80/155/EEC, indicating the minimum activities that midwives should undertake. The *Midwives' Rules and Standards* (NMC 2012d) also indicate that this directive must be met in educational programmes leading to registration as a midwife.

The law and the issue of consent

Consent is defined as a client's agreement for a healthcare professional to provide care. Consent may be given verbally, non-verbally (such as a woman holding out her arm in order to have her blood taken) or in writing (DH 2009).

The NMC *Code: standards of conduct, performance and ethics for nurses and midwives* (NMC 2008) clearly states healthcare professionals' responsibilities in relation to obtaining consent before any treatment or intervention is undertaken. This is a general legal and ethical principle and reflects the fundamental right of all individuals to decide for themselves what is to happen to their bodies (DH 2009).

All adults are presumed to have the mental capacity to give consent or refuse treatment unless they are unable to take in information about the treatment, are unable to understand the information given and are unable to consider the information given as part of the decision-making process (NMC 2012a). Issues relating to minors are discussed later in this chapter.

There are two areas of the law relating to consent:

1. The actual giving of consent by the client.
2. The duty of the midwife to give appropriate information before the client gives consent.

If consent is not given but treatment is undertaken, the client may have grounds to sue the practitioner for trespass to the person. An assault is when a person perceives that there is a threat that she may be touched without her consent. On the other hand, if she is actually touched without giving consent, this is battery. For example, threatening verbal behaviour without any physical contact is assault while a vaginal examination undertaken without a woman's consent is battery (Dimond 2011).

The person who has suffered the trespass can sue for compensation in the civil courts. In these cases the individual does not have to prove that harm has occurred as a result of the interaction, just that touching occurred without her consent. However, it is worth remembering that the touching behaviour must refer to care or treatment being undertaken by the practitioner. An arm around the shoulder of a distressed person would not count as trespass to the person in these cases.

A healthcare professional also has a duty to give the client all information relating to the treatment, including risks, benefits and alternative treatments. If this is not undertaken, then a woman could sue if she suffers harm as a result of accepting a treatment but then claims that the healthcare professional did not alert her to the possibility that harm could occur. A charge of negligence could then be brought against the healthcare professional.

Consent is valid only if it is given voluntarily by an individual who is fully informed and has the mental capacity to consent to the treatment or care (DH 2009). A midwife attempting to gain consent from a woman for any particular procedure should consider whether the woman has the capacity to give consent, whether she has been given enough information, with time to consider her options and discuss them with a healthcare professional. It is suggested that 'seeking consent' should be considered as a joint decision-making process between the client and the healthcare professional (DH 2009). Once consent has been given, the midwife should consider whether consent was given voluntarily or whether the woman was under pressure from her partner, family or others to make a particular decision (Jones & Jenkins 2004).

Usually the healthcare professional who is proposing to undertake the procedure will obtain consent (NMC 2012a). However, in certain circumstances this may be delegated to another healthcare professional who has been appropriately trained for that specific area of practice (NMC 2008). The midwife, according to the NMC (2012a), has three main professional responsibilities with regard to obtaining consent:

1. Always act in the best interests of the client.
2. Ensure that the process of establishing consent is rigorous and transparent.
3. Ensure that documentation is accurate and clearly records all discussions and decisions relating to obtaining consent.

Midwifery wisdom

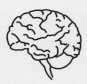

When giving information to a woman about a particular treatment or test, make sure you give her full details of advantages and disadvantages of what you are suggesting as well as possible alternatives.

There is further guidance concerning consent issued by the Department of Health, which includes key points for healthcare professionals to consider in relation to this issue (DH 2009).

Activity 15.2

Access the DH website for further guidance about the complex issues relating to consent: www.dh.gov.uk.

Emergency situations

An adult who is unable to give consent because she is unconscious may receive whatever treatment is required in order to save her life, provided it is in her best interests (NMC 2012a). In such cases the health-care professionals would not be committing a trespass to the person (Dimond 2011).

Exceptions to this are when the client has already issued an advance directive (sometimes referred to as a 'living will') indicating that any further treatment is refused (NMC 2012a). Another exception would be if a woman had made a decision while she was still mentally competent and alert. A Jehovah's Witness, for example, may refuse a blood transfusion or the use of any blood products and it would be unlawful for midwives or doctors to administer these even if she loses consciousness and her condition becomes critical.

It is not possible for anyone to give consent for treatment for another adult. In this case the practice of midwives asking a partner or another next of kin for consent is unlawful (Jones & Jenkins 2004).

Case study 15.1

Gina is 38 weeks pregnant and expecting her first baby. She has high blood pressure and has been diagnosed as suffering from pre-eclampsia. The doctor advises urgent admission to hospital with a view to inducing her labour. The concern is that as her condition worsens, her life and the life of her baby will be at risk. Gina fully understands all the risks involved and after careful consideration decides that she does not want to be induced. She would prefer to wait a few more days to see if labour starts naturally...

Despite the fact that the law states that a mentally competent person has the absolute right to consent to or refuse medical treatment for any reason (or even no reason at all), it is suggested that in the past this has not been fully understood by healthcare professionals in relation to maternity care. There seems to have been an assumption that pregnant women are obliged to give consent to various procedures and interventions for the sake of their unborn baby (Jones & Jenkins 2004).

A case illustrating this is *Re F (in utero)* [1988]. A woman with a history of drug abuse and mental illness went missing late in her pregnancy. The local authority was concerned for the welfare of the unborn baby and sought to make the fetus a ward of court, which would mean that the woman would be found, housed and required to attend for hospital appointments. The judges in this case, although sympathetic to the concerns of the local authority, rejected the application. They stated that the fetus had no legal rights and that a court order of this kind would over-ride the rights of the woman.

Another controversial case, *St George's Health Care Trust v S* [1998], highlights similar issues. In this instance, a woman refusing a caesarean section was detained under section 2 of the Mental Health Act, 1983 and a caesarean section was carried out without her consent. The woman later sought a judicial review of her case and the Court of Appeal ruled that she had been unlawfully detained under the Mental Health Act. Although her thinking processes were unusual and contrary to the views of most other people, she was not suffering from a mental disorder which warranted her detention in hospital. Furthermore, a woman detained under the Act for mental disorder could not be forced into a procedure (in this case, a caesarean section) unconnected with her mental condition. S was not held to be mentally incompetent and so the compulsory caesarean section was a trespass to her person.

The cases above illustrate the position of the law in relation to the fetus: the fetus as an unborn child is not a separate person from its mother. The need of the fetus for medical assistance to save its life does not over-ride the rights of the mother. In the case of Gina described in the previous scenario, as long as she has the mental capacity to make an informed decision, she cannot be forced to be induced against her will just because the health practitioners believe that it might be better for her baby.

267

Consent of minors

Case study 15.2

 Renuka, a community midwife, visits a young mother at her home. Katrina is 14 years old and has a 7-day-old baby. Renuka wants to undertake the neonatal blood spot screening test on the baby but Katrina is on her own as her parents are both out.

Renuka asks Katrina if she has heard about the blood test and if she knows what it is for. Katrina shows Renuka a leaflet which the teenage support midwife had given her when she had attended a preparation for parenthood session with some other young mothers. Katrina tells Renuka that she has discussed the procedure with her friends in the class. While they had all agreed that they were not keen on their babies having the test because it would hurt them to be pricked, they also knew it was important and meant that if their babies had any of the conditions listed then this would be picked up early so that the right treatment could be started straight away.

Renuka is particularly impressed that Katrina knows the names of most of the conditions being screened for and where on the baby's foot the blood would be taken from. She also knows that the blood obtained is dripped as four large spots onto an absorbent card and then sent away for analysis.

Renuka confirms this and then also gives Katrina information about when she can expect to receive the results. After this discussion, Renuka is satisfied that Katrina is fully aware of what the test is for and why her baby should have it. Renuka carefully records details of their discussion in

Katrina's medical records and signs the entry. This is her evidence that the relevant information was given and that in her opinion was fully understood by Katrina. Renuka goes ahead to prepare to take the sample. Katrina asks Renuka if she can cuddle her baby while she is obtaining the sample. She tells Renuka that it is a good job her Mum is out at the shops as she is very squeamish about blood and might faint if she was there to see the blood being taken!

In England, Wales and Northern Ireland, adulthood is deemed to start from 18 years of age (in Scotland this legal capacity is reached at 16 years of age). However, young people between 16 and 18 years have been given the absolute right to consent to or refuse treatment in relation to diagnostic investigations, care and treatment in the same way as a competent adult (Family Law Reform Act 1969). This does not apply to certain areas though, such as the donation of blood or organs which are not being used in the treatment of the young person him/herself. Parents or those with parental responsibility may over-ride the refusal of a young person up to the age of 18 years.

Until 1986, consent by parents or those with parental responsibility was always needed for children and young people under 16 years. Following the court ruling in the case of *Gillick v West Norfolk and Wisbech Area Health Authority* [1986], the law was changed. Victoria Gillick was concerned that the government was going to allow doctors to give family planning advice and treatment to girls under 16 years without parental consent if it was considered to be in the best interest of the girl. Mrs Gillick claimed that to do so was unlawful. The House of Lords eventually ruled that it was lawful in those cases where the girl possessed sufficient understanding and intelligence to understand fully the proposed treatment. This level of understanding was termed Gillick competence, but is now more likely to be referred to as following the Fraser Guidelines. The principles apply to all areas of healthcare, not only contraceptive advice, and were incorporated into the Children Act 1989.

The test for Gillick competence involves the healthcare professional considering three key questions:

1. Does the client understand the situation she is in?
2. Have the options available to her been explained and does she understand them?
3. Does she understand the possible consequences of these options?

Although midwives' clients will have reached physical maturity, there is a great deal of variation between the emotional and mental maturity of young people between the ages of 12 and 16. A 13 year old may pass the test while a 15 year old may not. In either case, it is just as lawful to act on the wishes of the 13 year old as it is to seek parental consent for the 15 year old (Jones & Jenkins 2004).

Accurate record keeping (NMC 2009) is extremely important in these cases, so that the midwife can clearly demonstrate that the young person has passed the test and that all aspects of care have been discussed. The competence principle described here also applies to decisions which a young mother may need to make regarding treatment for her baby, as highlighted in the scenario describing the young mother Katrina and her midwife Renuka.

Parental consent for babies

There may be times when the parents will not give consent for their baby to undergo a medical procedure which doctors believe is essential to the well-being of the child. In these cases, healthcare practitioners may need to apply for a judicial ruling in the best interests of the baby (DH 2009, Jones & Jenkins 2004). This scenario is illustrated in the practice dilemma described in Case study 15.3.

Case study 15.3

Sextuplets were born to a Canadian couple who were Jehovah's Witnesses. The six babies were born nearly 3 months prematurely. Two died within a week and the doctors told the parents that the remaining four babies needed urgent blood transfusions if they were to stand any chance of survival. The parents refused to give their consent as their religion strictly forbids the use of blood products. The hospital in Vancouver applied to the British Columbia government to take the surviving babies into protective custody so that the transfusions could be given. The authorities complied and the babies were transferred to the care of the state. Two of the babies received blood transfusions. The parents were devastated and accused the doctors of violating their children (Philp 2007).

Legislation used by the midwife in her practice

There are numerous Acts which may govern midwives' actions in their everyday practice. This chapter will consider some of the most relevant. The following will be discussed:

- The Human Rights Act 1998
- Equal Opportunities legislation (e.g. Sex Discrimination Act 1975)
- Access to patient records (Data Protection Act 1998, Access to Health Records Act 1990)
- Abortion Act 1967
- Births and Deaths Registration Act 1953
- Human Fertilisation and Embryology Acts 1990, 1991, 1992
- Criminal law and attendances at birth (Nurses, Midwives and Health Visitors Act 1997, Nursing and Midwifery Order 2001)
- Children Act 1989
- Congenital Disabilities (Civil Liability) Act 1976

Human Rights Act 1998

Under the Human Rights Act, the following articles are pertinent in midwifery:

- Article 2: the right to life
- Article 3: the right not to be tortured or subjected to inhumane or de grading treatment or punishment
- Article 5: the right to liberty and security
- Article 6: the right to a fair trial
- Article 8: the right to respect privacy and family life

There is some debate surrounding prisoners being handcuffed to a bed whilst attending for antenatal care or actually giving birth in relation to article 3: 'being subjected to inhumane or degrading treatment' (McShane & Wiseman 2010).

Guidance from the Royal College of Midwives (RCM 2008) in relation to the care of pregnant prisoners recommends that midwives should ensure that the dignity of every prisoner who is pregnant or in labour is maintained, regardless of her situation. It is the midwife's responsibility to ask for handcuffs or any other restraints to be removed prior to consultations and examinations, including during labour. Indeed, the fact that a woman is a prisoner does not mean that she loses her right to a confidential consultation with a midwife. Midwives should insist on maintaining confidentiality and privacy during examinations, otherwise prison officers will expect to be present. This could be seen as contravening article 8 of the Human Rights Act.

Equal opportunities legislation

In relation to midwifery practice, the following equal opportunities legislation is of some relevance:

- European Communities Act 1972
- Sex Discrimination Act 1975
- Employment Rights Act 1996
- Employment Act 2002

This legislation gives the pregnant woman certain rights which protect her against discrimination. It is against the law for employers to treat pregnant women unfairly, dismiss them or select them for redundancy for any reason connected with pregnancy, childbirth or maternity leave.

A pregnant woman:

- does not have to tell a potential employer if she is pregnant when going for an interview
- does not have to tell her employer that she is pregnant until the 15th week before her baby is due
- is entitled to take time off for antenatal appointments and other appointments without loss of pay.

In addition, if a pregnant woman is:

- made redundant whilst on maternity leave, her employer must offer her any suitable alternative employment that is available; if there is none, they must give the woman notice and redundancy pay
- dismissed when she tells her employer of her pregnancy, she has 3 months to go to an employment tribunal.

The pregnant woman must inform her employer that she is pregnant in writing. Regarding returning to work,

- she should give her employer 28 days' notice before returning to work
- her employer can write from 15 weeks into the woman's maternity leave asking if she is coming back to work and her expected date of return. A reply must be given by the woman within 21 days, although the date of return can be changed.

Access to patient records

Patients have a right to access health information about themselves (DH 2004) as governed by the Data Protection Act 1998. The data controller (e.g. a GP)is usually responsible for giving the patient access to their records. However, the following principles apply before access can be granted:

- A request has to be made in writing.
- The access request should be verified.

- Enough data are present to check that the identification matches with the record.
- If a previous request has been made, a second request can be refused unless a significant change has occurred in the condition of the patient.
- A patient can be charged to gain access to their records.
- The request must be logged appropriately.
- The health professional responsible for the clinical care must be con sulted (this might be a GP, a hospital consultant or in maternity cases, a midwife).

There are two reasons why the information does not have to be disclosed:

1. Where the information could cause significant harm to the mental or physical well-being of the patient or another party.
2. Where the information has been disclosed by a third party who does not give consent for the information to be made available.

Activity 15.3

In your trust, find out the process if a woman who delivered at the maternity unit a few years earlier requests a copy of her records. Is this something that can be arranged and how might a woman going about doing this?

Abortion Act 1967

This Act requires two medical practitioners to agree to a termination of pregnancy and the following stipulations apply with regard to the procedure:

- The pregnancy is less than 24 weeks' gestation, and to continue it would involve a greater risk to the woman's physical or mental health, or that of her existing children, than would a termination; or
- The termination is necessary to stop permanent damage to the physical or mental health of the woman; or
- If the pregnancy were to continue it would involve a greater risk to the life of the pregnant woman than if it were terminated; or
- If the child were born there would be a substantial risk of it being seri ously handicapped, mentally or physically.

However, in an emergency situation the necessity to have the agreement of two medical practitioners can be waived, provided that the medical practitioner holds the opinion that a termination is immediately necessary to save the life of the pregnant woman or prevent her from being permanently mentally or physically injured.

Article 4 of the Abortion Act 1967 gives healthcare practitioners with a conscientious objection, including midwives, the right to refuse to have direct involvement in abortion procedures. An individual who has a conscientious objection to undertaking a procedure contained within this Act shall not be under any duty to do so. However, it should be noted that in any subsequent legal proceedings, the responsibility of proving their conscientious objection (that is, the 'burden of proof') shall lie solely with the individual claiming to rely on it.

The Abortion Act 1967 also highlights the duty of nurses and midwives to participate in any treatment which is deemed necessary to save life or prevent 'grave, permanent injury to the physical or mental health of a pregnant woman' regardless of a conscientious objection.

The NMC (2012c) recommends that midwives and nurses should give careful consideration to whether or not to accept employment in an area that carries out treatment or procedures to which they have a conscientious objection.

Registration of births and stillbirths

By law, every birth has to be registered (Births and Deaths Registration Act 1953). This applies to births and stillbirths taking place after 24 weeks' gestation (as amended by the Stillbirth Definition Act 1992). Where the neonate is born alive (whatever the gestation, even if prior to 24 weeks) and then dies, the birth and death must both be registered. Where a miscarriage occurs before 24 weeks' gestation, there is no requirement to register it and the fetus shows no signs of life. However, the wishes of the parents must be taken into consideration along with public decency when disposing of the body.

272

Human Fertilisation and Embryology Acts 1990, 1991 and 1992

Following the 1990 Act, the Human Fertilisation and Embryology Authority (HFEA) was set up to issue licences, oversee the clinics managing infertility and monitor them accordingly. The 1991 Act influenced the Abortion Act, changing the gestation for a legally induced abortion to the end of the 24th week. Previously it had been to the 28th week. The time limit for a legal abortion continues to be a contentious issues as technological advances in neonatal care mean that fetuses of an earlier gestation are surviving more frequently. However, the current time limit remains at 24 weeks' gestation.

The law allows for a selected reduction of fetuses if one or more of the fetuses is seriously abnormal or if to continue with that number of fetuses would cause the woman ill health or threaten her life.

The 1990 and 1992 Acts influence where fertility treatment can take place.

The HFEA has since 1991 kept a confidential register of information about donors, patients and treatments. From 2008, anyone over 16 who is thinking about getting married, or anyone over 18, who asks the HFEA will be told whether or not they were born as a result of licensed assisted conception treatment and, if so, whether they are related to the person they want to marry.

Since 2005, the HFEA has also asked all gamete donors to provide identifying information via the clinic where they are donating eggs or sperm. Any child born as a result of sperm, egg or embryo donation now has the right to this information once they reach the age of 18. The HFEA will not divulge any information, however, without first contacting the donor (HFEA 2012).

In the event that a donor of sperm or egg does not disclose any relevant genetic or medical history and a child is born with a disability, a court can require the HFEA to disclose the donor's identity under the Congenital Disabilities Act (Civil Liabilities) Act 1976 (HFEA 2012). See p.274.

Further information about this topic can be found by visiting the HFEA website: www.hfea.gov.uk.

Criminal law and attendances at birth

Under the Nurses, Midwives and Health Visitors Act 1997, section 16, it is a criminal offence for someone other than a midwife or registered medical practitioner (or their students) to attend a woman in childbirth. The exception to this is in an emergency.

This legislation is reiterated in the Nursing and Midwifery Order 2001, article 45. However, it should be noted that attending a woman in childbirth in a professional capacity implies delivering actual midwifery care (such as performing an abdominal examination, a vaginal examination or listening to the fetal heart). This is the aspect that is considered illegal. In fact, an unqualified individual (such as the woman's partner, friend or relative) may be with a woman during childbirth for support. As long as midwifery and/or medical care is not provided by that unqualified individual, then no crime has been committed (NMC 2012b). If you do suspect that an unqualified person has been involved in a woman's care during birth or intends to be involved and administer midwifery care, then you should seek further guidance from a supervisor of midwives (SOM) and/or your line manager (NMC 2012b) in the first instance.

Freebirthing or unassisted birth means that a woman gives birth without professional or medical assistance of any kind. In the UK, it would appear that this type of birthing experience is increasing in popularity (NMC 2012b). It is not illegal unless, as has been highlighted above, the unqualified individual supporting the woman delivers medical or midwifery care and assumes responsibility for the birth. In the case of freebirthing, the woman herself assumes full responsibility for the birth. A midwife has no legal right to be present at any birth and if a woman chooses to give birth without medical or midwifery support then that is her choice and she has a legal right to make that decision for herself.

273

Midwifery wisdom

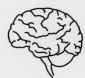

As a midwife, you have no legal right to insist that you are present at a birth. This is always the woman's decision. It is, however, illegal for an unqualified individual to assume responsibility for a birth as if she/he were a midwife.

Children Act 1989

The midwife must be familiar with child protection, taking immediate action to inform the appropriate person if they suspect that a child or minor in the care of one of their clients is being physically, emotionally or sexually abused. The nature of child protection dictates that different professionals will be working together in these instances so good interdisciplinary relations need to be fostered. It is imperative that the midwife has contact details of local agencies. Interagency communication is of the utmost importance. In the case of Victoria Climbié (Laming 2003), interagency working broke down. Victoria had come into contact with various aspects of healthcare provision and other professionals but no-one had taken the lead to deal with the problems that subsequently led to her death.

In cases of child protection it is everybody's responsibility and where there is any doubt about whether neglect or abuse is taking place, healthcare professionals must not assume that another professional has raised concerns. We must remember that the main priority is the safety of the child. (See Chapter 6 for more information on interprofessional working.)

Many healthcare professionals worry about the consequences if they suspect that a case of child abuse or neglect is taking place but their concerns are unfounded. In cases such as these, the name of the professional who raised the concerns will not be divulged.

The underlying principles of the Children Act 1989 are as follows:

- The welfare of the child is the main consideration in court proceedings.
- Children should be brought up by and cared for in their own families wherever possible.
- Courts should make an order only where it is better than making no or der at all and should ensure that any delay is avoided.
- Children should be kept informed of the proceedings and should be in volved with the decision-making processes about their future.
- When the children no longer live with their parents, the parents contin ue to have parental responsibility. They should therefore be included in the decision-making process in relation to their children's future (it is only if children are adopted that the birth parents lose parental responsibility which then becomes the responsibility of the adopted parents).
- Parents with children in need should be facilitated to bring up their children themselves. The help that the parents receive to enable them to do this should:
  - be provided in partnership with them
  - meet the identified needs of each child
  - appropriately address the child's race, culture, religion and language
  - be open to 'effective independent representation and complaints proce dures'
  - use effective partnerships between the local authority and other agencies, including voluntary organisations.

Midwifery wisdom

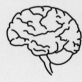

Try to foster good working relationships with other professionals you come into contact with during the course of your work, such as general practitioners, social workers and health visitors. In this way you can help to facilitate a holistic approach to the care of women and their families.

Congenital Disabilities (Civil Liability) Act 1976

This Act enables children who are born with a disability due to a negligent act before birth to claim compensation from the person who was negligent, which potentially could be a midwife or medical practitioner. In the case of a road traffic collision where the mother has been negligent, it is her insurance company which pays any compensation. This is the only scenario in which a child can sue its mother. Recently, provisions have been made in relation to children who have been disabled during *in vitro* fertilisation (IVF) treatment.

Conclusion

This chapter has considered the practice of midwifery within a contemporary legal framework. It has introduced the reader to the law and its principles, exploring what the law is, and the differences between criminal and civil law, and statutory, case and European law. It has raised key areas for discussion such as consent and the rights of the fetus and highlighted the legislative requirements in which the midwife is expected to practise in relation to obtaining consent for examinations and treatment. The chapter then looked in more detail at specific legislation which midwives need to be familiar within order to ensure that they practise within the law.

The importance of team working along with clear and contemporaneous record keeping has been referred to throughout this chapter. By ensuring that these factors are maintained, the midwife will be enabled to provide the best care for her clients. The Supervisor of Midwives (SOM) is a good source of further guidance and support should the midwife require this when dealing with some of the more challenging dilemmas discussed here.

Word Search

Use the clues below to solve the puzzle.

A test for minors
A test of general medical opinion?
Keeping records
A paper setting out Government strategy
Allows Parliament to make amendments to Acts
Law decided by judges
A Court for criminal cases
An Act giving us rights
Agreeing to a procedure
Lacking capacity
Living will
Unaided birth

```
A P O N T E W R I C A T A H A H E B R
R D N L R F M L R O T P E U O M O E S
M P V E A O R O W T A T C M N M N T S
I N D A B R W E C C E E N A E A C T G
R H E O N N T I T L T P E N F W T A P
G M I B C C I H E T I H T R R T L C O
P S S O R U E C D D H A E I A E W C W
A N U L E I M D T O L E P G G C S I T
D R R A N E I E D I B D M H N T B O A
T N E M U R T S N I Y R O T U T A T S
K R P T C E E C R T R A C S W N P S H
T A A E T N A T A C A E K A E L T M E
B C P S C P H E E H R T C C U G R A E
N N E T A I E A P W N W I T S A E C E
C H T C N A C E N E A C L O I I S A Y
P O I G C T D A S R A V L I N V V N I
S T H E T H T N C T N C I A U C E T H
Y N W A L N O M M O C A G T M A T M I
T E O T M C R I I T T O R E R R A M A
```

References

Department of Health (DH) (1998) *Our Healthier Nation: A Contract for Health*. London: HMSO.

Department of Health (DH) (1999) *Saving Lives: Our Healthier Nation*. London: HMSO.

Department of Health (DH) (2004) *Confidentiality and Disclosure of Information: General Medical Services, Personal Medical Services and Alternative Provider Medical Services Code of Practice 2004*. London: HMSO.

Department of Health (DH) (2009) *Reference Guide to Consent for Examination or Treatment*, 2nd edn. London: Stationery Office. Available at: www.dh.gov.uk/en/Publicationsandstatistics/Publications/PublicationsPolicyAndGuidance/DH_103643 (accessed January 2013).

Department of Health (DH) (2010) *Healthy Lives, Healthy People: our strategy for public health in England*. Available at: www.dh.gov.uk/en/Publicationsandstatistics/Publications/PublicationsPolicyAndGuidance/DH_121941 (accessed January 2013).

Dimond B (2006) *Legal Aspects of Midwifery*, 3rd edn. Edinburgh: Books for Midwives.

Dimond B (2011) Law and the midwife. In: Macdonald S, Magill-Cuerden J (eds) *Mayes' Midwifery: a textbook for midwives*, 14th edn. London: Baillière Tindall.

House of Commons (2007) Statutory Instruments. Information sheet L7. London: House of Commons.

Human Fertilisation and Embryology Authority (HFEA) (2012) Information for existing and potential donors. Available at: www.hfea.gov.uk/egg-and-sperm-donors.html (accessed January 2013).

Jones S, Jenkins R (2004) *The Law and the Midwife*, 2nd edn. Oxford: Blackwell Publishing Ltd.

Laming WH (2003) *The Victoria Climbié Inquiry*. Report of an Inquiry by Lord Laming. London: Stationery Office.

McShane C, Wiseman E (2010) Born Behind Bars. Observer, 21st February. Available at: www.guardian.co.uk/lifeandstyle/2010/feb/21/pregnant-women-in-prison (accessed May 2013).

Nursing and Midwifery Council (NMC) (2002) *Code of Professional Conduct*. London: Nursing and Midwifery Council.

Nursing and Midwifery Council (NMC) (2008) *The Code: Standards of conduct, performance and ethics for nurses and midwives*. London: Nursing and Midwifery Council.

Nursing and Midwifery Council (NMC) (2009) *Record Keeping: guidelines for nurses and midwives*. London: Nursing and Midwifery Council. Available at: www.nmc-uk.org/Publications/Guidance/ (accessed May 2013).

Nursing and Midwifery Council (NMC) (2012a) *Regulation in Practice: consent*. Available at: www.nmc-uk.org/Nurses-and-midwives/Regulation-in-practice/Regulation-in-Practice-Topics/consent/ (accessed January 2013).

Nursing and Midwifery Council (NMC) (2012b) *Regulation in Practice: freebirthing*. Available at: www.nmc-uk.org/Nurses-and-midwives/Regulation-in-practice/Midwifery-New/Free-birthing/ (accessed January 2013).

Nursing and Midwifery Council (NMC) (2012c) *Regulation in Practice: conscientious objection by nurses and midwives*. Available at: www.nmc-uk.org/Nurses-and-midwives/Regulation-in-practice/Regulation-in-Practice-Topics/Conscientious-objection-by-nurses-and-midwives-/ (accessed January 2013).

Nursing and Midwifery Council (NMC) (2012d) *Midwives' Rules and Standards*. London: Nursing and Midwifery Council.

Philp C (2007) Babies seized after Jehovah's Witness mother refuses blood for sextuplets. *The Times* 23rd February: 3.

Royal College of Midwives (RCM) (2008) *Position Statement: caring for childbearing prisoners*. Available at: www.rcm.org.uk/college/policy-practice/guidelines/rcm-position-statements/position-statements/ (accessed January 2013).

Legislation

Births and Deaths Registration Act 1953. London: HMSO.

Congenital Disabilities Act (Civil Liabilities) Act 1976. London: HMSO.

Data Protection Act, 1998. London: HMSO.

Human Fertilisation and Embryology Acts 1990, 1991 and 1992. London: HMSO.

Nurses, Midwives and Health Visitors Act 1997. London: HMSO.

Abortion Act 1967. London: HMSO.

Children Act 1989. London: HMSO.

Family Law Reform Act 1969. London: HMSO.

Human Rights Act 1998. London: HMSO.

Mental Health Act 1983. London: HMSO.

Cases

Bolam v Friern Hospital Management [1957] 2 All ER 118.

Gillick v West Norfolk and Wisbech Area Health Authority [1986] CLR 113 (HL)

Re F (in utero) [1988] 2 All ER 193, [1988] Fam 122 (CA)

St George's Health Care Trust v S [1998] 3 All ER 673 (CA)

16

Decision Making

Sandy Wong

Aim

The aim of this chapter is to introduce you to the extremely complex concept of decision making, and to help you develop and/or improve your skills in this area by proposing principles to foster a systematic approach to the process.

Learning outcomes

By the end of this chapter you will:

1. have an increased awareness of the importance of appropriate decision making, both in the clinical setting and in management
2. have a better understanding of the scale of decision-making errors, and their underlying causes
3. have learned the appreciation of evidence in the decision-making process
4. be able to exercise your knowledge and skills, and expand your cognitive faculty in making decisions
5. have some guiding principles to help you develop and/or improve your judgement and decision-making skills.

Introduction

Within this book, midwives are reminded of the importance of effective communication, interdisciplinary working and legislation in order to provide high-quality care. Chapter 18 on evidence-based practice further reinforces the importance of understanding research principles and methods. This helps to appraise the quality of reported studies and therefore to judge whether or not the conclusions of such studies should be taken into consideration in practice.

The Student's Guide to Becoming a Midwife, Second Edition. Edited by Ian Peate and Cathy Hamilton.
© 2014 John Wiley & Sons, Ltd. Published 2014 by John Wiley & Sons, Ltd.

Decision making is closely linked to the appreciation of evidence. However, it needs to be seen in the context in which women, midwives and other healthcare professionals, as well as economists, politicians and ethicists, live, practise and relate to each other. The concept of decision making is extremely complex and brings to bear a multitude of aspects that can only be partly considered in this chapter.

The management and prioritising of competing demands through all aspects of midwifery practice will be given consideration. This will include decisions relating to referral to appropriate healthcare professionals when interventions to maintain the safety of the woman and her baby are required.

This chapter considers some fundamental principles of decision making as they complement or challenge evidence, experience or accepted practice. Two main areas are explored: clinical decision making and managerial decision making. Principles are then offered as guidance for midwives to follow in order to improve their judgement and decision-making skills.

Decision making

As individuals, we make a multitude of decisions every day. These decisions can be wide-ranging, from simple things like what time to get up in the morning, to major decisions on career choice, getting married, moving house or starting a family. The examples are endless, but essentially there are two main areas of decision making that midwives face in their day-to-day practice: clinical decision making and managerial decision making. Clinical decision making includes diagnostics and treatment. Examples of diagnostic choices in midwifery may be that a woman is or is not in labour or that a baby suffers or does not suffer from neonatal jaundice. Examples of treatment choices include the recommendation to use active management with Syntometrine or to apply physiological approach for the third stage of labour, or to use or not to use an epidural for a woman diagnosed with pregnancy-induced hypertension or pre-eclampsia.

Midwifery wisdom

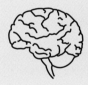

Managerial decision making ranges from organising one's own workload to managing others and service provision.

The decisions or choices one makes are not necessarily always correct. Even though the majority of healthcare professionals aim to do the best they can for the people they care for, errors can occur with alarming frequency. This is highlighted in the publication of enquiries into maternal mortality (CMACE 2011a) and perinatal mortality (CMACE 2011b). Indeed, the Confidential Enquiry into Maternal Deaths (CMACE 2011a) refers to 'substandard' care that could be classified as either 'major' or 'minor'.

In this context, major substandard care is defined as care that contributed significantly to the death of the woman, i.e. different management would reasonably have been expected to alter the outcome. Minor substandard care is defined as a relevant contributory factor, in that different management might have made a difference although the woman's survival was unlikely (CMACE 2011a). In most cases, the midwives and doctors caring for these women were doing their best, yet some of the women died. This demonstrates that even with the best of intentions, errors can and do occur. Fortunately, the majority of these errors do not lead to major problems, but occasionally they do.

Errors

Maternal death is the most negative outcome of pregnancy in midwifery and obstetric practice. Some maternal deaths are inevitable because of severe pathology. Examples are women with severe congenital heart malformation or cancer during pregnancy, but these events are rare. However, the majority of maternal deaths in the developed world are not associated with inevitable causes, they mostly result from human errors (CMACE 2011a). These errors can be broadly classified as:

- *underdiagnosis*: originates from a failure to recognise risk factors or a failure to appreciate the significance of presenting signs and symptoms; hence, the real pathology is not detected and action is not taken swiftly and correctly
- *overdiagnosis*: this is when a condition that does not exist is diagnosed, usually instead of the correct diagnosis, leading to inappropriate treatment and/or care management.

Clinical expertise is closely linked to clinical experience. Severe maternal pathology is by definition rare as pregnancy is usually a physiological state. Most midwives and obstetricians will never come across a maternal death or if they do, their experience will be very limited because this untoward event is very rare.

Therefore, it is easy to underestimate the severity of symptoms in a condition that most practitioners will not have encountered. This may go some way to explaining the poor interpretation of some of the presenting symptoms, and hence the delay in action, which lead to a catastrophic outcome. Evidence shows that more experienced practitioners, and those who are more certain of their diagnosis, are often right. However, some conditions are more difficult to diagnose. The misdiagnoses can at times be associated with ineffective or even harmful treatments (Ermenc 1999, McKelvie 1993; Roosen et al. 2000, Roulson et al. 2005, Sarode et al. 1993). An example of this is the administration of an anticoagulant to a person misdiagnosed as having a myocardial infarction, but who is in fact suffering from a gastric ulcer. The anticoagulant may lead to severe haemorrhage and subsequent death. It is easy to think that this is far-fetched and would not happen, but the literature clearly demonstrates that such errors are not uncommon (Cameron & McGoogan 1981). Sometimes an incorrect diagnosis is arrived at because practitioners rely too much on intuition and gut feeling instead of factual analysis of hard data.

Poor understanding and interpretation of statistics may lie at the root of many errors, leading to devastating consequences. This was clearly demonstrated in Sally Clark's case by Professor Sir Roy Meadow, as his statistical interpretation of the likelihood of a second infant death from natural causes occurring in one family was flawed (Rozenberg 2006). Therefore, an understanding of some statistical terminology may help midwives question and interpret diagnostic tests more accurately. This may also help them to be better able to explain the significance of screening tests offered. For example, information on statistical values can be useful in supporting women and their partners to make informed decisions about screening for Down's syndrome (also known as trisomy 21).

Moreover, midwives are regularly required to make decisions based on observations only. Questions may then be raised as to whether observations are diagnostic of a particular condition or not, as it is likely that the presentation of the information and its analysis are not always clearly identified. Sometimes, a positive test is taken as confirming the existence of a condition without analysing the likelihood of a false-positive test. Indeed, the steady rise in caesarean section is causing concern because this increase in maternal morbidity does not correlate with a corresponding fall in neonatal problems. When a baby has been delivered by emergency caesarean section he may cry loudly at birth; this should not be interpreted as fetal distress as this would be a misdiagnosis.

Midwifery wisdom

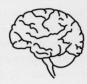

Midwives and obstetricians must do better if unnecessary interventions, including caesarean sections, are to be avoided.

Using heuristics

The art of midwifery, like medicine, is the skilled application of medical science (Chapman & Sonnenberg 2003, Connolly et al. 2000), the processing of information (Lilford 1990) or the choice of decisions (Thornton 1990). However, as seen when examining the quality of judgement or diagnoses, common decisions can also appear quite complex when they are translated into a statistical model or framework, or if other factors are involved. The choice between active and physiological management of the third stage of labour provides a relatively simple example. If one considers only the lower risk of a postpartum haemorrhage (PPH), there is little doubt that the active management of the third stage of labour should be favoured. However, this is not without side-effects, in particular nausea, vomiting and hypertension. This information renders the choice more complex, particularly if the midwife or obstetrician is confronted with a situation of increased risk of PPH in a woman who has a phobia of vomiting or of injections.

Judgement or decision making often involves the manipulation of large amounts of information, yet evidence shows that the human brain can only manipulate small amounts at any one time. In order to simplify the process, one often uses rules of thumb or cognitive shortcuts, otherwise known as heuristics, to explain phenomena and come to decisions or solve problems (Bursztajn et al. 1990, Cioffi & Markham 1997). However, rules of thumb cannot be accurate, and heuristics fail systematically to process information that is necessary to make sense of the whole issue under consideration. It follows that any heuristic decision has a higher chance of being the result of only partial consideration of all the dimensions of a problem.

Human beings are extremely prone to these shortcomings. In midwifery, as in medical practice, decision making relies heavily on human judgement. Therefore, many mistakes are inevitable. The underdiagnosis of conditions such as thrombosis and/or thromboembolism, in pregnancy or in the postnatal period, offers a good example of the application of heuristics in maternity care where the severity of symptoms is not always recognised or the symptoms are attributed to other causes. Such cases have been highlighted by the Report on Confidential Enquiry into Maternal Deaths (RCOG 2004). The rarer an event, the less likely it is to be recognised by health professionals due to their lack of experience in putting all the pieces of the jigsaw puzzle together.

Midwifery wisdom

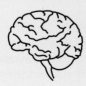

In order to avoid unnecessary errors, midwives should use a more systematic approach to decision making.

Clinical decision making

Diagnoses and clinical judgement are the subject of a multitude of errors. These errors sometimes arise because of poor understanding of statistical principles. The same can be said of clinical choices or decision making, and often for the same reasons: inadequate or inaccurate weighing of options and their consequences. When a systematic approach is used to make a choice, it is said to be subjected to decision analysis. This analytical framework originates mostly from psychology as psychologists have for some time been preoccupied with how and why people make mistakes. One such psychologist is Arthur Elstein and he defined decision analysis as:

> a formal analytic framework that is increasingly being applied to the problem of selecting an action in clinical situations in which the optimal choice is not intuitively clear or the judgments of competent physicians differ. These situations often involve complex combinations of uncertainty, values, risks, and benefits, precisely where human judgment may encounter difficulty in reaching an optimal solution and where a decision aid may be useful.
>
> (Elstein et al. 1986)

Some decisions are relatively easy to make, whilst others are more complex and difficult. As human beings, healthcare practitioners make mistakes. Fortunately, most of these lead to no significant consequences for their service users, but some do. In an effort to avoid errors, formal analytical models have been developed to guide good decisions. One of the best known is Bayes' theorem. Bayes based his theorem on the fact that people hold basic beliefs about various phenomena, but these can be altered in the presence of new probabilistic information (Thompson 1999). Decision analysis combines probabilities of the potential outcomes such as:

- the prior probability of this outcome based on experience (Rayburn & Zhang 2002) or on epidemiological studies (Haynes de Regt et al. 1986, Spiegelhalter et al. 1999)
- the conditional probability of a positive test, a concept that is similar to the true positive rate or sensitivity of a test
- the posterior probability that combines the prior probability and the condition probability.

Bayes' theorem expresses this as:

$$P(\text{disease} / \text{findings}) = \frac{P(\text{findings} / \text{disease}) \times P(\text{disease})}{P(\text{findings})}$$

where:
P(disease/findings)=probability of a disease given a positive test, i.e. the posterior probability or odds
P(findings/disease)=probability of a positive test given the presence of the disease
P(disease)=probability of the disease, i.e. the prior probability or odds
P(findings)=probability of the findings.

Bayes' theorem provides an answer to the question: 'What is the probability of a particular outcome given a particular action?'. For example, what are the chances of someone having a car accident given that they are over the alcohol limit?

$$P(\text{car accident} / \text{over the alcohol limit})$$

$$= \frac{P(\text{over the acohol limit} / \text{car accident}) \times P(\text{car accident})}{P(\text{over the alcohol limit})}$$

The chance of a car driver having an accident if he is over the alcohol limit is not the same as the chance of the driver being over the limit given that he has had a car accident. In other words, the majority of people who are over the limit do not (fortunately for the innocent others) have car accidents but a sizeable proportion of people who have a car accident are over the alcohol limit. This explains why the police breathalyse all drivers involved in an accident or those who are driving erratically, but not all drivers who are driving apparently normally.

An example closer to midwifery is: 'What are the chances of a woman becoming pregnant given that she has had sexual intercourse?'. Clearly, the majority of women who are pregnant have had sexual intercourse but the majority of women who have intercourse do not get pregnant every time.

$$P(\text{pregnancy} / \text{intercourse})$$

$$= \frac{P(\text{intercourse} / \text{pregnancy}) \times P(\text{pregnancy})}{P(\text{intercourse})}$$

These examples explain why we can only say that there is an increased chance or risk that one action will lead to a consequence, i.e. people who are over the alcohol limit are more likely to be involved in accidents and women who have sexual intercourse are more likely to get pregnant. However, statistically, one does not *cause* the other because if it did, that same action would *always* be followed by the same consequence. This is clearly not the case – increased risk, but not cause and effect.

Because of the elements that the Bayesian model takes on board, this process of decision making can sometimes be seen as too prescriptive. That is, if the Bayesian model is applied, the results should be accepted because the equation will have taken into consideration all the potential aspects of the problem. As the equation is used in the presence of uncertainty, and the model provides clarity, it would not make sense to dismiss the results because they do not quite match our *feelings*. It is presumed that the decision that combines the best chances and the best values for the outcome will be the decision of choice. This model of decision making would only be ideal if the level of information required in such a process was readily available to midwives and obstetricians, but in reality that is not necessarily so. Thompson (1999) suggests that there is a need for 'middle ground' where the intuitive-humanistic approach as a cognitive continuum should be taken into account in order to enhance the decision-making process.

Principles in clinical decision making

There is now evidence that using the internet search engine Google may help physicians identify diagnoses in some difficult cases (Tang & Ng 2006). One might be forgiven for thinking that it is a straightforward process to formulate a care management plan once the correct diagnosis is made. However, this is far from the truth. The cost-effectiveness of each treatment alternative and the increasing emphasis on service user empowerment and shared decision making have necessitated the need for 'trade-offs', thus rendering the decision-making process much more complex. Therefore, following a framework by applying some basic principles may help clinicians make better decisions. Bordley (2001) identifies the following principles:

- The problem must be correctly defined.
- Values, preferences and trade-offs must be clearly articulated.
- A wide range of creative solutions to the problem must be explored.
- Credible relevant data must be used for evaluating these alternatives.
- Logically correct reasoning must be used to evaluate alternatives.
- All the stakeholders need to be involved to ensure commitment to acting on the results of the analysis.

Most of the steps are relatively self-explanatory and are common sense. It is essential that a problem or a question should be framed correctly if it is to be answered efficiently in order to find the most suitable solution. It is equally important that all the potential answers ought to be stipulated so that they can be explored in turn. As seen when referring to Bayes' theorem, it is vital that accurate data should be available not only on the likelihood of a condition, but also on the likelihood of treatment success or failure for each of the considered alternatives. All stakeholders must be involved in the decision-making process, including clinicians, health economists, policy makers, service providers and above all service users. The inclusion of service users and the exploration of their views will enable the identification of values, preferences and trade-offs during the decision-making process. The inclusion of values in the equation is called the maximising of utilities (O'Leary et al. 1995, Schackman et al. 2002).

The example of active management of the third stage of labour has already been identified as a potential clinical decision-making situation. To be able to make a decision about how best to manage this situation for a specific woman, information must be available, i.e. the incidence of postpartum haemorrhage generally, the specific risk assessment for this woman, bearing in mind her own specific risks, the alternatives available and the likelihood of outcomes given each alternative. Maximising utilities by adding the values that this woman would attach to each outcome would ultimately help to make the decision pertinent to this specific situation.

Other principles which may also come into play when making decisions are:

- clinicians' (midwife/obstetrician) expertise
- policy or guidelines (national and local), e.g. National Institute for Health and Clinical Excellence (NICE) guidelines
- legal frameworks such as legislation and Nursing and Midwifery Council (NMC) regulations
- research evidence
- available resources.

The clinician's experience in decision making is of course central in the whole process. Her understanding of the various principles involved is vital in arriving at the appropriate decision. The adoption of clinical guidelines, rather than the more rigid protocols, enables midwives to include the values of the women they care for in the equation. In the example of the management of the third stage of labour, the incidence of postpartum haemorrhage can be gathered from epidemiological data and calculated according to the various decision options. The risk can then be more specifically calculated bearing in mind the specific risk factors of the woman. Finally, given that any choice will involve both potentially positive and negative outcomes, e.g. a reduced blood loss but an increased chance of nausea and vomiting (Prendeville et al. 2000), the midwife can now present the likelihood of the various outcomes with the given choices and then ask the woman to provide her own values on the outcomes. Including the woman's values in the equation means that the final decision is tailor-made for the individual. It is essential to note that the likelihood of the outcome does not effect a change in the values of the woman.

Figure 16.1 illustrates these principles more clearly.

283

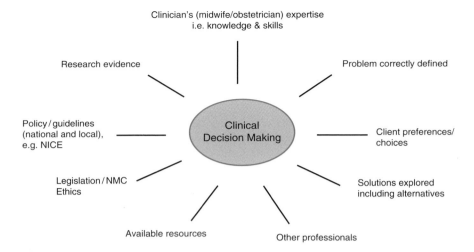

Figure 16.1   Issues to be considered during the decision-making process.

Application of principles

The following case studies demonstrate how these principles can be applied in practice. However, one must beware of thinking that these principles are simple and easy to follow. In fact, nothing could be further from the truth. Nonetheless, they provide guidance for better judgement.

Case study 16.1

A 30-year-old primigravida, Sasha, and her partner had chosen to deliver their first baby in the birth centre, partly because they were keen to embrace midwife-led care and a natural childbirth. Sasha had regular antenatal care with her midwife in the community, and her pregnancy had been uncomplicated. Sasha came to the maternity day assessment unit (MDAU) at term + 3 days (i.e. 40 weeks + 3 days) with her partner as she had felt a reduction in fetal movements. Sasha was to have a cardiotocograph (CTG) to monitor her baby's heart rate and her uterine activity, if any, as per local guidelines.

The CTG trace recorded a reduced variability of the fetal heart rate of less than 5 beats per minute (bpm) with a baseline rate of 140 bpm. An unprovoked deceleration of the fetal heart rate down to 110 bpm was noted after 35 min. There was no uterine activity recorded on the CTG. The MDAU midwife called the obstetric registrar on duty to review Sasha's CTG. The obstetrician, having reviewed the CTG and conducted a vaginal examination with Sasha's consent, spoke with Sasha and her partner about induction of labour in the delivery suite (DS), which they both consented to.

Decision analysis
Midwifery decision – the first principle that supported the midwife's decision to call for an obstetric opinion was her clinical experience (i.e. knowledge and skills). Using her knowledge and clinical skills, the MDAU midwife recognised (i.e. diagnosed) that the CTG was pathological. As this is a deviation from the norm which is outside her sphere of practice, applying other principles such as

clinical guidelines (NICE 2008a) and the *Midwives' Rules and Standards* (NMC 2012), the midwife was able to make the appropriate decision of calling the obstetrician to review Sasha and the CTG.

Obstetric decision – again, the relevant principle was the obstetrician's knowledge and skills, and the application of research evidence and clinical guidance. In view of the gestation and the presence of a pathological CTG, the obstetrician used her clinical judgement to decide that induction of labour was the best course of action as this was more beneficial to both mother and child (NICE 2008b). Although Sasha was booked to give birth in the birth centre and had an uncomplicated pregnancy, in the presence of a pathological CTG, it was deemed that induction of labour and subsequent interpartum and delivery care would be more appropriately carried out in the DS (NICE 2007, 2008b).

Service users' decision – when the obstetrician spoke with Sasha and her partner, she explained the situation to them. Although Sasha's preference was to have a natural childbirth in the birth centre, the value she attached to the outcome was to have a healthy baby delivered safely; hence her decision to consent to induction of labour and delivery in the DS.

Case study 16.2

Michelle, a 34-year-old multipara, who had an uncomplicated normal delivery of a healthy full-term son weighing 3500 g 3 years ago, was booked to have her second baby at home. At 39 weeks' gestation, Michelle's labour started in the morning. Her husband, John, had taken the day off work to stay with her. Her mother, who lived nearby, was also there to help look after their 3-year-old son. By lunchtime, her contractions had established a regular pattern of one in every 7–8 min. Michelle called her community midwife and informed her of the situation.

Midwife Ann arrived at Michelle's home half an hour later to assess her labour. Michelle was found to be in established labour with regular contractions one in every 7 min. Fetal heart rate was satisfactory at 140 bpm. All other observations and vital signs were found to be within normal limits. On abdominal palpation, Ann found nothing untoward except that the presenting head was not engaged, but this is not an uncommon feature for multiparous women at this stage. Ann then carried out a vaginal examination with Michelle's consent to assess labour progress. Michelle's cervix was found to be 4 cm dilated; cephalic presenting at 1 cm above the ischial spines; membranes were intact. Ann went about organising her equipment to prepare for the delivery. Observations on maternal and fetal condition were carried out at regular intervals and they were all within normal limits. Michelle was allowed to labour on without undue intervention.

Three hours later, Michelle's membranes ruptured spontaneously and clear liquor was seen. Ann explained to Michelle and John that it was important for her to carry out another vaginal examination, in order to exclude cord prolapse and to assess labour progress, for which Michelle gave her consent. Ann was shocked to find that the presenting part was in fact a breech rather than cephalic as she originally thought. The cervix was now 7 cm dilated, membranes still intact (i.e. Michelle was having 'hindwater' leak and the 'forewaters' were still intact). She apologised to Michelle and John for her failure to diagnose a breech early on. Ann also explained to them that she had to make arrangements for Michelle's care to be transferred to the obstetric team as this was a deviation from the norm and that it would now be safer for the baby to be delivered in the DS at the hospital. Both Michelle and John agreed to the transfer. Ann contacted the DS and spoke with the co-ordinator as per local guidelines. The DS co-ordinator agreed to liaise with the obstetric team whilst Ann made the necessary arrangements with the paramedics for a swift transfer.

Michelle and John arrived at the hospital 40 min later. Michelle's labour had progressed further during the transfer and she was now 8–9 cm dilated. Fetal heart rate and other observations were all satisfactory. In view of her gravid status (i.e. multigravida) and the duty obstetrician's experience, the decision was made to allow Michelle's labour to progress to a vaginal breech delivery which occurred 2 hours later. Both Michelle and her new daughter were doing well and were subsequently discharged home the following afternoon.

Decision analysis

Ann's decision to transfer care – although Ann failed to diagnose the breech presentation in the first place, this may be partly due to her inexperience in clinical practice, or that the breech was just difficult to diagnose due to bulging membranes or the presenting part being too high. However, once the diagnosis of a breech was made and a deviation from the norm was identified, Ann was correct to refer Michelle to the obstetric team. This was in accordance with the NMC (2012) *Midwives' Rules and Standards* as the situation was now outside her sphere of practice.

Obstetrician's decision to aim for a vaginal breech delivery – this was made after consideration of the following:

- weighing up the risk of a vaginal breech delivery for a multiparous woman who was already 8–9 cm dilated on admission to the DS
- risk of complications following an emergency caesarean section
- the couple's preference for a 'normal birth' (hence the choice of homebirth), and the obstetrician's experience in vaginal breech delivery.

The obstetrician's decision was supported by her clinical experience and skills and by guidelines (NICE 2007).

Service users' perspective – once again, the value the service users attached to the outcome was to have a healthy baby delivered safely. Hence their readiness in agreeing to the transfer.

Midwifery wisdom

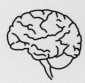
The fundamental principle of clinical decision making must be consideration of the health and safety of mother and child.

The interpersonal skills and information needed to successfully share decisions are major challenges, but they are vital elements within interprofessional working such as during a transfer of care. The benefits of service user involvement and the skills required to achieve this approach need to be given much higher priority at all levels, i.e. policy making, education and within further professional development strategies.

Managerial decision making

Most organisations operate by people making decisions. Within the health services, clinicians such as midwives, doctors and other health professionals plan their workloads; managers plan, organise, lead and control their staff by executing decisions. The effectiveness and quality of those decisions often determine the success (or otherwise) of an organisation. Managerial decision making is frequently concerned with using limited resources to maximise outcomes (Block 2006). This may be the selection of a course of action from available alternatives (i.e. making choices), setting priorities and allocation decisions such as staff deployment and budgeting. Many of these decisions involve an ethical component (Jones 1991), which is one of the most important considerations in healthcare management.

Healthcare management, in the main, is not about profits but rather cost-effectiveness of treatment outcomes (Detsky & Naglie 1990). Block (2006) advocates that there are generally four dimensions to healthcare evaluation.

- The first is measuring effectiveness by looking at the benefits of health services demonstrated by the improvement of health in a given population.
- The second is the study of efficiency by comparing the cost of health intervention to the benefits gained by the individuals or population being studied (i.e. the degree of health gained).
- The third is being humane (i.e. being able to share service users' feelings as they interact with clinicians).
- The fourth is concerned with equity, i.e. being fair in terms of distribution of both benefits and burdens of healthcare services amongst the population; in other words, availability (Detsky & Naglie 1990).

Therefore, any managerial decision-making process must encompass all the dimensions of healthcare evaluation where cost-effectiveness, cost-benefits and cost-utility analysis are taken into consideration (Block 2006). For midwives, with their ever-increasing workloads, ensuring smooth running of a clinical area (i.e. the delivery suite or an inpatient ward), under the current economic constraints and with completing demands, is no mean task.

Midwifery wisdom

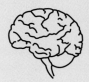
Midwives must develop skills in setting priorities in order to maximise outcomes in relation to limited resources.

Managerial decision-making skills are obviously required when midwives work in triage, manage a team or have the responsibility of setting service provision. As with clinical decision making, the midwife's experience plays a crucial role in this process. Having the knowledge and skills would certainly help her to decide what is more urgent or important (i.e. to prioritise); hence, it is logical to say that the more experienced the midwife, the better she is equipped to manage but this is not always the case. However, by adopting a more systematic approach to problem solving and some guiding principles (as mentioned in the section on clinical decision making), midwives should be in a better position to develop their skills in this area.

The following activities provide an illustration as to how this systematic approach can be applied.

Activity 16.1

Sarah is a community midwife who has a very heavy workload. On this particular day, on top of her usual workload, there is also a very important meeting that Sarah would like to attend. What should Sarah do in order to accomplish all her tasks?

Decision-making process

Sarah needs to exercise her clinical knowledge and skills to prioritise her workload. She should ask herself whether all the women on her visiting list really require a visit that day. Or would a phone call suffice? What does legislation say about this action? Consider also the NMC regulations (NMC 2012), and any national or local guidelines in relation to this decision. If the above was not possible, how about enlisting the help of another colleague to share out the workload?

Are there any other alternatives, e.g. working with other colleagues to share out attendance at important meetings and feedback to each other, i.e. using available resources to maximise outcomes?

Seek help from the management team as appropriate.

Activity 16.2

Wendy is the DS co-ordinator. She comes on duty one morning and takes over a very busy ward with all the labour rooms filled with women in different stages of labour. All except two of these women have high-risk factors attached to them. Although Wendy has the right number of midwives on duty, she only has one Band 7 midwife to support her. The rest of the team is made up of Band 6 midwives of varying experience, amongst them two very junior midwives who only qualified recently and an agency midwife (Band 6) who has never worked in this hospital before. What action, if any, should Wendy take to ensure that she manages her DS efficiently and safely?

Decision-making process

Wendy needs to have the knowledge and skills to ascertain the 'skills mix' of her team and be able to allocate workload accordingly.

As the DS is so busy, ideally Wendy could do with someone who has more experience and local knowledge of the DS than the agency midwife in order to support the team. This is especially relevant to support for the two newly qualified midwives. She could work with her manager to explore the option of redeployment of the agency midwife to the antenatal or postnatal ward and swap one of the unit's own midwives whoknows the DS well to support the team.

Alternatively, Wendy, in conjunction with the appropriate managers, may request help from other areas that are not as busy, should the situation in the DS worsen.

The basic principles of Wendy's decision and action must be to ensure the efficient running of the DS and equity of support for her staff to provide safe and high-quality care to women and their babies.

It can be seen from these activities that the fundamental principles of managerial decision making are equity, ethics and safety. In exercising their managerial decision-making skills, midwives must learn to think 'outside the box' and be 'creative'. However, with some guiding principles, midwives should be able to handle most of the day-to-day demand of their own workload, some lower and/or middle management issues.

Conclusion

The process of decision making is extremely complex. The proposed guidance on clinical judgement and managerial decision making might lure the reader into thinking that these principles are simple and easy to follow. In fact, nothing could be further from the truth. The process requires midwives not only to exercise their clinical knowledge and skills, but to expand their cognitive faculty. A better understanding of the scale of clinical errors and their underlying causes should motivate midwives and other clinicians to challenge poor judgement and bring about changes.

As far as the decision-making process is concerned, this chapter has only scratched the surface. However, even the briefest of introductions to the subject should be enough to whet the appetite of many midwives as the ultimate aim of the care they provide is to maximise normality and reduce unnecessary risk and intervention. At a time when the caesarean section rate is at its highest, with no obvious benefit for either women or their babies, it is time for midwives, with their medical colleagues, to adopt a systematic approach to decision making in providing maternity care, together with the elicitation of the values of women, leading to more individualised and safer care.

Quiz

1. Midwives should develop decision-making skills in:

    a. deciding whether to wear make-up or not when going on duty
    b. choosing their holiday destinations
    c. clinical practice and in managing own workload and others
    d. telling others what to do
    e. all of the above.

2. In the developed world, maternal deaths are mainly due to:

    a. accidents on the road
    b. human errors
    c. inevitable causes of severe pathology
    d. mothers not looking after themselves
    e. all of the above.

3. Reports on maternal deaths define major substandard care as:

    a. care that would have made a difference in management, but would not have necessarily saved the woman
    b. care being a significant contributory factor that could have changed the management and prevented the death of the woman
    c. care that would have made no difference in the management and outcome
    d. poor care that is the direct cause of the woman's death
    e. all of the above.

4. Midwives should based their decision making largely on:

   a. human judgement
   b. their intuition or gut feeling
   c. clinical observations only
   d. hard data supported by clinical manifestations
   e. all of the above.

5. Heuristics is a decision-making process:

   a. that uses a systematic approach to solve problems
   b. relying on rules of thumb or cognitive shortcuts to solve problems
   c. best used to make sense of the whole issue under consideration
   d. all of the above
   e. none of the above.

6. Thompson (1999) suggests that there is a need for 'middle ground' in the decision-making process because it has become much more complex due to:

   a. the cost-effectiveness of each treatment alternative
   b. the increasing emphasis on service user empowerment
   c. shared decision making which has necessitated the need for 'trade-offs'
   d. all of the above
   e. none of the above.

7. A systematic approach to decision making means:

   a. inclusion of service users' values, preferences and trade-offs to maximise utilities
   b. that a wide range of creative solutions to the problem, including alternatives, must be explored
   c. all the stakeholders need to be involved
   d. the problem must be correctly defined
   e. all of the above.

8. Decision making in healthcare management is often concerned with:

   a. utilising limited resources to maximise outcomes
   b. setting priorities, i.e. making choices
   c. staff deployment and budgeting
   d. all of the above
   e. none of the above.

9. Midwives are required to exercise their managerial decision-making skills when:

   a. prioritising their own workload
   b. managing a team of staff
   c. working in triage
   d. setting service provision
   e. all of the above.

10. The processes of decision making require midwives to:

    a. read more books on decision making
    b. take on more management roles
    c. exercise their clinical knowledge and skills, and expand their cognitive faculty
    d. be familiar with their professional body's rules and regulations
    e. all of the above.

References

Block DJ (2006) *Healthcare Outcomes Management: strategies for planning and evaluation*. London: Jones and Bartlett.

Bordley R (2001) Naturalistic decision-making and prescriptive decision theory. *Journal of Behavioral Decision-making* **14**(5): 355–357.

Bursztajn H, Feinbloom R, Hamm R, Brodsky A (1990) *Medical Choices, Medical Chances: how patients, families and physicians can cope with uncertainty*. London: Routledge.

Cameron HM, McGoogan E (1981) A prospective study of 1152 hospital autopsies: II. *Analysis of inaccuracies in clinical diagnoses and their significance. Journal of Pathology* **133**(4): 285–300.

Centre for Maternal and Child Enquiries (CMACE) (2011) *Saving Mothers' Lives: reviewing maternal deaths to make motherhood safer: 2006–2008*. The 8th Report of the Confidential Enquiries into Maternal Deaths in the UK. London: Centre for Maternal and Child Enquiries.

Centre for Maternal and Child Enquiries (CMACE) (2011) *Perinatal Mortality 2009*. London: Centre for Maternal and Child Enquiries.

Chapman GB, Sonnenberg FA (2003) *Decision Making in Health Care: theory, psychology, and applications*. Cambridge: Cambridge University Press.

Cioffi J, Markham R (1997) Clinical decision-making by midwives: managing case complexity. *Journal of Advanced Nursing* **25**(2): 265–272.

Connolly T, Arkes HR, Hammond KR (2000) *Judgment and Decision Making: an interdisciplinary reader*. Cambridge: Cambridge University Press.

Detsky AS, Naglie IG (1990) A clinician's guide to cost-effectiveness analysis. *Annals of Internal Medicine* **113**: 147–154.

Elstein AS, Holzman GB, Ravitch MM et al. (1986) Comparisons of physicians' decisions regarding estrogen replacement therapy for menopausal women and decisions derived from a decision analytic model. *American Journal of Medicine* **80**(2): 246–258.

Ermenc B (1999) Minimizing mistakes in clinical diagnosis. *Journal of Forensic Science* **44**(4): 810–813.

Haynes de Regt R, Minkoff H, Feldman J, Schwartz R (1986) Relation of private or clinic care to the caesarean birth rate. *New England Journal of Medicine* **315**(10): 619–624.

Jones TM (1991) Ethical decision making by individuals in organizations: an issue-contingent model. *Academy of Management Review* **16**(2): 366–395.

Lilford R (1990) Limitations of expert systems: intuition versus analysis. In: Lilford R (ed) *Baillière's Clinical Obstetrics and Gynaecology*. London: Baillière Tindall.

McKelvie PA (1993) Medical certification of causes of death in an Australian metropolitan hospital. Comparison with autopsy findings and a critical review. *Medical Journal of Australia* **158**(12): 816–818, 820–821.

National Institute for Health and Clinical Excellence (NICE) (2007) *Intrapartum Care: management and delivery of care to women in labour*. Clinical Guideline No. CG55. London: National Institute for Health and Clinical Excellence.

National Institute for Health and Clinical Excellence (NICE) (2008a) *Antenatal Care: routine care for the healthy pregnant woman*. Clinical Guideline No. CG62. London: National Institute for Health and Clinical Excellence.

National Institute for Health and Clinical Excellence (NICE) (2008b) *Induction of Labour* Clinical Guideline No. CG70. London: National Institute for Health and Clinical Excellence.

Nursing and Midwifery Council (NMC) (2012) *Midwives' Rules and Standards*. London: Nursing and Midwifery Council.

O'Leary JF, Fairclough DL, Jankowski MK, Weeks JC (1995) Comparison of time-tradeoff utilities and rating scale values of cancer patients and their relatives: evidence for a possible plateau relationship. *Medical Decision-Making* **15**(2): 132–137.

Prendeville WJ, Elbourne D, McDonald S (2000) Active versus expectant management in the third stage of labour. *Cochrane Database of Systematic Reviews* **3**: CD000007.

Rayburn W, Zhang J (2002) Rising rates of labor induction: present concerns and future strategies. *Obstetrics and Gynecology* **100**(1): 164–167.

Roosen J, Frans E, Wilmer A et al. (2000) Comparison of premorten clinical diagnoses in critically ill patients and subsequent autopsy findings. *Mayo Clinic Proceedings* **75**(6): 562–567.

Roulson J, Benbow EW, Hasleton PS (2005) Discrepancies between clinical and autopsy diagnosis and the value of post mortem history: a meta-analysis and review. *Histopathology* **47**: 551–559.

Royal College of Obstetricians and Gynaecologists (RCOG) (2004) *Why Mothers Die 2000–2002*. Report on Confidential Enquiries into Maternal Deaths in the United Kingdom.London: RCOG Press.

Rozenberg J (2006) Sir Roy Meadow, the flawed witness, wins GMC appeal. *The Telegraph*. Available at: www.telegraph.co.uk/news/uknews/1510798/Sir-Roy-Meadow-the-flawed-witness-wins-GMC-appeal.html (accessed May 2013).

Sarode VR, Datta BN, Banerjee AK et al. (1993) Autopsy findings and clinical diagnoses: a review of 1,000 cases. *Human Pathology* **24**(2): 194–198.

Schackman BR, Goldie SJ, Freedberg KA et al. (2002) Comparison of health state utilities using community and patient preference weights derived from a survey of patients with HIV/AIDS. *Medical Decision-Making* **22**(1): 27–38.

Spiegelhalter D, Myles J, Jones D, Abrams K (1999) An introduction to Bayesian methods in health technology assessment. *British Medical Journal* **319**: 508–512.

Tang H, Ng JHK (2006) Googling for a diagnosis – use of Google as a diagnostic aid: Internet-based study. *British Medical Journal* **333**(7579): 1143–1145.

Thompson C (1999) A conceptual treadmill: the need for 'middle ground' in clinical decision-making theory in nursing. *Journal of Advanced Nursing* **30**(5): 1222–1229.

Thornton J (1990) Decision analysis in obstetrics and gynaecology. In: Lilford R (ed) *Baillière's Clinical Obstetrics and Gynaecology*. London: Baillière Tindall.

17

Health, Safety and Environmental Issues

Lisa Nash

Aim

The aim of this chapter is to enhance your knowledge and understanding of the midwife's role in maintaining health and safety in the working environment.

Learning outcomes

By the end of this chapter you will be able to:

1. demonstrate your understanding of key legislation, including the Health and Safety at Work Act 1974, the Workplace (Health, Safety and Welfare) Regulations 1992, the Management of Health and Safety at Work Regulations 1999, Control of Substances Hazardous to Health Regulations 2002, and Reporting of Injuries, Diseases and Dangerous Occurrences regulations 1995
2. demonstrate the knowledge and understanding required to carry out a risk assessment, enabling you to reduce the risks of slips, trips, falls, dealing with violence and aggression and the vulnerability of working in isolation
3. identify signs of poor mental health and stress, equipping you with useful tools
4. understand the importance of looking after your back and posture
5. discuss key issues concerning infection prevention and control and reduction of sharps injuries along with the requisite knowledge and understanding.

The Student's Guide to Becoming a Midwife, Second Edition. Edited by Ian Peate and Cathy Hamilton.
© 2014 John Wiley & Sons, Ltd. Published 2014 by John Wiley & Sons, Ltd.

Introduction

This chapter will look at some of the common issues in relation to health and safety and the environment in the workplace. The legislation that has been put in place to protect employees will be discussed, along with practical advice about assessing and avoiding risks in the first place. There are activities throughout the chapter along with weblinks which you will find useful.

Assessing risk

A risk assessment ensures that everything possible has been done to stop anything harmful occurring. It is a legal requirement for employers to assess all potential risks in the workplace. It is equally important that we each take responsibility by routinely carrying out risk assessments in our work environment to prevent injuries, accidents and ill health. The Health and Safety Executive (HSE) (2006, 2011) has a simplified five-step guide to carrying out risk assessments, which should be used in any area in which you work. Use the acronym HAZDERR to help you remember these:

1. Look for any **ha**zards.
2. **D**ecide who might be affected by them.
3. **E**valuate the risks and decide whether the existing precautions are adequate or whether more should be done.
4. **R**ecord your findings.
5. **R**eview your assessment, revising it if necessary.

Activity 17.1

 Follow steps 1 and 2 above, looking out for areas where hazards could exist and therefore what you need to check. It is not anticipated that you will identify risks but the exercise should enhance your observations of potential risks. An example of avoiding a potential risk would be the testing of all electrical devices and plug sockets.

Within the maternity services there are potential risks everywhere, as there are in any workplace, for example a blocked emergency exit; equipment left in corridors, such as beds; a hostile partner; lone working; or driving in poor weather conditions for those working in the community. Those at risk include:

- midwives
- healthcare assistants/team support workers
- domestic or portering staff
- new and expectant mothers
- all visitors
- any contractors working in the environment
- doctors and other allied healthcare professionals.

In the event of a fire or for any other reason to evacuate any healthcare premises, an obstructed exit will impede the safe evacuation of those present and could be life-threatening. This is a high risk and the emergency exit will need to be unblocked as legislated by the Regulatory Reform (Fire Safety) Order 2005 which dictates the responsibilities of the employer and employees in prevention of fire hazards.

Equally all of the other examples above will need to be considered with solutions to limit the risks they pose.

You need to reduce the possibility of any risk occurring, therefore you may wish to think of measures to prevent the same event recurring by educating staff, finding suitable storage for the object(s) blocking the area and putting up notices. You may be able to think of other ways to achieve this.

To control risks, the following principles should be applied:

- Try an alternative option which will be less risky.
- Prevent access to the hazard, for example by guarding.
- Reduce exposure to the hazard by organising work accordingly.
- Issue personal protective equipment (including goggles and gloves).
- Provide facilities to aid welfare in the event of an occurrence, for example first aid and washing facilities to enable the removal of substances on the skin.

You need to record what you found during your risk assessment and what you did about it. You must tell your employer/the employees about your findings. Adverse incidents are usually caused by a chain of events so by completing risk assessments competently, you are reducing the risk of these happening. There are risks in everyday life and they cannot all be completely removed, but every possible means should be taken to reduce any risk.

295

Midwifery wisdom

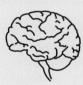

Wearing the protective goggles you are issued with will stop any splashes from amniotic fluid (that you may not even be aware of) getting into your eyes. Glasses do not offer the same degree of protection. Next time you facilitate a birth, take a look at the goggles afterwards.

Activity 17.2

Find out who conducts the risk assessment in your clinical area. You may find it helpful to discuss with them how they conduct the risk assessment and look at any paperwork that they use.

Slips, trips and falls

Slips and trips account for a third of all accidents in the workplace (HSE 2002). Avoiding them is everyone's responsibility so we need to ensure that our working environment is as safe as it can be. Often where serious accidents or falls occur, someone else has first slipped or tripped in the same place.

Although avoiding slips and trips may seem like common sense, it may be easy at times to overlook these when we are in a hurry.

All members of staff and students are responsible for:

- attending any training sessions that are offered
- following health and safety procedures and policies within their working environment
- tidying up as they go.
- being aware of potential hazards at all times.

Activity 17.3

 Follow the link below to complete an online package devised by the Health and Safety Executive:www.hse.gov.uk/slips/step/

You should:

- look at what is going on around you and be aware of where you are going and what you are doing
- look where you are going and never run or rush
- use any safety equipment provided
- be especially careful on uneven ground and steps, using handrails where provided (for example, when you are walking down stairs)
- follow safety guidelines in your area
- use lighting in dark areas (it is surprising how many people walk around in dark or dimly lit storage areas)
- not attempt to carry out any activity beyond your capability; ask for assistance if you need it
- conduct yourself in an appropriate fashion. Playing a practical joke on colleagues may seem like fun, but can be a serious risk to you and your colleagues if it results in an accident.

Activity 17.4

 Find out how you would deal with a blood spillage in your area, including where you would go to find cleaning equipment.

Preventing slips

- Deal with any spillage (e.g. blood, liquor or vomit) immediately; do not wait for someone else to clear it up, it's everyone's responsibility.
- Take care on slippery surfaces, including those which have recently been waxed or washed.

- Non-skid mats should be used around washing areas, such as showers and baths.
- Ensure that mats and carpets are secured to the floor surface; maintain any areas which are frayed, worn or curled up.
- Flooring may have uneven surfaces or be damaged in some way; take extra care when walking on these surfaces. Similar hazards exist on pavements and walkways around your workplace, so take care here too.
- Be aware of your footing as the level may change unexpectedly, for example when you go round a corner.
- Be cautious when walking on icy surfaces and alert your employer to enable precautions to be implemented.
- Wear shoes that are fit for your job. They should offer support, have enough grip on them and should not be open-toed.

Activity 17.5

 As newly cleaned surfaces have caused so many slips in the past, the HSE (2009a) has put together a leaflet examining a case study and discussing appropriate methods of cleaning. To find out more, follow the link below:www.hse.gov.uk/pubns/web/slips02.pdf

Preventing trips

- Get into a daily routine of ensuring that your working environment is kept tidy, with items returned to where they belong.
- Keep floors free from rubbish and any other debris such as swabs, incontinence pads, wrappers, and so on.
- Do not leave anything on the stairs.
- Keep drawers and cupboard doors closed.
- Store equipment such as cardiotocograph machines, stools and ventouse apparatus safely out of the way.
- Make sure that electrical leads and cables attached to resuscitaires, cardiotocograph machines and ventouse apparatus do not trail across walkways or where anyone can trip over them.
- Have a place for everything and keep it there. Do not store anything in corridors.
- Be mindful of where any furniture is placed, allowing easy access for anyone needing to come into the area.
- Move obstacles out of the way; do not attempt to step over them.

Preventing falls

- When going up or down stairs, do not carry anything that obscures your vision and use the handrail.
- Ensure that adequate lighting is available. Stair lighting especially should be bright.
- Ask for help when carrying heavy loads.

- Do not stand on chairs. If you need a stepladder, use one.
- Make sure that chairs are fit for purpose and use them appropriately, for example not standing on them or rocking.
- Use a ladder to get down from a height, such as when getting out of a store room or closing a high window.
- If you are using a ladder, for example to get to equipment out of your reach, know how to use it properly.

Remember, it is your responsibility to:

- dress appropriately. You should not wear jewellery, long hair should be tied back and you should ensure that your footwear is sturdy with closed toes
- only carry out the work that you are trained to do
- take time to organise and plan how you are going to do your work. For example, if you need anything which is out of reach, ensure that you can reach it safely using the appropriate equipment.

Activity 17.6

Reflect on your work in the last week. Can you recall any incidents when you took unnecessary risks? If so, think about how you could reduce the risk in future. If not, think of a risk activity that you have undertaken in the past and how you would prevent yourself being in that situation in the future. An example could be using a chair to get something that is out of your reach.

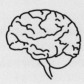

Midwifery wisdom

Don't be tempted to take short cuts to save time – it could change your life forever.

Activity 17.7

Visit the following link for the HSE's 'Shattered Lives' campaign: www.hse.gov.uk/shatteredlives/index.htm

Mental health and stress

Under the Disability Discrimination Act 1995, employers may not discriminate against people with a mental health disorder (including depression or schizophrenia). This means that they cannot deny someone a job or career progression on the grounds of mental ill health. It also means that the employer is legally obliged to make 'reasonable adjustments' to prevent the employee being disadvantaged by their illness.

Activity 17.8

Reflect on a time when you experienced a stressful situation – a new job, a house move, bereavement or a busy day at work when you felt pulled in many directions. Think through the following points.

- How did you deal with the situation?
- Did you feel that you dealt with it adequately?
- How did you feel about it?
- Who supported you?
- Were you able to take time out for yourself?
- Did the situation change your perceptions in any way?

It is recognised that stress affects the smooth running of any business, including an increase in staff turnover, and is therefore costly. Thus, it makes good business sense to reduce stress in the workplace. The employer has a legal obligation to protect employees against ill health, including the effects of stress. A risk assessment should be conducted and precautions taken to avoid unnecessary stresses (Amicus 2006). Stressors in the workplace include:

- boring or repetitive work
- too little to do
- too much to do or too little time to do it in
- inadequate or excessive work-based training
- uncertainty about roles within the team
- having responsibility for others
- lack of flexible work schedules
- the threat of violence
- poor working conditions
- lack of control over work activities
- lack of communication and consultation between managers and staff
- negative culture, for example a blame culture
- lack of developmental support.

Many of us experience stress outside work, which will equally have an impact on our health and standard of work. When dealing with stress, it is important for the employer to listen to staff. The following measures can be taken to prevent stress from becoming a problem (Amicus 2006):

- Take stress seriously.
- Show an understanding attitude to those affected.
- Make sure that staff have the appropriate skills, training and resources to enable them to carry out their job confidently and competently.
- Allow staff to have a say in how they do their work.
- Where possible, vary working conditions.
- Treat all staff fairly and consistently.
- Deal effectively with bullying and harassment.
- Ensure good communication in the workplace between managers and staff, paying particular attention in times of change.
- Design and implement an effective mental health policy, taking into account the view of all sectors of staff.

Within the maternity unit, many pressures are put on staff which may cause stress. In current practice, the massive changes that maternity units are undergoing, such as hospital mergers, are a good example. Mergers cause anxiety due to the uncertainty that they cause and changes within the team, such as a change of management; shift times; working environment; and working with different staff who may have different working practices.

300

Activity 17.9

Reflect on a recent change which has affected you. This could be relatively small, such as a change in hospital policy, or major, such as a change in job role.
   How did you feel about the change and how did you adapt to it? Did you find anything particularly difficult? Did you adapt quickly or was it a slow process?

Stress at work can lead to mental and physical ill health, including depression. Stress is caused when you are under excessive pressure for some time. You may notice the following signs in someone suffering from stress (HSE 1998b):

- increased sick leave
- more unexplained absences
- poor time-keeping
- poor performance
- increased intake of alcohol, drugs, tobacco or caffeine
- social withdrawal
- frequent headaches or backaches
- indecisiveness
- poor decision making
- fatigue or low energy levels
- mood changes (irritability, tearfulness).

Activity 17.10

Visit the following link to the HSE to find more information on stress: www.hse.gov.uk/stress/index.htm

Midwifery wisdom

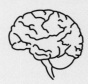

Finding out what support is available now will ensure that you will know where to go when you do need it (and when it may feel all too difficult to find out what support is available).

Looking after your back

In midwifery practice we use and abuse our backs in all manner of ways. All staff are required to attend mandatory moving and handling sessions on an annual basis. As midwives and allied healthcare professionals, we unnecessarily put strain on our backs in many different scenarios, including the following:

- conducting deliveries
- moving beds around bays or to the operating theatre
- conducting a postnatal examination on the mother and baby
- conducting antenatal examinations on the women in our care
- attaching a cardiotocograph machine
- collecting equipment from store rooms.

We should all do the following in our everyday lives to look after our backs (NHS Choices 2012).

- Exercise regularly.
- Make sure we bend at knees and hips (rather than stooping over).
- Hold heavy objects close to us when we lift and carry them.
- Use rucksacks instead of over-the-shoulder bags.
- If you smoke, stopping will help increase the blood supply to the discs (smoking is believed to reduce the blood supply and cause degeneration of the discs).
- Ensure that you maintain a healthy weight; excessive weight will put more of a strain on your back.
- Maintain a good posture at all times.
- When you are sitting, make sure that your back is well supported in a chair with a backrest, placing your feet firmly on the floor.
- Make sure that your bed suits your age, height and sleeping position.
- Avoid twisting and lifting at the same time.

Activity 17.11

Reflect on the following.

- In which situations do you rush without thinking of the damage that you are potentially doing to your back?
- How do you ensure that you maintain a good posture when auscultating the fetal heart when the mother is immersed in water?
- Do you ensure that you take a 'hands off approach when facilitating mothers to breastfeed?
- How do you ensure that you protect your back when you are facilitating a standing delivery?

Do you need to alter your behaviour in order to care for your back?

Infection control

Infection control is important to prevent cross-infection and thereby maintain our clients' as well as our own well-being. Midwives can be contaminated with human immunodeficiency virus (HIV) or hepatitis C, or women and their babies can be contaminated with methicillin-resistant *Staphylococcus aureus* (MRSA) or group B streptococcus (GBS).

Infection control has been the focus of publicity recently with various campaigns running to highlight this basic but essential aspect of healthcare. Cases of MRSA are frequently reported, along with other organisms. The Royal College of Nursing (RCN) and the Infection Prevention Society have published *Infection Prevention and Control: minimum standards* (2009), something which the RCN had been campaigning on for some time. The standards include the following:

- Access for all to appropriate hand decontaminants
- Availability of 24 hours, sufficiently trained cleaning services
- The development of a tool for nurses to measure environmental cleanliness
- Establishment of systems to enable nurses to maintain ward standards
- Dedicated decontamination services
- Mandatory training of all health and social care staff in infection prevention and control
- Ongoing training updates
- The introduction of a standardised infection prevention and control module in all pre-registration programmes
- Establish a system enabling staff to demonstrate and record their ongoing competence at managing infection control
- Recruit sufficient practice educators to ensure that the theory–practice gap is supported

As healthcare professionals, we are the most prolific carriers of infection; by always using the correct hand-washing technique between client contacts, we will be ensuring that infection rates are significantly reduced (RCN 2012). We all play a vital role in maintaining standards for the prevention of infection and should follow the standard precautions (RCN 2012), ensuring that we:

- maintain appropriate hand-washing techniques to maintain hand hygiene
- use personal protective equipment
- handle and dispose of sharps safely

- handle and dispose of clinical waste safely
- manage blood and bodily spillages appropriately
- decontaminate equipment
- keep the clinical environment clean and well maintained
- use indwelling devices appropriately
- manage accidents effectively
- communicate well with our colleagues, patients and visitors
- attend training and educate those around us.

Activity 17.12

Examine your own actions when dealing with these areas of clinical practice. For example, do you wash your hands before and after *every* client contact? Do you educate parents about maintaining hand hygiene before and after changing their baby's nappy?

Dealing with sharps

Midwives deal with sharps on a regular basis, including amniocentesis hooks, needles, fetal scalp electrodes and drug vials. It is vital that you use and dispose of sharps appropriately to prevent infection of hepatitis B, hepatitis C and HIV. After back injuries, sharps injuries are the second most common injury in the NHS. The RCN (2005) reports that over the 5-year period 1997–2002, there were 1550 incidences of exposures to blood-borne viruses in healthcare workers, 42% of whom were nurses or midwives.

To ensure that the risks of sharps injuries are kept to the minimum, you should maintain the following practice (RCN 2012):

- Never pass sharps from hand to hand. Always use a receiver.
- Keep the handling of sharps to a minimum. There should be no unnecessary handling.
- Check that needles are not damaged before use or disposal.
- Never dismantle syringes and needles but dispose of them as a single unit.
- Never resheath needles.
- Take responsibility for the disposal of your own sharps. Always dispose of them appropriately when you have finished with them – do not ask someone else to do it.
- Sharps containers must comply with British Standard 7320 and UN standard 329.
- Never fill a sharps box more than two-thirds full to ensure that injuries are not caused by sharps sticking out.
- Sharps boxes must be stored away from the public to prevent them being tampered with.
- Sharps trays should have integral sharps bins.
- Sharps should be disposed of immediately after they are used.
- Be aware of your local sharps policy.

In the event of a sharps injury you must (RCN 2012):

- encourage the wound to bleed (but do not suck)
- wash well with running water
- cover with a plaster
- report the injury to occupational health (A & E if out of hours) and to your manager
- complete an accident report form
- if the injury is from a used needle, you should seek advice from a microbiologist, infection control doctor or consultant for communicable disease control.

In the event of contamination with body fluids you should:

- wash the mouth out with water if fluids enter the mouth
- irrigate the eyes if fluids enter them.

Activity 17.13

Read through your local policy on sharps injuries, ensuring that you know what to do in the event of an injury.

Working in isolation

We will all be working alone at some point in our career. For some, it will mean being in a delivery room on our own, for others it will be mean being in someone's home on our own. Although many of us will only need to call for help to a colleague, those of us working in the community are very isolated and therefore the potential risks are greater as generally your location will be unknown, no one will know that you are in trouble and when help is summoned it will not be immediately available.

Under the Health and Safety at Work Act 1974 (HSE 1998a, 2009b), employers are required to assess risks to those working in isolation and minimise them. Of course, as an employee it is our responsibility to take precautions too. As with any area covered by the Act, employers must discuss this aspect with the employees that it affects and put in place controlling measures. These can include instruction, training, supervision and protective equipment.

Considerations for lone workers include the following:

- Emergency situations, such as maternal collapse in the home.
- Physical activities/situations. For example, you may have to consider how you would transfer a labouring woman down five flights of stairs.
- Mental stressors. For example, you might walk into a stressful situation, such as a couple having a row, or find that you have too much work to do.
- Adequate training to ensure that the lone worker can practise safely. For example, being able to deal with emergency situations such as a postpartum haemorrhage.

Activity 17.14

Take time to consider any vulnerable situations that you may find yourself in when working alone, for example, attending a born before arrival to find that the woman is having a postpartum haemorrhage and you are the only person there, or conducting a delivery where the partner becomes aggressive (in the home or in hospital).

- What would be your immediate actions?
- How would you raise an alarm for help?
- What other considerations might you have to take into account?

Precautions to be taken to increase your safety include the following (HSE 1998a, 2009b):

- Identify exits when entering a building.
- Ensure that you can handle all your equipment safely.
- Do not work alone if you have a medical condition that would make it dangerous or impractical to do so.
- Consider which tasks can be carried out on your own and which require assistance. For example, in case of an emergency during a home delivery, it is standard practice to have a second midwife in attendance.
- Undertake any training offered, including any that helps you handle an aggressive situation.
- Seek advice from a manager as and when necessary.
- Maintain regular contact with colleagues.
- Ensure that someone (e.g. a colleague) knows where you are due to go each day.
- Use your judgement. Walk away if you feel threatened, you can return later with the police or a colleague.
- Consider whether you need to take a colleague with you, for example, if there has been an aggressive incident on the premises in the past.
- Consider whether you are the most suitable person. If you have already had some degree of misunderstanding/altercation with the client or their partner, it may be wise for another colleague to attend who may be able to handle the situation differently (for example, they may be perceived differently by the client and/or their partner).
- Ensure that you have the equipment necessary to deal with emergency situations.
- Check in with colleagues when you return to your base site or home.
- An alarm system should be used which will send an alert out when you have had periods of inactivity.

There are alternatives to alarm systems which are discussed by the Suzy Lamplugh Trust (2010) which also recommends that a lone-working system is put in place. This can be relatively low tech and inexpensive, for example a midwife could have a movements sheet in the office and a contact (for example, a community clerk) who she contacts regularly throughout the day to confirm arrival and departure from visits and destinations. There are many more technological systems available. It is important to remember that when a member of staff needs assistance, the police will need as much information as possible about the location and who they were visiting.

Violence and aggression

People working in a healthcare setting are up to four times more likely to experience violence in the course of their work than anyone else. Periodic inspections are carried out by the HSE to check what arrangements are in place to deal with workplace violence (HSE 2004).

305

The HSE (2004) reports that the following factors increase the risks of violent or aggressive situations:

- impatience
- frustration
- anxiety
- resentment
- alcohol, drugs or mental instability.

Activity 17.15

Reflect on how these factors could manifest in your clinical environment. It may help to talk to colleagues about their experiences of dealing with violent or aggressive clients, partners or visitors.

As with any other health and safety issue, the employer has to assess the risk and put appropriate measures in place. These measures may include:

- providing training and information
- reviewing and improving the environment in which you work
- altering staff roles.

It is disturbing to note that a surprisingly high number of nurses and midwives (84%) do not carry out routine risk assessments when conducting lone visits in the community around their personal safety (Brennan 2010).

Activity 17.16

It would be useful to do this activity when you are working in the community, either alone or with a mentor.

Brennan (2004) devised a rapid risk assessment tool which is worth considering, covering the following areas:

- Do you know the person you are visiting?
- If not, where can you find out about them?
- Is there a known history of violence or harassment?
- Is the area that you are visiting known to be unsafe?
- Do you use a lone-worker system?
- Do you have a mobile phone and a personal alarm?
- Is there a colleague who could accompany you on a visit?
- Are you trained in de-escalation skills?
- Would you be able to 'break away' from a violent person?
- Could the visit you are going to undertake trigger violence?

Working with visual display units

However infrequently we work on a computer, using one incorrectly can result in health risks. These need to be addressed. Some users report getting upper limb disorders, including aches and pains in the hands, arms and neck. Under the Health and Safety (Display Screen Equipment) Regulations 1992, the employer has an obligation to ensure that these risks are minimised by the effective design of the workplace and jobs.

Good practice when working with a computer includes the following points (HSE 2011):

- Take frequent breaks or change your activity.
- Ensure that there is adequate lighting.
- Sit in a comfortable position with knees at right angles (adjusting the height of your chair accordingly).
- Your eyes should be positioned level with the top of the screen
- If you straighten your arm out, the screen should sit an arm's length away,
- The keyboard should be at the correct height; ensure that your arms are bent at 90º.
- Make sure that you have adequate space for documents that you are working on.
- Your mouse should be relatively near you, so that your wrist is straight and your forearm is supported whilst using it.
- You should maintain an upright posture and sit near the desk.
- Make sure that the screen is free from glare and bright reflections.
- You should have plenty of room to move your legs under the desk.
- Ensure that your knees and back of your legs are not experiencing excessive pressure.
- Consider where your keyboard is placed. It should be relatively near you, although some room in front of it may be useful for resting your hands when not typing.
- Good keyboard technique is essential – your fingers should not be overstretched and you should touch the keys softly.
- Make sure the screen is clean.
- Ensure that the text is large enough to read and that the characters do not flicker.
- Be mindful of the colours that you are working with on the screen, ensuring that they are easy on the eye.
- Avoid using a laptop where possible.
- When using a laptop, you must take extra precautions to ensure that the keypad is at the correct height.
- Employers should have a designated person who assesses workstations. Ensure that you have yours assessed as various equipment can be provided to improve your comfort.
- Have your eyes tested regularly. Employees regularly using computers are entitled to get their employers to pay for their eye examinations.

Reporting of Injuries, Diseases and Dangerous Occurrences Regulations 1995

Under RIDDOR, some work-related accidents, dangerous occurrences and diseases must be reported (HSE 2008, 2012):

- The reported incident will be investigated by the HSE, along with local authorities, to ascertain the causes of serious incidents.
- They will identify where and how risks arise.
- They will give advice on the reduction of injury, ill health and accidental loss.

The following need to be reported (HSE 2012):

- death or major injury
- an injury which is not serious but causes you to be absent from work for 7 days or more
- disease
- any dangerous occurrence.

The midwife may suffer from a major injury due to equipment failure, equipment falling over or splashes, etc. A major injury includes the following (HSE 2012):

- fractures (excluding to fingers, thumbs or toes)
- amputation
- dislocation of the shoulder, hip, knee or spine
- loss of sight (temporary or permanent)
- chemical or hot metal burn to the eye or any penetrating injury to the eye
- injury resulting from an electric shock or electrical burn leading to unconsciousness; or requiring resuscitation; or admittance to hospital for more than 24 hours
- any injury that leads to hypothermia, heat-induced illness or unconsciousness; or requiring resuscitation; or requiring admittance to hospital for more than 24 hours
- unconsciousness caused by asphyxia or exposure to a harmful substance or biological agent
- acute illness requiring medical treatment, or loss of consciousness arising from absorption of any substance by inhalation, ingestion or through the skin
- acute illness requiring medical treatment where there is reason to believe that this resulted from exposure to a biological agent or its toxins or infected material.

The HSE (2008, 2012) describes dangerous occurrences as follows:

- Collapse, overturning or failure of load-bearing parts of lifts and lifting equipment.
- Explosion, collapse or bursting of any closed vessel or associated pipe work.
- Electrical short-circuit or overload, causing fire or explosion.
- Dangerous occurrence at a well (other than a water well).
- Failure of any load-bearing fairground equipment, or derailment or unintended collision of cars or trains.
- A dangerous substance conveyed by road involved in a fire or released.
- Unintended collapse of any building or structure under construction, alteration or demolition where over 5 tonnes of material fall; a wall or floor in a place of work; any false work.
- Explosion or fire causing suspension of normal work for over 24 hours.
- Sudden, uncontrolled release in a building of:
  - 100 kg or more of a flammable liquid; or
  - 10 kg or more of a flammable liquid above its boiling point; or
  - 10 kg or more of a flammable gas; or
  - 500 kg of these substances if the release is in the open air.
- Accidental release of any substance which may damage health.

Diseases which are reportable include the following:

- some poisonings
- some skin diseases, including occupational dermatitis
- infections, including leptospirosis, hepatitis, tuberculosis, anthrax, legionellosis and tetanus
- other conditions, for example occupational cancer and some musculoskeletal disorders.

What to do when an incident occurs

- Notify the HSE area office immediately by telephone in the event of a death, major injury or dangerous occurrence.
- Complete an accident report form whenever there is an accident.
- A record of any occurrence must be kept for 3 years and should include:
  - the date and method of reporting
  - the date, time and place of the event
  - personal details of those involved
  - a brief description of the nature of the event or disease.

Control of Substances Hazardous to Health Regulations 2002

Under the COSHH Regulations, the employer has certain obligations regarding hazardous substances:

- those used directly in work activities (such as cleaning agents)
- biological agents (such as bacteria and other micro-organisms).

Substances which are hazardous to health (e.g. bleach, drugs and chemicals) carry a warning label (see Figure 17.1), and as such they should be treated appropriately according to COSHH.
   Effects of hazardous substances include:

- skin irritation/dermatitis
- asthma
- unconsciousness
- cancer
- infections.

Activity 17.17

Identify hazardous substances in your workplace which could cause an adverse effect. For example, latex gloves cause an allergic reaction in some people, leading to dermatitis.

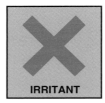

Figure 17.1   An example of a warning label.

The COSHH Regulations require you to undertake the following eight steps in relation to substances which can be hazardous to health (HSE 2005):

1. Assess the risks – who is likely to be at risk and how likely a risk does the substance pose?
2. Decide what precautions are needed.
3. Prevent or adequately control exposure.
4. Ensure that control measures are used and maintained.
5. Monitor the exposure.
6. Carry out appropriate health surveillance.
7. Prepare plans and procedures to deal with accidents, incidents and emergencies.
8. Ensure that employees are properly informed, trained and supervised.

Conclusion

This chapter has examined some of the common issues surrounding health and safety and environmental issues in the workplace. Legislation which has been put in place to protect employees has been brought to the attention of the reader to expand their knowledge and understanding. Together with the activities, this should have increased awareness of the issues. Throughout the chapter some common principles have become apparent which the midwife should follow. These include using common sense when dealing with anything; not rushing unnecessarily; planning your work before you carry it out; attending any training that is offered; taking responsibility for your actions; looking out for hazards; seeking advice from your supervisor of midwives, manager or colleagues; and documenting everything.

Quiz

1. What are the five steps of risk assessment?
2. What are the causes of stress in the workplace?
3. Why is it important to deal with stress in the workplace?
4. What measures can you take to look after your back?
5. What measures should you put in place when working in isolation to protect yourself?

References

Amicus (2006) *Stress*. Bromley: Amicus.
Brennan W (2004) Lone Rangers. *Occupational Health* **56**: 9.
Brennan W (2010) Safer lone working: assessing the risk to health professionals. *British Journal of Nursing* **19**: 22.
Health and Safety Executive (HSE) (1998a) *Working Alone in Safety*. Sudbury: HSE Books.
Health and Safety Executive (HSE) (1998b) *Help on Work-Related Stress*, Sudbury: HSE Books.
Health and Safety Executive (HSE) (2002) *Preventing Slips, Trips and Falls at Work*. Sudbury: HSE Books.
Health and Safety Executive (HSE) (2004) *Work-Related Violence*. Sudbury: HSE Books.
Health and Safety Executive (HSE) (2005) *COSHH: a brief guide to the regulations*. Sudbury: HSE Books.
Health and Safety Executive (HSE) (2006) *Five Steps to Risk Assessment*. Sudbury: HSE Books.
Health and Safety Executive (HSE) (2008) *RIDDOR in Detail*. Sudbury: HSE Books.

Health and Safety Executive (HSE) (2009a) *Slips and Trips: the importance of floor cleaning* . *Slips and Trips* 2. Sudbury: HSE Books.

Health and Safety Executive (HSE) (2009b) *Working Alone. Health and safety guidance on the risks of lone working.* Sudbury: HSE Books.

Health and Safety Executive (HSE) (2011) *Working with VDUs*. Sudbury: HSE Books.

Health and Safety Executive (HSE) (2012) *Reporting Accidents and Incidents at Work. A brief guide to Reporting Injuries, Diseases and Dangerous Occurrences Regulations in the workplace (RIDDOR)*. Sudbury: HSE Books.

NHS Choices (2012) *Top Ten Back Care Tips*. Available at: www.nhs.uk/Livewell/Backpain/Pages/Topbacktips.aspx (accessed May 2013).

Suzy Lamplugh Trust (2010) *Guidance on Choosing a Lone Worker System*. London: Suzy Lamplugh Trust.

Royal College of Nursing (RCN) (2005) *Good Practice in Infection Control*. London: Royal College of Nursing.

Royal College of Nursing (RCN) (2009) *Infection Prevention and Control: minimum standards*. London: Royal College of Nursing.

Royal College of Nursing (RCN) (2012) *Essential Practice for Infection Prevention and Control: guidance for nursing staff*. London: Royal College of Nursing.

18

Evidence-Based Practice

Maxine Offredy

Aim

This chapter focuses on the midwife's role in contributing to the development and evaluation of guidelines and policies to ensure the best care for women and babies, including discussions on research and best available evidence in contemporary midwifery practice.

Learning outcomes

After reading this chapter, the student will be able to:

1. summarise the major points of best available evidence
2. explain what is meant by evidence-based practice
3. explain the importance of evidence-based practice in midwifery
4. discuss the steps involved in searching the literature
5. evaluate the quality of research studies using established criteria
6. discuss the tasks required to implement change in midwifery practice.

Introduction

One of the guiding principles of pre-registration midwifery education is the requirement of knowledge and the use of best available evidence to inform practice. The *Standards for Pre-registration Midwifery Education* emphasise that this must be achieved through searching, analysing, critiquing the evidence and using it in practice. The need to change and adapt practice as well as disseminating research findings are key aspects of the student's education (NMC, 2009) as well as being a focus in ongoing professional

The Student's Guide to Becoming a Midwife, Second Edition. Edited by Ian Peate and Cathy Hamilton.
© 2014 John Wiley & Sons, Ltd. Published 2014 by John Wiley & Sons, Ltd.

development of the midwife. Furthermore, the commitment in contemporary maternity policies to pro-vide quality service within an evidence-based environment underscores the necessity for a cadre of midwives knowledgeable in both research and evidenced-based midwifery practice.

This chapter focuses on the midwife's role in contributing to the development and evaluation of guidelines and policies to ensure the best care for women and babies. It will include a discussion on research and best available evidence concerning midwives, women and babies. The importance of the critical appraisal of knowledge and research evidence will be emphasised as well as keeping up to date with evidence, applying evidence to practice and the dissemination of new evidence to others. In particular, the chapter aims to address Domain IV of Standard 17 of *Standards for Pre-registration Midwifery Education* (NMC 2009). Domain IV relates to advancing quality care through evaluation and research. This is to be achieved by the application of relevant knowledge to the midwife's own practice in structured ways which are capable of evaluation. This entails:

- a short reminder of some research methods that midwives might encounter that are relevant to their practice
- a discussion of best available evidence
- steps involved in searching the literature
- hierarchy of evidence
- appraising the literature
- guidelines in midwifery practice.

Research methods

The purpose of research is to increase the body of knowledge available to practitioners, consumers, managers, economists and educationalists. It is a systematic scientific approach characterised by (1) order and control, (2) empiricism, and (3) generalisation (Polit & Beck 2006). Research evidence can be viewed as a continuum, going from a purely qualitative perspective at one end to the purely quantitative at the other end. The methods used depend on the question(s) to be addressed. Several classifications of research methods are available, e.g. quantitative or qualitative, prospective or retro-spective, descriptive, exploratory or explanatory, phenomenology or positivism, holistic or reductionist, to cite but a few.

Research methods situated at the more qualitative or phenomenological end of the research contin-uum are more likely to be associated with the social sciences because the questions they answer are based on an assumption that the world in which events occur is socially constructed. This type of research does not aim to test a hypothesis, but rather to generate one based on the understanding of the values and meanings of observed phenomena, from the perspective of participants. Qualitative research approaches typically include methods such as in-depth interviews, focus groups, case studies, non-participant observations and ethnography.

At the other end of the continuum, quantitative or positivist research methods are based in the natural sciences, and aim to test a stated hypothesis. This area of research is reductionist rather than holistic, e.g. measuring the level of cortisol in the presence of stress but not how the individual experiences/feels about stress which would be addressed via a more holistic qualitative approach. Hypothesis testing will be based on empirical, objective and measured observations. Measurements will be statistically tested so that the initial hypothesis can be either supported or rejected. This type of research is concerned with the testing of cause-and-effect relationships, or at least correlations.

Each research method has its own specific aims, characteristics, strengths and limitations. Numerous textbooks on research methods exist. Many have been written more specifically for different professional groups, e.g. nurses, doctors or psychologists, but the principles are the same whatever the discipline for which they are intended. We turn now to exploring best evidence followed by appraisal of research evidence.

Best available evidence

The student may begin by asking: What is meant by best available evidence to inform practice? Given that practice should be informed by evidence, evidence-based practice is one in which the midwife's approach to decision making incorporates a number of factors such as the best evidence that is available (which may or may not be research based), that is appropriate and includes the patient's views as well as clinical expertise about the topic under review.

Three definitions of evidence-based practice are provided below: Sackett et al.'s (1996, pp71–72) frequently cited definition of evidence-based practice is from a medical perspective and states that evidence-based practice is:

> ... the conscientious, explicit, and judicious use of current best evidence in making decisions about the care of individual patients. The practice of evidence-based medicine means integrating individual clinical expertise with the best available external clinical evidence from systematic research ... and compassionate use of individual patients' predicaments, rights, and preferences in making clinical decisions about their care.

DiCenso's (2003, pp21–22) definition is from a non-medical point of view and is applicable to midwifery.

> "Best research evidence" refers to methodologically sound, clinically relevant research about the effectiveness and safety of nursing (and midwifery) interventions, the accuracy and precision of nursing assessment measures, the power of prognostic indicators, the strength of causal relationships, the cost-effectiveness of nursing (and midwifery) interventions and the meaning of illness or patient experiences. Research evidence alone, however, is never sufficient to make a clinical decision. As nurses (and midwives), we must always trade the benefits and risks, inconvenience and costs associated with alternative management strategies, and in doing so consider the patient's values.

A less rigid definition of evidence-based practice is offered by Muir Gray (1997, p9) who suggests that it is:

> ... an approach to decision making in which the clinician uses the best evidence available, in consultation with the patient, to decide upon the option which suits the patient best.

You will note that the definitions give attention to the patient's views in the decision-making process. Further, the emphasis on systematic research as the best quality evidence may not always be available. There may be areas in midwifery practice which remain under-researched. For example, transcutaneous electrical nerve stimulation (TENS) is a method of pain relief that has been used in childbirth since the 1970s. The precise physiological mechanisms whereby TENS relieves pain are not well understood but some women have used it on more than one occasion. There is a paucity of methodologically robust evidence on which to provide women with informed choices but nevertheless it is used based on experience in practice. Thus the 'best available evidence' may not always be research based in that it has been subjected to the rigours of systematic research. Midwives need to be aware that the type of evidence they may need to integrate into their practice may prove to be difficult and time consuming to find. It is, however, an essential skill to have in order to implement evidence to improve practice. Furthermore, midwives will be expected to present the evidence on which their decision was based. In an economic climate where cost-effectiveness is a factor in resource allocation, the midwife will have to find and apply the best available evidence for women and babies in their care.

An important consideration for evidence-based practice is the culture of the organisation (Offredy et al. 2009). Parahoo (2000) suggests that organisational characteristics of healthcare settings are overwhelmingly the most significant barriers to research use among nurses. These views include whether or not the organisation is a learning one with a memory (Offredy et al. 2009), which encourages continuing education of staff, thus valuing people, or one with low staff morale and low regard for individuals. Thus organisational support is crucial if midwives are to be proactive in extending the boundaries of care.

Sackett et al.'s (1996) definition of evidence-based practice has meant that there has been a tendency to view 'evidence' in terms of quantitative research such as randomised controlled trials and systematic reviews. Potts et al. (2006) acknowledge the importance of randomised controlled trials whilst stating that evidence that may be used to improve maternity and child care will come from a variety of sources as some of the issues encountered in practice are not always quantifiable, for example, women's experience of being in labour, the effects of treatment or choice of treatment. Thus, the type of evidence used will depend on the clinical situation, the question to be answered and the type of decision being made.

To be able to adopt an evidence-based approach to practice, midwives must ensure that they understand how to appraise the quality of the evidence presented in published work and decide if research findings should or should not be implemented. The next section provides a step approach to searching the literature followed by appraisal of the literature.

315

Steps in searching the literature

The flow diagram in Figure 18.1 takes you through the steps you need to undertake in order to identify and obtain the relevant literature.

Inclusion criteria

Inclusion criteria are characteristics which are essential to the problem under scrutiny (Polit & Beck 2008). They are sometimes referred to as eligibility criteria; in other words, the sample population must possess the characteristics. Examples of inclusion or eligibility criteria are:

- age groups (for example, you may wish to have inclusion criteria for primigravida women aged 25–35 years of age to compare their experiences of labour)
- language (for example, English)
- location (for example, France, United States or a local area)
- date/time period (for example 2010–2013)
- (possibly) evidence-based medicine.

The inclusion criterion of evidence-based medicine will mean that the results of the search will be limited to articles reviewed in databases such as Health Technology Assessment (HTA), the Cochrane Database of Systematic Reviews (CDSR) and Databases of Abstracts of Reviews of Effectiveness (DARE). DARE complements the CDSR by providing a selection of quality-assessed reviews in those areas where there is currently no Cochrane review (Polit & Beck 2008).

```
┌──────────────┐          ┌────────────────────────────────┐
│   Keyword    │─────────▶│ Decide on the keywords of your  │
└──────┬───────┘          │ topic and include alternative   │
       │                  │ terms that may be used. These   │
       │                  │ are known as synonyms. Acronyms │
       │                  │ are abbreviations using the     │
       │                  │ capital letter of the word, for │
       │                  │ example, PICO                   │
       │                  │ You should also bear in mind    │
       │                  │ United States and United Kingdom│
       │                  │ spellings, for example program  │
       │                  │ (US) and programme (UK)         │
       │                  └────────────────────────────────┘
       │
       ▼
┌──────────────────────┐   ┌────────────────────────────────────────────┐
│ Boolean operators are:│──▶│ These allow precision in finding information:│
│ AND                   │   │                                              │
│ OR                    │   │ The use of AND allows you to narrow your     │
│ NOT                   │   │ search by combining words using AND.         │
│ AND NOT               │   │                                              │
└──────────┬───────────┘   │ OR lets you broaden your search to include   │
           │               │ similar or other information connected by OR. │
           │               │                                              │
           │               │ NOT or AND NOT allow you to exclude specific │
           │               │ information from the search.                 │
           │               └────────────────────────────────────────────┘
           ▼
┌──────────────────┐   ┌──────────────────────┐   ┌──────────────────────┐
│ Word combination │──▶│ In addition to the use│──▶│ These include        │
└──────────────────┘   │ of Boolean terms, you │   │ setting of dates,    │
                       │ can also combine words│   │ language, location,  │
                       │ to broaden or narrow  │   │ gender, ethnicity,   │
                       │ your search           │   │ age and so on        │
                       └───────────┬──────────┘   └──────────────────────┘
                                   ▼
                       ┌──────────────────────┐   ┌──────────────────────┐
                       │ Read relevant         │──▶│ Discard irrelevant   │
                       │ references and take   │   │ material             │
                       │ notes                 │   └──────────────────────┘
                       └───────────┬──────────┘
                                   ▼
                       ┌──────────────────────┐   ┌──────────────────────┐
                       │ Organise material    │──▶│ Analyse and          │
                       └───────────┬──────────┘   │ integrate material   │
                                   │              └──────────────────────┘
                                   ▼
                       ┌──────────────────────┐
                       │ Write review         │
                       └──────────────────────┘
```

Figure 18.1 Steps in the literature search. Adapted from Hart 1998; Burns & Grove 2007; Polit & Beck 2008.

Table 18.1   Hierarchy of evidence

Level	Evidence
1	Systematic reviews/meta-analyses
	Randomised controlled trials (RCTs) Experimental designs
2	Cohort control studies Case–control studies
3	Consensus conference
	Expert opinion
	Observational study
	Other types of study, e.g. interviews, local audits
	Quasi-experimental, qualitative design
4	Personal communication, expert opinion

Exclusion criteria

Exclusion criteria are characteristics that you specifically do not wish to include in your search, such as multigravida if the problem pertains to primigravida with diabetes. The inclusion and exclusion criteria are important characteristics of a research study as they have implications for both the interpretation and generalisability of the findings (Polit & Beck 2008).

Having obtained the literature, you will need to decide on the worth of the material found. This can be done by assessing the information by using a hierarchy of evidence (Table 18.1) or by reviewing the literature using the research process.

Midwifery wisdom

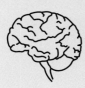

By reading and assessing a wide variety of studies, you will begin to form an impression of the important aspects of your topic, identify whether any diverse or conflicting viewpoints exist and how these have been interpreted.

Appraising the literature

Reviewing or appraising the literature requires developing a complex set of skills acquired through practice. A comprehensive review of the literature is important because it:

- provides an up-to-date understanding of the topic and its significance to midwifery practice
- identifies the methods used in the research

- helps in the identification of significant controversies
- identifies inconsistencies in findings relating to your area of midwifery practice
- helps in the formulation of research topics, questions and direction
- sharpens your ability to identify and peruse the relevant literature efficiently and effectively
- enhances your ability to apply analytical principles in identifying unbiased and valid research in midwifery practice
- provides a basis on which the subsequent research findings can be compared.

A key principle when appraising research is to have a structured, systematic approach. It is useful to keep a record of how the review is conducted to ensure that the strategy is explicit, thorough/comprehensive, transparent and avoids replication and/or omission of references.

Before you begin your search, you should have a well-structured question: what is it that you would like to find out about? This will give a guide as to the type of research methods you may wish to explore.

Writers such as Burns & Grove (2003), Grbich (1999) and Polit & Beck (2008) suggest that a review of the literature can be divided into several sections. The subdivisions discussed below are an adaptation of the ideas and writings from these authors.

The structure of the report

Is the organisation of the report logical? Does it make sense/is it understandable? Does the report follow the sequence of steps of the process of research, such as these?:

- Introduction
- Identification of the research problem
- Planning of the research study
- Data collection methods
- Data analysis methods
- Discussion of the study and its results
- Conclusions obtained from the study
- Recommendation as a result of the findings from the study.

The organisation of the report may vary, but in all cases it should be logical. It should begin with a clear identification of what is to be studied and how, and should end with a summary or conclusion recommending further study or application. Different journals may require a different layout, but the key issue is a logical progression. As a general rule, a research report should comprise the following.

The abstract

The abstract of a research paper provides a summary of the question and the most important findings of the study. It outlines how these differ from those of previous studies and gives some indication of the methodology undertaken. It is usually about 200–300 words long, depending on the guidelines for specific journals and the thesis format of the relevant university. The abstract provides the reader with an overview of what the research has found. It is the first part of a paper that is read and if it does not include the relevant information that is being sought, it is unlikely that the remainder of the paper will be read as it may not be relevant to the reader.

Does the abstract, in a concise paragraph, describe:

- what was studied?
- how it was studied?
- how the sample was selected?
- how the data were analysed?
- the main findings of the research?

The introduction

The introduction serves to explain 'why' and 'how' the research problem was defined in a particular way. It should include the rationale for undertaking the research. It should also review critically the previous literature that the researcher has reviewed, pointing out any limitations in findings, methodology or theoretical interpretation. In addition, it provides a pathway to the methodology section by clarifying the need for research to be undertaken in the chosen topic, especially with regard to the methodological orientation or techniques chosen by the researcher.

The problem statement/purpose of the research

The introduction should be followed by a statement and discussion of the problem the researcher has investigated in the study. In this section you should consider whether:

- the general problem has been introduced and stated promptly
- the problem under investigation has been supported by evidence with adequate discussion of the background to the problem and the need for the study
- the general problem has been narrowed down to a specific research problem or to a problem that contains relevant sub-problems as appropriate
- if it is an experimental quantitative research study, the hypothesis directly answers the research problem
- if it is any other type of research study, that the research question directly addresses the problem identified.

The literature review and theoretical rationale for the study

This subsection relates to your own literature review. In a review of previous literature (including a theoretical rationale for the study to take place) you should aim to consider whether this section is relevant, clearly written, well organised and up to date and whether the reliability of the methods and data collection has been addressed. Your reasons should be substantiated.

- Was there a sufficient review of the literature and theoretical rationale associated with the previous research to assure you that the authors considered a broad spectrum of all the possibilities there were for investigating the present research problem?
- Is it clear how the study will extend previous research findings?

Midwifery Wisdom

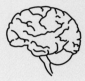

You should be aware that a full report on a research study or an academic thesis requires an extensive literature review, whilst in a journal article/paper the author will usually cite the major pieces of work that are relevant to the study in hand.

Methodology

The methodology section must fully inform readers of the step-by-step processes undertaken in conducting the study. In this section you should consider the appropriateness of the research methods chosen, including:

- the sampling approach
- the data collection methods
- the validity and reliability of observations or measurements.

In order to assist you to understand this section of a research paper, it is important that you consider the following subheadings and questions under each heading.

The population and sample

Ask yourself the following questions:

- Is the study population specific enough so that it is clear to which population the findings can be generalised? In other words, have the researchers defined their population and is it closely linked to the topic being investigated?
- Is the sample representative of the population defined?
- Would it be possible for you or others to replicate the study population?
- Is the method of sample selection appropriate?
- Was any bias introduced by this method? (See Pannucci & Wilkins' (2010) definition in Box 18.1.)
- Is the sample size appropriate and how is it substantiated?
    - Is it large enough for a quantitative research study?
    - Are the statistics significant?

Box 18.1   Bias

Bias is defined as any tendency which prevents unprejudiced consideration of a question. In research, bias occurs when 'systematic error [is] introduced into sampling or testing by selecting or encouraging one outcome or answer over others'. Bias can occur at any phase of research, including study design or data collection, as well as in the process of data analysis and publication (Pannucci & Wilkins 2010).

  ○   Is the rationale for the size of the sample given and is it adequate?
  ○   Is the method of determining the sample stated?
  ○   Is it adequate for a qualitative research study and is the rationale given?

Instrumentation – method of data collection

- Are the data collection methods used appropriate to the study?
- Did they obtain the data that the researcher was searching for in order to answer the research question/hypothesis?
- Has the author discussed the validity and reliability of the instruments used within the context of the research study?

The procedure for data collection

- Were steps taken to control extraneous variables?
- Are the collection methods used replicable in a similar type of research?

Ethical considerations to be addressed

You should ask yourself these questions whilst reading the section on ethics in the research paper:

- Were the rights of participants involved in the research addressed?
- Has the researcher included in the report any discussion of ethical considerations?
- Is there discussion of the impact of any ethical problems on the merit of the study and the wellbeing of the participants?
- Has the researcher presented any evidence to suggest that the rights of the study's participants have been protected (e.g., is there a discussion of informed consent with examples?)
- Are the steps that were introduced to protect the participants discussed and are they appropriate?
- Has the researcher discussed any violations of ethical principles that occurred and made suggestions as to how these could have been avoided?

Polit & Beck (2006) suggest useful points to consider when critiquing the ethics of research studies:

- Was undue influence or coercion used in the recruitment of the participants?
- Were vulnerable groups included?
- Were participants deceived in any way?
- Was the study fully explained to the participants?
- Were they given sufficient time to consider whether or not they wished to take part in the study?
- Were appropriate consent procedures followed?
- Was there adherence to consent procedures?
- Was privacy ensured fully?
- Did the benefits outweigh the risks?
- Was the study approved and monitored by an ethics committee?
- Was reporting of the results accurate and unbiased (e.g. were any data omitted or changed to fit the findings?)?
- Was the hypothesis changed?
- Was there acknowledgement of funding?
- Was any conflict of interest revealed?

Midwifery Wisdom

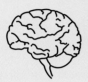

It should be noted that due to space restrictions, research reports frequently do not provide detailed information about adherence to ethical principles. This does not necessarily mean that adherence did not take place.

The pilot study

You should ask yourself the following questions:

● Was a pilot study undertaken?
● Were any changes made following the pilot study? If not, why not? If there were, were these discussed and rationalised, and evidence produced for the changes?

Analysis of data

When reading the section on data analysis, you should bear in mind that analysis of the data will differ according to whether the research was undertaken using a qualitative or quantitative design. Depending on the type of research being reported, ask yourself the following questions, as appropriate:

● Was the analysis of the data clear and is it related to the hypothesis or research question?
● Have the researchers made it clear which statistical methods they used and what values were obtained? Have they given a rationale for the choice of their statistical test?
● Is there a statement to indicate whether or not the data support the hypothesis?
● Has a thorough examination of each hypothesis been included, including the use of appropriate statistical analysis and the decision to accept or reject the hypothesis?
● Have the researchers indicated whether the data have answered the research question?
● Have the researchers explained how and why the data collected and analysed have answered the research question?
● Have the researchers shown how the data have given rise to 'themes' that will answer the research question?
● Have the researchers provided a comprehensive discussion of the data?
● Have the researchers given an explanation of how missing data (if any) were handled?
● Have experts been used to assist in the analysis of the data?
● Was computer software used in the analysis of the data?
● Has the analysis of the data been verified by an expert?

Discussion

This section of the research paper is very important because it draws together the main threads of the research and the findings are discussed and put into context. You should ask yourself the following questions.

- Have the researchers presented a discussion of the research study critically, particularly the analysis and the findings?
- If it is a quantitative research study, can the findings be generalised?
- Have the researchers made sense of the findings within the context of the study?

Conclusions and limitations

At the end of the research paper, ask yourself the following questions:

- Have the researchers related their findings to the theoretical proposition underlying the study?
- Have the researchers identified any methodological problems?
- Have the researchers overgeneralised, or are they specific about what the results have shown?
- Are the implications of the findings for practice identified? If not, have the researchers discussed why not?
- Are there any suggestions for further research?

References and bibliography

If a reference and bibliography section is included, ask yourself the following questions:

- Are all the references cited relevant to the study? If not, has a rationale been given for their inclusion?
- Do the references and bibliography reflect the review of the literature?
- Do they relate to the search for and/or development of valid and reliable instruments/methodology?
- Are any references missing?

Midwifery wisdom

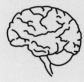
You will see that there is a lot of work to be done when reviewing the literature and you should allocate sufficient time for the task. This will be time spent well when it comes to undertaking your own research study. Hart (1998) reminds us that when reading or undertaking a review, we should be aware of our own value judgement and try to avoid personal, destructive comments.

Literature review frameworks

Since the mid-1990s, a variety of frameworks have been available to assist in clarifying the question and reviewing the literature:

- *CASP (Critical Appraisal Skills Programme)*: has developed a number of tools for different types of studies, for example, randomised controlled trials, systematic reviews, cohort studies and others, which are available free for personal use on the internet at www.casp-uk.net/.
- *SPICE (Setting, Population, Intervention, Comparison, Evaluation) (Booth 2004)*: this framework may be useful in questions relating to general health.

- ECLIPSE (Expectation, Client Group, Location, Impact, Professionals, Service, Evaluation) (Wildridge & Bell 2002): this may be used for some questions relating to health policy/management.
- PICO (Patient, Intervention, Comparison, Outcome) (Richardson et al. 1995): this framework may be used with questions relating to evidence-based practice.

Implementation of evidence-based midwifery

Recent developments in midwifery practice and management have seen the emergence of consultant midwives or research and development midwives, and this demonstrates an eagerness on the part of the NHS to see evidence-based midwifery in practice. This does not mean that individual midwives are no longer responsible for their personal updating, far from it; it simply demonstrates an additional commitment that ought to support midwives in their continuous professional development. It is an expectation that midwives will contribute to the development of evidence-based guidelines, policies and standards for midwifery practice (NMC 2009).

Engagement with evidence-based midwifery can be seen at two levels: the individual practitioner and the clinical environment. Midwives who are looking after individual women must ensure that the care they provide is based on evidence. Women should not be advised to follow treatments that are not based on sound evidence, unless they are told that no evidence is currently available and that this is therefore the best suggestion that can be put forward. At the same time, midwives ought to keep information about the areas of care where they find a lack of evidence to support their practice. This would be an initial step for personal and/or group reflection, literature searching, assessment of the available evidence and the setting up of personal or unit guidelines.

Midwives should not feel that the responsibility for providing evidence-based care rests solely on their individual shoulders. Networking is important and there are a number of interest lists that midwives can subscribe to in order to meet like-minded people and exchange ideas. One of the most useful internet sites is www.jiscmail.ac.uk where midwives can search the many interest lists. A keyword search of 'midwi' or 'birth' will identify a number of lists of potential interest and enable anyone who joins any of these lists to identify colleagues who have similar interests and therefore foster a community that can develop evidence-based midwifery practices.

Dunning et al.'s (1999) report for the King's Fund, *Promoting Action on Clinical Effectiveness (PACE)*, explored issues of change in 16 clinical settings across the NHS in England. Their analysis defined 10 distinct but often overlapping tasks that require attention if success in implementing change in clinical practice is to be achieved:

1. Choose your initiative and ensure support for the proposal.
2. Engage clinicians and secure their support for the proposed initiative.
3. Involve patients after careful consideration about why patients need to be involved.
4. Define and agree the intended standard of practice.
5. Communicate clearly with those affected as the work is taken forward.
6. Change is the key aspect of the work and involves a range of activities with multidisciplinary teams.
7. Assess the service and resource consequences of the initiative. Provide services to fill any gaps in clinical practice.
8. Measure impact to demonstrate achievement.
9. Sustain change to ensure that the changes become routine practice.
10. Learn lessons and manage the work as a learning experience.

Midwifery guidelines

Recent developments by NICE have seen the publication of guidelines for antenatal and postnatal care, as well as the use of electronic fetal monitoring and induction of labour (NICE 2001a,b, 2003, 2006). These developments include the following:

- NICE (2007a) Intrapartum care of healthy women and their babies during childbirth.
- NICE (2007b) Care of women and their babies during labour.
- Department of Health (2006) National guidelines for maternity services liaison committees (MSLCs).
- NICE (2008) Guidance for midwives, health visitors, pharmacists and other primary care services to improve the nutrition of pregnant and breastfeeding mothers and babies in low income households.

In 2010 NICE provided a suite of evidence-based guidance on maternity care, which addresses:

- antenatal care for the healthy pregnant woman (NICE 2010a)
- hypertension in pregnancy (NICE 2010b)
- quitting smoking in pregnancy and following childbirth (NICE 2010c)
- weight management before, during and after pregnancy (NICE 2010d)
- pregnancy and complex social factors(NICE 2010e).

Other guidelines have been developed by midwives (for example, Spiby & Munro 2001) and by international bodies (for example, WHO 2011); the *State of the World's Midwifery Report* (UN Population Fund 2011) confirms the critical role midwives play in improving maternal and newborn health and survival.

325

Conclusion

Evidence-based practice has evolved from the principles of research-based practice and has taken into consideration the huge developments in the production of scientific publications, access to electronic facilities such as the internet and, perhaps more importantly, electronic databases and electronic journals.

Midwives are now required to ensure that their practice is based on evidence wherever possible, and where this is not the case, it makes sense that midwives should generate questions that can be answered empirically. This requires them to develop the skills necessary for retrieving relevant material and a sound knowledge of research methods to enable them to appreciate the strengths and limitations of various publications. Midwives, however, do not live in isolation from other practitioners and more facilities are becoming available to ensure that midwives can work in collaboration with other practitioners and develop networks of specialist interest. The situation is becoming more complex but the tools are also developing to ensure that all midwives can have access to knowledge and to colleagues.

Midwifery Wisdom

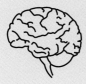

The application of sound evidence-based principles in the maternity services, by midwives and other healthcare professionals, should in the long term be in the interest of mothers and babies as this approach should ensure that the care proposed is the best and most cost-effective care that can be achieved.

Quiz

The following multiple choice questions are designed to check your understanding of selected issues in this chapter. Select all that you think are relevant to the question/statement.

1. Implementing evidence-based midwifery practice can be made possible by:

   a. promoting a learning environment to help midwifery practitioners to make decisions based on best available evidence
   b. accepting diversity
   c. inclusion of patients' and carers' views
   d. valuing and promoting a culture of inquiry
   e. all of the above.

2. As a student midwife on the delivery suite, you would like to get involved in the research being proposed. Your unit encourages all grades of staff to participate in evidence-based midwifery practice. Which aspects of evidence-based practice are important for you to have?

   a. sound bedside midwifery skill
   b. knowledge of key roles of staff on your unit
   c. methods of assessing published information
   d. knowledge of health and safety regulations.

3. Evidence-based midwifery practice provides the midwife with the ability to:

   a. select practice activities based on evidence
   b. analyse published research results
   c. solve all midwifery problems
   d. identify gaps in the literature
   e. all of the above.

4. What barriers are there to evidence-based practice?

   a. resistance to change
   b. conflicting evidence
   c. communication
   d. all of the above
   e. none of the above.

5. A literature review is important because it:

   a. helps you for formulate your research topics/questions
   b. provides an up-to-date understanding of the topic
   c. identifies the significance in midwifery practice
   d. helps in the identification of significant controversies
   e. all of the above
   f. none of the above.

6. When reviewing ethical considerations in a research study, it is important to consider:

   a. whether the rights of the participants have been protected
   b. discussion of the impact of any ethical problems
   c. whether the researcher has included discussions of ethical considerations in the report
   d. all of the above
   e. none of the above.

7. The abstract of the research paper tells you:

   a. what was studied
   b. how it was studied
   c. how the sample was selected
   d. how the data were analysed
   e. none of the above.

8. The unit in which you work is organising a lunchtime seminar for the wider midwifery staff about evidence-based practice. You are invited to do a brief presentation of four key points about evidence-based practice in midwifery. What would you include as your key points?

   a. Evidence-based practice is a problem-based approach where research evidence is used to inform clinical decision making. It involves the integration of the best available research evidence with clinical expertise, clients'/carers' views and circumstances, as well as consideration of the clinical environment.
   b. Evidence-based practice is important because it aims to improve midwifery outcomes. It also has a role in facilitating professional accountability and guiding decisions about the funding of health service provision.
   c. Evidence-based practice is used in areas such as policy formulation and implementation, purchasing and management as midwives are involved in these areas of healthcare.
   d. Not all research evidence is of sufficient quality that midwives can confidently use it to inform their clinical decision making. Thus a knowledge of how to appraise the literature critically before deciding whether to use it is of importance.
   e. All published work is of high quality so it is unnecessary to appraise the literature.

9. Demonstrating evidence-based competence is a complex task – there is only one assessment method which provides all of the necessary data to assess the complexity.

   a. True
   b. False

10. The highest level of evidence is said to be:

   a. randomised controlled trial
   b. meta-analysis of descriptive studies
   c. systematic review of level II studies
   d. expert opinion
   e. none of the above.

References

Booth A (2004) Formulating answerable questions. In: Booth A, Brice A (eds) *Evidence Based Practice For Information Professionals: a handbook*. London: Facet Publishing, pp61–70.

Burns N, Grove SK (2003) *Understanding Nursing Research*, 3rd edn. Philadelphia: Saunders.

Burns N, Grove SK (2007) *Understanding Nursing Research: building an evidence-based practice*. Philadelphia: Saunders.

Department of Health (DH) (2006) *National Guidelines for Maternity Services Liaison Committees (MSLCs)*. London: Department of Health.

DiCenso A (2003) Evidence based practice: how to get there from here. *Nursing Leadership* **4**: 20–23.

Dunning M, Abi-Aad G, Gilbert D, Hutton H, Brown C (1999) *Experience, Evidence and Everyday Practice*. London: King's Fund.

Grbich C (1999) *Qualitative Research in Health*. London: Sage.

Hart C (1998) *Doing a Literature Search*. London: Sage.

Muir Gray JA (1997) *Evidence-based Health Care: how to make health policy and management decisions*. London: Churchill Livingstone.

National Institute for Health and Clinical Excellence (NICE) (2001a) *Induction of Labour*. London: National Institute for Health and Clinical Excellence.

National Institute for Health and Clinical Excellence (NICE) (2001b) *The Use of Electronic Fetal Monitoring*. London: National Institute for Health and Clinical Excellence.

National Institute for Health and Clinical Excellence (NICE) (2003) *Antenatal Care – routine care for the healthy pregnant woman*. London: National Institute for Health and Clinical Excellence.

National Institute for Health and Clinical Excellence (NICE) (2006) *Routine Postnatal Care of Women and Their Babies*. London: National Institute for Health and Clinical Excellence.

National Institute for Health and Clinical Excellence (NICE) (2007a) *Intrapartum Care of Healthy Women and Their Babies During Childbirth*. London: Royal College of Obstetricians and Gynaecologists.

National Institute for Health and Clinical Excellence (NICE) (2007b) *Care of Women and Their Babies During Labour*. London: National Institute for Health and Clinical Excellence.

National Institute for Health and Clinical Excellence (NICE) (2008) *Guidance for Midwives, Health Visitors, Pharmacists and Other Primary Care Services to Improve the Nutrition of Pregnant and Breastfeeding Mothers and Babies in Low Income Households*. London: National Institute for Health and Clinical Excellence.

National Institute for Health and Clinical Excellence (NICE) (2010a) *Antenatal Care for the Healthy Pregnant Woman*. London: National Institute for Health and Clinical Excellence.

National Institute for Health and Clinical Excellence (2010b) *Hypertension in Pregnancy*. London: National Institute for Health and Clinical Excellence.

National Institute for Health and Clinical Excellence (NICE) (2010c) *Quitting Smoking in Pregnancy and Following Childbirth*. London: National Institute for Health and Clinical Excellence.

National Institute for Health and Clinical Excellence (NICE) (2010d) *Weight Management Before, During and After Pregnancy*. London: National Institute for Health and Clinical Excellence.

National Institute for Health and Clinical Excellence (NICE) (2010e) *Pregnancy and Complex Social Factors*. London: National Institute for Health and Clinical Excellence.

Nursing and Midwifery Council (NMC) (2009) *Standards for Pre-Registration Midwifery Education*. London: Nursing and Midwifery Council.

Offredy M, Rhodes M, Doyle Y (2009) The anatomy, physiology and pathogenesis of a significant untoward incident. *Quality in Primary Care* **17**(6): 415–421.

Pannucci CJ, Wilkins EG (2010) Identifying and avoiding bias in research. *Plastic and Reconstructive Surgery* **126**(2): 619–625.

Parahoo K (2000) Barriers to, and facilitators of, research utilization among nurses in Northern Ireland. *Journal of Advanced Nursing* **31**: 89–98.

Polit DF, Beck CT (2006) *Essentials of Nursing Research: methods, appraisal and utilisation*, 6th edn. Philadelphia: Lippincott Williams and Wilkins.

Polit DF, Beck CT (2008) *Nursing Research: generating and assessing evidence for nursing practice*, 8th edn. Philadelphia: Lippincott Williams and Wilkins.

Potts M, Prata N, Walsh J, Grossman A (2006) Parachute approach to evidence-based medicine. *British Medical Journal* **333**(7570): 701–703.

Richardson W, Wilson M, Nishikawa J, Hayward R (1995) The well-built clinical question: a key to evidence-based decisions. *ACP Journal Club* **123**: A12–13.

Sackett D, Rosenberg W, Muir Gray J, Haynes R, Richardson W (1996) Evidence based medicine: what it is and what it isn't. *British Medical Journal* **312**: 71–72.

Spiby H, Munro J (2001) Evidence-based midwifery in action: an introduction. *British Journal of Midwifery* **9**(9): 549.

United Nations Population Fund (2011) *State of the World's Midwifery Report*. New York: United Nations Population Fund.

Wildridge V, Bell L (2002) How CLIP became ECLIPSE: a mnemonic to assist in searching for health policy/management information. *Health Information and Libraries Journal* **19**(2): 113–115.

World Health Organization (WHO) (2011) *Strategic Directions of the Department of Maternal, Newborn, Child and Adolescent Health*. Geneva: World Health Organization.

19

Statutory Supervision of Midwives

Kath Mannion

Aim

To inform the reader about statutory supervision of midwives in the United Kingdom, its origins and current functions.

Learning outcomes

By the end of this chapter you will be able to:

1. define the current legislations surrounding midwifery practice in the UK
2. describe the process for a registered midwife notifying her intention to practise
3. have a critical awareness of the evolution of statutory supervision
4. identify how a supervisor of midwives can help support your midwifery practice.

Introduction

The United Kingdom is unique in that it is the only country where midwifery supervision is enshrined in legislation. The Local Supervising Authorities (LSAs) are responsible for the provision of statutory supervision of midwives in their area. They appoint supervisors of midwives to undertake statutory supervision and ensure that every midwife in the LSA area has a named supervisor of midwives. Every midwife who practises in the UK needs to notify her intention to practise to a supervisor of midwives.

The Student's Guide to Becoming a Midwife, Second Edition. Edited by Ian Peate and Cathy Hamilton.
© 2014 John Wiley & Sons, Ltd. Published 2014 by John Wiley & Sons, Ltd.

The supervisors of midwives pass on the notification of intention to practise to the LSA, which in turn informs the Nursing and Midwifery Council (NMC) that the midwife is practising within the LSA area. The LSAs also ensure that all midwives have access to a supervisor of midwives for support and guidance at all times. Through this system safe and effective midwifery practice is facilitated. By enabling safe and effective practice, supervisors of midwives protect the public and ensure that midwives are supported in their everyday work.

History

In order to understand what statutory supervision of midwifery in the UK is today, it is essential to understand how the midwifery profession and statutory supervision have evolved over time.

Supervision is not a new concept. In their book on the history of midwifery, Towler & Bramall (1986) reported that in the 1500s the chief physician of the city of Frankfurt supervised midwives. The earliest records of midwifery show that medicine and men have attempted to control midwifery practice (Donnison 1977, Witz 1992).

The drive to legislate midwifery practice in the UK arose from a desire to reduce the high perinatal and maternal morbidity and mortality evident in Victorian England, and 'protect' the public from untrained midwives. Midwives were characterised as ignorant, drunk and lazy, and ridiculed in the guise of Sairey Gamp in Charles Dickens' *Martin Chuzzlewit* (Heagerty 1996). Heagerty (1996), however, notes that most midwives were hard-working and skilled. With the founding of the Midwives' Institute (the forerunner of the Royal College of Midwives), a number of prominent women began to push for legislation which would legalise the practice of midwifery and gain greater recognition for the profession (Towler & Bramall 1986).

Statutory supervision of midwives came into effect when the Midwives Act was enacted in England and Wales in 1902. Scotland followed in 1915 and Ireland in 1918 (Jenkins 1995). Midwives were recognised legally and appropriate training had to take place before registration with the Central Midwives Board (CMB). Registration was not without its opposition as many saw that this was putting midwives under the control of men/doctors (Donnison 1977, Kirkham 1995, Robinson 1990, Witz 1992). Kirkham (1995) notes that men and non-midwives dominated the composition of the CMB. It was not until 1920 that the CMB was required to include midwives, although several notable nurses and members of the Midwives' Institute were already members. LSAs were responsible for enacting statutory supervision of midwives and reporting to the CMB. The CMB was the statutory body that was to rule midwifery for the next 70 years until the formation of the United Kingdom Central Council of Nursing and Midwifery in 1983.

Statutory supervision of midwives

1902–1937

Supervisors of midwives were known as inspectors of midwives until 1937. Inspectors were selected from women, for example middle-class and wealthy women, who had undergone nurse training but did not go on to work in nursing (Kirkham 1995). Towler & Bramall (1986) note that the focus was on the social and moral aspect of the midwives being supervised rather than their clinical skills. This finding is supported by Heagerty (1996), who recorded that these inspectors of early midwifery had little or no education in midwifery supervision. Almost all were from the middle or upper class and their knowledge and inspection methods were more concerned with cultural and moral issues than actual clinical practice. With little or no background knowledge apart from what was available to them in largely medical textbooks and the *Midwives' Rules*, there was no possibility of these inspectors being able to offer constructive comment on clinical issues.

Reports to inspectors from other sources such as doctors were often made without any substantive evidence (e.g. the midwife being drunk at a birth), even though this could result in midwives being struck off the register or severely censured (Heagerty 1996). The midwife had no leave to appeal and Kirkham (1995) reports that many were struck off simply because of 'offences' relating to the poverty of their clients when the rules required the midwife to summon medical aid but the family would not and could not as they had no means to pay the doctor's fee. This left the midwife in a dilemma between the rules that governed her practice and the wishes of her clients.

Donnison (1977) regards the Midwives Act 1902, along with all subsequent Acts, as a disadvantage for midwifery on several counts compared to other professions. She regards midwives as subjected to supervision and likens it to controls on tradesmen; it therefore did not promote the profession. Investigations of misconduct, which included review of the private life of the midwife, were defined under strict criteria with no recourse to appeal if the midwife was struck off. Leap & Hunter (1993) describe the fear many midwives experienced as unannounced visits from an inspector were common.

1937–1974

In 1937 the term 'inspector' was dropped in favour of 'supervisor', and a two-tier system of medical and non-medical supervisors came in. The medical supervisor was usually the Medical Officer for Health for the area, with the non-medical supervisor being a midwife, nurse or health visitor. Strangely, although it was recommended that the non-medical supervisors of midwives should have some experience in midwifery practice, it did not recommend that those who were currently in clinical practice should be supervisors of midwives (Kirkham 1995).

Towler & Bramall (1986) report that the creation of medical and non-medical supervisors was an acknowledgement of unsuitable appointments in the past. As the medical supervisor of midwives was usually the Medical Officer for Health and was therefore aware of the social and public health issues of the area, supervision was more knowledgeable and demonstrated understanding of the everyday issues that midwives encountered in their practice (Allison & Kirkham 1996).

Allison & Kirkham (1996) describe how non-medical supervisors were community based during the 1940s. These supervisors were practising midwives and worked in the community as part of the domiciliary maternity service. They knew the conditions in which the midwives worked and therefore were much more supportive than the previous inspectors. They formed a valuable resource and were also responsible for recording and passing on to the medical supervisor statistics that enabled information on birth and maternity outcomes to be produced (Allison 1996).

Jenkins (1995) and Kirkham (1995) believe that the changes that took place in statutory supervision of midwives in 1937 sowed the seeds for what supervision should be today, i.e. the supervisor being the supporter and friend of the midwife.

Throughout the 1940s and 1950s most women continued to give birth at home. A small number chose to give birth in hospital and midwives were employed to provide care for women who delivered there and also to assist doctors. Supervisors did not have any control over hospital midwives until 1942, when it became mandatory for these 'institutional' midwives to notify their intention to practise to the LSA (Bent 1993). Statutory supervision was provided to hospital midwives by senior community-based supervisors (Robinson 1990).

Kirkham (1995), in a consensus conference report, discussed the 1951 Midwives Act and noted that supervision continued to be linked with issues of control. This Act stipulated that midwives were required to attend a refresher course every 5 years, and it was in the remit of the supervisor to check that midwives adhered to this.

331

1974–1985

Jenkins (1995) notes that despite major consolidation of midwifery legislation in 1951, there were no changes to the requirements for supervision until 1974. The changes in legislation, when they came, were a result of the reorganisation of the National Health Service. This transferred the powers of the LSAs from local authorities to regional health authorities (England), area health authorities (Wales), health boards (Scotland) and health and social services boards (Northern Ireland).

All midwives were now employed by the NHS and supervision was transferred from community-based supervisors to hospital-based midwives, with the supervisor usually being the head of midwifery services (Jenkins 1995).

Medical supervisors of midwives also became obsolete with the reorganisation of the NHS in 1974 and this finally ended with an order in 1977 that all supervisors had to be experienced practising midwives, which also dropped the criterion that a supervisor required a year's experience of domiciliary practice (Jenkins 1995).

1985–2002

The *Midwives' Rules* (UKCC 1993) saw the addition of Rule 45, which detailed how a LSA must discharge its functions. One of the features of this rule was that for the first time, each LSA had to make available to all midwives practising in its area a list of all supervisors and how contact could be made with a supervisor on a 24/7 basis. This was to facilitate support to midwives whenever they needed it and to heighten awareness of who the supervisors in each LSA were. A more comprehensive definition of the role of the supervisor of midwives was considered by the UKCC for inclusion in the revised *Midwives' Rules* of 1998. This, according to Steene (1996), was an effort to improve the understanding and purpose of supervision.

The Association of Radical Midwives held a consensus conference in April 1995 following the publication of *Draft Proposals for Midwifery Supervision* (ARM 1994). The consequences of this conference were far-reaching with the spotlight being firmly placed on supervision and its relationship in supporting changes in midwifery practice, as described in *Changing Childbirth* (DH 1993). The conference proceedings were to become one of the first books on statutory supervision of midwives and this was followed shortly afterwards by Kirkham's *Supervision of Midwives* (1996).

In 1996 consortia of LSAs were organised in England and Wales as a result of the abolition of regional health authorities. The reason behind the consortium arrangements was that there were technically 127 LSAs in England alone, which hardly fostered equity of supervision standards across the country. The LSAs were amalgamated into eight regions with one or two LSA midwifery officers being appointed to each region on a full-time basis. This provided equity of approach in the provision of support and advice to supervisors and midwives alike (Sauter 1997).

Activity 19.1

 How have the *Midwives' Rules* impacted on the health and well-being of women?

2002 to present day

The Nursing and Midwifery Order (HMSO 2001) led to the establishment of the Nursing and Midwifery Council (NMC) and the continuing recognition and support for statutory supervision of midwives. The NMC came into being on 1 April 2002 and has developed many standards for statutory supervision. Statutory supervision of midwives was recognised as being a pivotal part of maintaining good midwifery services.

Enquiries such as Northwick Park (NMC 2005) and more recently Morecambe Bay (NMC 2011) highlighted that where statutory supervision was not adequately recognised and supported within a service, poor standards of maternity care were unlikely to be escalated and acted upon. *Safe Births: everybody's business* (King's Fund 2008) recognised the value of statutory supervision of midwives and supported its continuance in that it promoted safe and effective practice ensuring safety of women and their babies. *Midwifery 2020: delivering expectations* (DH 2010) likewise extolled the virtues of statutory supervision and how it is an essential prerequisite for all midwives in practice.

The NMC developed *Standards for the Supervised Practice of Midwives* (NMC 2007), ensuring that such programmes had equitable standards across the UK. Although the *Midwives' Rules and Standards* (NMC 2012c) revoke the 2007 standards, programmes supported by the LSAs which address individual midwives' poor practice continue and provide support and an opportunity for remedial action rather than direct referral to the fitness to practise directorate of the NMC.

Previous consortium arrangements for England and Wales were adopted across the UK and in 2006 all LSAs had a practising midwife holding the post of LSA Midwifery Officer. The LSA Midwifery Officers formed the LSA Midwifery Officers Forum (UK) and meet on a regular basis to develop and implement the NMC standards. They work with key stakeholders such as the NMC, Royal College of Midwives, Independent Midwives UK and Departments of Health from all four countries of the UK. Outputs from the Forum include national guidelines, strategic direction and an annual report.

Activity 19.2

A dedicated LSA Midwifery Officer Forum website is available at:
http://www.lsamoforumuk.scot.nhs.uk/

Access this site to see what information is available to support both midwives and supervisors in their roles.

All LSAs are required to submit an annual report defined within Rule 13 of the *Midwives' Rules and Standards* (NMC 2012c). Since 2009 the NMC has compiled an analysis of all LSA annual reports. These publications, entitled *Supervision, Support and Safety* (NMC 2012b), form part of the NMC's quality assurance process of the LSAs.

Activity 19.3

Where would you go to access your LSA's annual report? What would you expect to see in that report?

The NMC also developed a system for reviewing LSAs and ensuring that the rules and standards for statutory supervision have been met in each LSA. These reviews are available on the NMC website at: www.nmc-uk.org/Nurses-and-midwives/Midwifery-New/NMC-Review-of-LSA-reports/.

Midwives' Rules and Standards

The *Midwives' Rules and Standards* (NMC 2012c) is the legislation under which every midwife practises in the UK. Supervisors of midwives use the *Rules* alongside *The Code: standards of conduct, performance and ethics for nurses and midwives* (NMC 2008) to guide midwives through the principles of professional, safe and effective midwifery practice.

One criticism of previous editions of the *Midwives' Rules* is that until the 2004 edition, they had passed down virtually unchanged from the first *Rules* issued following the passing of the Midwives Act 1902.

The early *Rules* dictated clinical practice in an effort to stop the spread of infection, promote competent practice and safeguard the mother and baby. Something the modern-day midwife may find amusing is that the *Rules* did not confine themselves solely to professional practice and also specified, for instance, suppliers of official uniforms.

The *Midwives' Rules and Standards* (NMC 2012c) now provide midwives and supervisors of midwives with a framework in which safe and effective midwifery practice can be based. By providing rules, standards and guidance in one document, the NMC has combined legislation and practical advice for all midwives.

Role and responsibilities of a supervisor of midwives

Rule 8 of the *Midwives' Rules and Standards* (NMC 2012c) details the minimum role and responsibilities of a supervisor of midwives. However, this does not give a descriptive account of what the supervisor of midwives may encounter in her role. This has led the LSA Midwifery Officers Forum UK to develop role descriptions under three main categories of what is expected of supervisors of midwives (see Box 19.1).

Midwifery wisdom

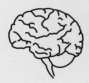 Get to know the supervisors of midwives in your area as they can help you through the provision of professional leadership, support, advice and guidance on practice issues.

The NMC has issued competencies for supervisors of midwives (NMC 2006) and these are reflected in the role description in Box 19.1. The suggested role description is not exhaustive but for the purpose of this chapter, the following key themes have been identified and will be explored briefly.

Named supervisor of midwives

Under Rule 9 of the *Midwives' Rules and Standards* (NMC 2012c), the LSA has to ensure that each midwife who submits her intention to practise has a named supervisor of midwives who will offer support on an individual basis.

Box 19.1 Advice and guidance. Source: LSAMO National Forum UK: www.lsamoforumuk.scot.nhs.uk/media/16959/nomination_selection_and_appointment_of_soms_policy.pdf

Statutory

1. Receiving and processing Notification of Intention to Practise forms to verify that the statutory requirements for practice have been met
2. Ensuring that midwives practise within the statutory *Midwives' Rules and Standards* (NMC 2012c) and that regulations for the supply, storage, administration and destruction of drugs used within the sphere of their role are met
3. Providing guidance on maintenance of registration and identifying updating opportunities in relation to statutory requirements
4. Investigating critical incidents to identify the action required, while seeking to achieve a positive learning experience for the midwives involved, liaising with the LSA as appropriate
5. Reporting to the LSA serious cases involving professional conduct where the NMC Rules and Codes have been contravened and, when it is considered that local action would not achieve safe practice, recommending referral to the NMC
6. Being available for midwives to discuss issues pertaining to their practice and to provide support. This includes those midwives who practise independently. Supervisors of midwives must participate in providing 24 hours supervisory cover
7. Arranging regular review meetings with individual midwives at least once a year to help them evaluate their practice and identify areas for development and agree the means by which their midwifery expertise can be maintained and developed
8. Ensuring that effective communication exists with all stakeholders engaged in determining health services policy, in order that relevant issues are appropriately addressed and resolved

Professional

1. Recognise own accountability to the LSA for all supervisory activities
2. Provide professional leadership to create a practice environment that supports the practitioner role and empowers professional practice through evidence-based decision making
3. Enhance knowledge of own role and individual professional development needs. Attend at least one meeting a year convened by the LSA Midwifery Officer to discuss relevant issues and share information and experience
4. Monitor the integrity of the service to ensure that safe and appropriate care is available to all women and neonates
5. Identify when peer supervisors are not undertaking the role to a satisfactory standard and take appropriate action
6. Audit the standards for statutory supervision (at least) annually. The LSA Midwifery Officer, through visits to practice sites, will validate standards. Validation of standards may also be achieved by external audits performed by other supervisors
7. Maintain records of all supervisory activities for at least 7 years. Records may be electronic or manual and must be stored in such a way as to maintain confidentiality. Participate in the safekeeping of all maternity and midwives' records for 25 years

Practice issues

1. Ensure that midwives have access to the statutory rules and guidance, evidence and local policies to inform their practice

2. Monitor the standards of midwifery practice through audit of records and assessment of clinical outcomes and take appropriate action
3. Contribute to activities such as confidential enquiries into maternal and child deaths, risk management strategies, frameworks for clinical governance or any other relevant enquiry relating to the maternity services
4. Lead activities such as standard setting, clinical audit and the development of evidence-based guidelines and protocols
5. Contribute to curriculum development of pre-registration and postregistration education programmes for midwives
6. Participate in the preparation and mentorship of new supervisors of midwives
7. Issuing of controlled drug authorities, if required, for midwives undertaking homebirths
8. Be available to guide and support midwives through difficult clinical situations

Activity 19.4

Discuss supervision of midwives with a midwife you are working with or have worked with. What are her experiences of statutory supervision? How did her relationship with her named supervisor work in practice?

Access to a supervisor of midwives

Rule 9 of the *Midwives' Rules and Standards* (NMC 2012c) determines that all practising midwives must have 24 hours access to a supervisor of midwives within the LSA area. This is facilitated throughout the UK in a variety of ways. For example, on-call rotas ensure that all midwives within an LSA area can speak to a supervisor of midwives for help and advice at any time of the day or night. This advice relates to midwifery practice and should not be confused with seeking advice from managers regarding organisational issues. Access to a supervisor of midwives is not just confined to midwives and women are able to access a supervisor by contacting their local maternity services (NMC 2012a).

Intention to practise

Rule 3 of the *Midwives' Rules and Standards* (NMC 2012c) stipulates that every midwife in the UK has to complete an Intention to Practise (ITP) form and hand this to a supervisor of midwives before she takes up employment or commences practice in an area. This includes midwives who are practising by virtue of their midwifery qualification, for example midwifery lecturers and health visitors. The practice year mirrors the financial year (April–March) and in January all midwives who have notified their intention to practise in the previous year are sent an ITP form by the NMC. The midwife must complete her ITP form and hand it to her named supervisor of midwives. The supervisor of midwives checks on behalf of the LSA that each midwife is eligible to practise and compliant with the NMC requirements to maintain midwifery registration. If the midwife is eligible to practise then the supervisor of midwives signs the ITP form and transmits the data electronically to the LSA via the national LSA database.

The LSA sends the ITP data electronically to the NMC and the information that the midwife has notified her intention to practise is included on the NMC register. Any employer, supervisor of midwives or member of the public can check with the confirmation service at the NMC to see if a midwife is 'live' on the register. Unless a midwife has submitted an ITP form, she may not practise anywhere in the UK except in an emergency. In an emergency, she may practise providing that she notifies her intention to practise within the next 48 hours to the LSA within whose area she provided the emergency care (NMC 2012c).

Choice of supervisor of midwives

Rule 9 of the *Midwives' Rules and Standards* (NMC 2012c) states that every practising midwife must have a named supervisor of midwives provided by the LSA. Although not a requirement within the current *Midwives' Rules*, previous guidance (NMC 2004) indicated that midwives must be offered a choice of supervisor of midwives. This also included that if either the midwife or supervisor found that the relationship was not beneficial, a change could be requested. LSA Midwifery Officers, as part of the annual audit of supervision within the LSA areas, continue to check that midwives are offered a choice of named supervisor of midwives and also have the opportunity to change supervisor if necessary. The LSA Midwifery Officers support the ideal of having a choice of supervisor of midwives and advise on how this can be achieved (LSAMO National Forum UK 2009).

Midwifery wisdom

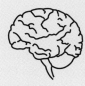

Supervision is a statutory responsibility which provides a mechanism for support and guidance to every midwife practising in the United Kingdom. The purpose of supervision of midwives is to protect women and babies by actively promoting a safe standard of midwifery practice.

Annual meeting with named supervisor of midwives

Rule 9 of the *Midwives' Rules and Standards* (NMC 2012c) states that at least once a year, a supervisor of midwives meets with each midwife for whom she is the named supervisor. The purpose of this meeting is to review the midwife's practice and to identify her training needs. The focus of the meeting is on the individual's needs and how both the supervisor and midwife can work to achieve the midwife's identified goals. Skoberne (2003) notes that statutory supervision of midwives aims to encourage learning by reflection, and all meetings with the named supervisor should adopt this approach. Yearly (2003) also recognises that a proactive approach to supervision can be facilitated by using guided reflection.

Although the *Midwives' Rules and Standards* (NMC 2012c) dictate that the midwife is expected to meet her supervisor at least once a year, in practice midwives may meet with and work alongside supervisors of midwives every day. Midwives recognise that such contact provides essential support and guidance in their everyday practice. Dimond (2006) recognises that the best approach to proactive supervision is when the supervisor of midwives adopts an open and accessible approach. She recommends that open contact and freely offered guidance encourage midwives to practise in a safe and effective manner.

Support for student midwives

Within the local supervising authority standard, set out in Rule 9 of the *Midwives' Rules and Standards* (NMC 2012c), student midwives must be supported by statutory supervision and have access to supervisors of midwives. This can take many forms, including student midwives being supported by a named supervisor of midwives in their practice placement area. Although there is no requirement for each individual student to have a named supervisor of midwives, the development of this mechanism has supported the concept of a proactive supervisory relationship for the newly qualified midwife (Mannion 1999).

Midwifery wisdom

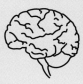

Even though there is no requirement for a student to have a named supervisor of midwives, you should begin as a student to learn about the roles and functions undertaken by the supervisor of midwives and how developing that relationship in the future can help you enhance your practice.

Statutory supervision and clinical governance

Clinical governance came into being in the NHS with the publication of *A First Class Service* (DH 1998), which described a framework which supported professional self-regulation, clinical standards, evidence-based practice, learning from critical incidents and poor performance. Kirkham (2000) recognises that the aims and dilemmas of clinical governance are the same as those of statutory supervision of midwives.

The NMC considers that the LSA Midwifery Officer holds a pivotal role in ensuring that standards of supervision of midwives and midwifery practice are met (NMC 2012c). By meeting all midwives practising in their area every year, supervisors of midwives ensure that not only are the *Midwives' Rules and Standards* (NMC 2012c) met but that statutory supervision can be used as a proactive tool which supports clinical governance.

Support for women and promoting normality

It is important that statutory supervision of midwives is recognised as a support mechanism for women accessing maternity services. Supervisors of midwives help women achieve their aims and support both women and midwives to meet challenges. Jones (2000) recognises that proactive statutory supervision is an enabling factor in establishing midwifery-led units. Mayes (1995) regards statutory supervision as supporting good practice and sees the supervisor as being the co-ordinator who enables midwives and mothers to achieve safe childbirth.

The NMC requires that supervisors of midwives promote childbirth as a normal physiological event by being involved in the development of strategies, guidelines and services based on sound evidence (NMC 2006). The NMC also promotes the supervisor of midwives to women and their families as being a support and advocate (NMC 2012a). Supervisors of midwives must demonstrate how they ensure that women influence the development of maternity services and also ensure that midwifery care is responsive to local needs (NMC 2012a). Supervisors also have a role in advising and supporting women who use midwifery services, advocating for the right of all women to make informed choices and providing additional advice to women who are experiencing difficulty in achieving care choices (NMC 2012a).

Suspension from practice

Suspension from practice by the LSA is a serious matter and can only be undertaken following an investigation (NMC 2012c). Supervisors of midwives investigate on behalf of the LSA serious incidents and allegations that individual midwives' fitness to practise may be impaired. The supervisors of midwives liaise closely with the LSA Midwifery Officer and report any concerns to her. Any midwife investigated under statutory supervision of midwives must be involved with the investigation and be informed of the outcome of the investigation. Although supervisors of midwives may recommend suspension from practice to the LSA, they cannot impose such a suspension.

Suspension from midwifery practice may only be enacted by two organisations within the UK. The LSA may suspend a midwife from practice in accordance with Rule 14 of the *Midwives' Rules and Standards* (NMC 2012c), and a Practice Committee of the NMC can suspend a midwife from practice under the powers of the Nursing and Midwifery Order (HMSO 2001).

The midwife must be informed of the suspension from practice and the reasons why this has been deemed necessary. The suspension from practice must also be notified immediately to the NMC, which through a Practice Committee will decide if the suspension is warranted and if there are grounds for imposing an interim suspension or interim conditions of practice order.

How to become a supervisor of midwives

Rule 8 of the *Midwives' Rules and Standards* (NMC 2012c) sets out the minimum requirements for eligibility for appointment as a supervisor of midwives. In addition to these statutory requirements, prospective supervisors must be nominated by their peers before being considered for appointment by the LSA. The current national guidelines issued by the LSA Midwifery Officers Forum UK advise on the many routes available for midwives seeking nomination to become a supervisor of midwives (LSAMO National Forum UK 2010).

This is a considerable change from the 1970s and 1980s when supervisors were mostly heads of midwifery/managers of midwifery services and were appointed because of their position within maternity services. In the 1990s appointment of midwives to the role of supervisor was opened up to all midwives providing they met the statutory requirements as in the *Midwives' Rules* of the time. The move to appoint supervisors of midwives at all levels of the profession was seen by Walton (1995) as a positive one. McCormick (1996) recognised that the qualities and person specification of midwives nominated as supervisors was very important. She advised that nominations should be sought by advertising, selecting and recruiting midwives capable of fulfilling the supervisor's entire role. Evidence suggests that where midwives are fully involved in the process of nomination, they nominate those peers who they feel will meet the needs of local midwives (Stapleton et al. 1998). Guidance issued by the LSA Midwifery Officers Forum continues to reflect this advice (LSAMO National Forum UK 2009).

There were no set ratios for the number of supervisors to midwives until the *Midwives' Rules* of 1993 stipulated a standard of 1:40. The ratio that is now recommended is no more than 1:15 (NMC 2012c) and the LSAs are charged with appointing sufficient numbers to ensure that statutory supervision can be effectively provided within the LSA area.

Supervisors of midwives must have credibility with the midwives they supervise and with trusts' senior management. They should be able to demonstrate ongoing professional development at a minimum of degree level. They must be experienced, academically able, perceived as approachable by their colleagues and able to communicate effectively with senior management so that they can contribute effectively to developments in midwifery practice (LSAMO National Forum UK 2009).

Midwifery wisdom

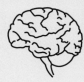

Supervisors of midwives have a statutory duty to promote childbirth as a normal physiological event, working together with women and creating opportunities for them to engage actively with the maternity services that you provide.

Education of supervisors of midwives

Early supervisors of midwives received little in the way of education on statutory supervision. The first main drive towards modern education for supervisors came about as a result of the English National Board developing *Preparation of Supervisors of Midwives* (ENB 1992). This invaluable tool formed the basis of many courses in all areas of the UK. Thomas & Mayes (1996) report that supervisors benefited from the structured format of the pack, which was based on a more educational and reflective mode than previous courses of preparation. They conclude that the pack was instrumental in informing both supervisors and midwives of the positive benefits of supervision, but that it should be updated regularly if it is to remain a live resource.

The pack was revised and reissued in 1997 and again in 2002 (NMC 2002). It was seen as an evolving resource and much valued by students on the preparation for supervisors of midwives course as well as established supervisors of midwives. The pack promoted reflective practice by the supervisor with each section encouraging the reader to examine her own thoughts on the subject covered as well as those of colleagues.

The NMC now sets the requirements of all preparation for supervisors of midwives courses in the UK (NMC 2006). The *Standards for the Preparation and Practice of Supervisors of Midwives* (NMC 2006) details the competencies expected of supervisors of midwives, based within four main domains:

1. theory, roles and responsibilities of a supervisor
2. statutory supervision in action with a focus on normality and evidence-based practice
3. working in partnership with women
4. leadership.

After appointment, supervisors of midwives have a minimum requirement of 6 hours' education relating to statutory supervision a year in addition to their PREP requirement (NMC 2006, 2012c). The NMC requires that the LSAs provide educational opportunities for supervisors of midwives (NMC 2012c). These activities can be undertaken in a variety of ways – conferences, study days and local activities around statutory supervision.

Resource packs for both student and appointed supervisors of midwives have been developed to reflect current needs (Kingscott 2010).

Debating the need for statutory supervision of midwives

Jenkins (1995) questions the need for supervision as midwives are now educated to diploma and degree level and as such should be able to determine their own learning needs. Cross (1996) questions whether supervision is really necessary as the professional accountability of each midwife obviates the need for supervision. However, the Royal College of Midwives, in a position paper on supervision (RCM 1996), saw statutory supervision as a cornerstone of the profession. The College viewed supervision as self-regulation of the profession coupled with the fostering of practice by reflection and development, and concluded that it supports the autonomous practitioner status of the midwife.

Flint (2002) suggests that statutory supervision, having being implemented as a means of control by the medical profession, now has the additional problem of being influenced by the personality of individual supervisors of midwives. However, Fraser (2002) also suggests that midwives are in the fortunate position of having the system of statutory supervision in place as it offers support, guidance, counselling and friendship.

Wells (2004) found that whilst midwives regard statutory supervision to be necessary, many voiced concerns that it needed reviewing. She reports that conflict was evident as managers within organisations are accountable for systems within their department but statutory supervision of midwives remained within the control of the profession via the LSA Midwifery Officers and supervisors of midwives.

Wells (2004) reports that supervisors perceived that organisational systems and supervision were seen as a duplication of work, rather than a reinforcement of systems. She urged supervisors to focus on statutory supervision as otherwise the supervisory system could be lost, with organisations fighting to take total control to ensure all staff are performing effectively (Wells 2004).

The NMC, by being more explicit about the expected role of the supervisor of midwives and the LSAs (NMC 2006, 2012a,c), also supports the continuation of statutory supervision in the UK.

The King's Fund (2008) recognised that statutory supervision was a rich source of learning at both local and national level and supported its continuance as being one way of ensuring safe care for women and babies.

Conclusion

Supervision of midwives continues to evolve and support both midwives and women in the shared goal of safe and effective midwifery care. Changes over the years now ensure that women are involved with their care and are seen as active partners in ensuring that statutory supervision remains fit for purpose. From the punitive and dictatorial role of yesteryear, the supervisor of midwives has emerged as the supporter of both women and midwives, ensuring good practice and enabling choice.

Quiz

1. The first Midwife Act in England came into being in:

   a. 1856
   b. 1902
   c. 1915
   d. 1918.

2. The first supervisors of midwives were called:

   a. matron
   b. supervisor of midwives
   c. inspector of midwives
   d. superintendent of midwives.

3. In relation to statutory supervision, the letters LSA mean:

   a. Local Safeguarding Authority
   b. Legal Supervising Authority
   c. Local Supervision Authority
   d. Local Supervising Authority.

4. Which item from the *Midwives' Rules and Standards* (NMC 2012c) defines the roles and responsibilities of a supervisor of midwives?

   a. Rule 3
   b. Rule 5
   c. Rule 8
   d. Rule 14.

5. Which item from the *Midwives' Rules and Standards* (NMC 2012c) defines the responsibility for a midwife to notify her intention to practise?

   a. Rule 2
   b. Rule 3
   c. Rule 4
   d. Rule 5.

6. A midwife can be suspended from practice by:

   a. her employer
   b. a head of midwifery
   c. a supervisor of midwives
   d. the LSA and the NMC.

7. Which item from the *Midwives' Rules and Standards* (NMC 2012c) legislates for the LSA to suspend a midwife from practice?

   a. Rule 3
   b. Rule 8
   c. Rule 14
   d. Rule 15.

8. A practising midwife must:

   a. care for at least 10 women every year
   b. notify her intention to practise on a yearly basis
   c. meet with her named supervisor of midwives every 3 years
   d. be a member of the Royal College of Midwives.

9. Which one of the following is not one of the four domains within which supervisor of midwives practise?

   a. theory, roles and responsibilities of a supervisor
   b. statutory supervision in action with a focus on normality and evidence-based practice
   c. planning and implementing duty rotas
   d. leadership.

10. Under the *Midwives' Rules and Standards* (NMC 2012c), a supervisor's caseload of midwives should not exceed a ratio of:

   a. 1:10
   b. 1:12
   c. 1:15
   d. 1:40.

References

Allison J (1996) *Delivered at Home*. London: Chapman and Hall.
Allison J, Kirkham M (1996) Supervision of midwives in Nottingham 1948–72. In: Kirkham M (ed) *Supervision of Midwives*. Hale: Books for Midwives Press.
Association of Radical Midwives (ARM) (1994) First draft proposals for future midwifery supervision. *Midwifery Matters* **Spring**: 26–27.
Bent EA (1993) Statutory control of the practice of midwives. In: Bennett VR, Brown LK (eds) *Myles' Textbook for Midwives*, 12th edn. Edinburgh: Churchill Livingstone.
Cross RE (1996) *Midwives and Management: a handbook*. Hale: Books for Midwives Press.
Department of Health (DH) (1993) *Changing Childbirth: Report of the Expert Maternity Group*. London: HMSO.
Department of Health (DH) (1998) *A First Class Service*. London: HMSO.
Department of Health (DH) (2010) *Midwifery 2020: delivering expectations*. London: Department of Health. Available at: www.gov.uk/government/publications/midwifery-2020-delivering-expectations (accessed May 2013).
Dimond B (2006) *Legal Aspects of Midwifery*, 3rd edn. Hale: Books for Midwives Press.
Donnison J (1977) *Midwives and Medical Men*. London: Heinemann.
English National Board for Nursing, Midwifery and Health Visiting (ENB) (1992) *Preparation of Supervisors of Midwives Open Learning Pack*. London: ENB. Revised edition, 1997.
Flint C (2002) Supervision of midwives. Are we celebrating our shackles? *Practising Midwife* **5**(2): 12–13.
Fraser J (2002) Time to celebrate supervision. *Practising Midwife* **5**(2): 13–14.
Heagerty BV (1996) Reassessing the guilty: the Midwives Act and the control of English midwives in the early 20th century. In: Kirkham M (ed) *Supervision of Midwives*. Hale: Books for Midwives Press.
HMSO (2001) *The Nursing and Midwifery Order*. London: HMSO.
Jenkins R (1995) *The Law and the Midwife*. Oxford: Blackwell Publishing Ltd.
Jones SR (2000) *Ethics in Midwifery*, 2nd edn. London: CV Mosby.
Kingscott A (2010) *Supervisor of Midwives Resource Pack*. Birmingham: Birmingham City University.
King's Fund (2008) *Safe Births: everybody's business. An independent inquiry into the safety of maternity services in England*. London: King's Fund.

Kirkham M (1995) The history of midwifery supervision. In: Association of Radical Midwives (eds) *Super-Vision Consensus Conference Proceedings*. Hale: Books for Midwives Press.

Kirkham M (ed) (1996) *Supervision of Midwives*. Hale: Books for Midwives Press.

Kirkham M (ed) (2000) *Developments in the Supervision of Midwives*. Hale: Books for Midwives Press.

Leap N, Hunter B (1993) *The Midwife's Tale*. London: Scarlet Press.

LSAMO National Forum UK (2009) *Modern Supervision in Action*. London: LSAMO National Forum UK.

Mannion K (1999) *Midwives' perception of statutory supervision and supervisors of midwives*. Unpublished MSc dissertation. Edinburgh: Queen Margaret University College.

Mayes G (1995) Supervision of midwives. In: Association of Radical Midwives (eds) *Super-Vision Consensus Conference Proceedings*. Hale: Books for Midwives Press.

McCormick C (1996) The chosen few. In: English National Board for Nursing, Midwifery and Health Visiting (eds) *Midwifery Supervision: a new perspective*. London: English National Board.

Midwives Act (1902) *The Public General Acts England and Wales* Edw VII C17 London.

Nursing and Midwifery Council (NMC) (2002) *Preparation of Supervisors of Midwives Open Learning Pack*, revised edition. London: Nursing and Midwifery Council.

Nursing and Midwifery Council (NMC) (2004) *Midwives' Rules and Standards*. London: Nursing and Midwifery Council.

Nursing and Midwifery Council (NMC) (2005) *Report on the Nursing and Midwifery Council's Extraordinary Visit to the Maternity Services at Northwest London Hospitals NHS Trust*. London: Nursing and Midwifery Council.

Nursing and Midwifery Council (NMC) (2006) *Standards for the Preparation and Practice of Supervisors of Midwives*. London: Nursing and Midwifery Council.

Nursing and Midwifery Council (NMC) (2007) *Standards for the Supervised Practice of Midwives*. London: Nursing and Midwifery Council.

Nursing and Midwifery Council (NMC) (2008) *The Code: standards of conduct, performance and ethics for nurses and midwives*. London: Nursing and Midwifery Council.

Nursing and Midwifery Council (NMC) (2011) *Review of University Hospitals of Morecambe Bay NHS Foundation Trust*. London: Nursing and Midwifery Council.

Nursing and Midwifery Council (NMC) (2012a) *Supervisors of Midwives: how they can help you*. London: Nursing and Midwifery Council.

Nursing and Midwifery Council (NMC) (2012b) *Supervision, Support and Safety: NMC quality assurance of the LSAs 2010–2011*. London: Nursing and Midwifery Council.

Nursing and Midwifery Council (NMC) (2012c) *Midwives' Rules and Standards*. London: Nursing and Midwifery Council.

Robinson S (1990) Maintaining the independence of the midwifery profession: a continuing struggle. In: Garcia J, Kilpatrick R, Richards M (eds) *The Politics of Maternity Care*. Oxford: Clarendon.

Royal College of Midwives (RCM) (1996) *Supervision of Midwives.The strength of the midwifery profession*. Position Paper 6. London: Royal College of Midwives.

Sauter S (1997) Supervision from a LSA officer's perspective. *British Journal of Midwifery* **5**(11): 697–699.

Skoberne M (2003) Supervision in midwifery practice. *Midwives Journal* **6**(2): 66–69.

Stapleton H, Duerden J, Kirkham M (1998) *Evaluation of the Impact of the Supervision of Midwives on Professional Practice and the Quality of Midwifery Care*. London: English National Board for Nursing, Midwifery and Health Visiting.

Steene J (1996) The Council's perspective and vision. In: English National Board for Nursing, Midwifery and Health Visiting (eds) *Midwifery Supervision: a new perspective*. London: English National Board.

Thomas M, Mayes G (1996) The ENB perspective: preparation of Supervisors of Midwives for their role. In: Kirkham M (ed) *Supervision of Midwives*. Hale: Books for Midwives Press.

Towler J, Bramall J (1986) *Midwives in History and Society*. London: Croom Helm.

United Kingdom Central Council (UKCC) (1993) *Midwives' Rules*. London: UKCC.

Walton I (1995) Conflicts in supervision of midwives. In: Association of Radical Midwives (eds) *Super-Vision Consensus Conference Proceedings*. Hale: Books for Midwives Press.

Wells D (2004) *Identification of the core competencies for supervisors of midwives within the Northern Consortium*. Unpublished MALIC Course dissertation. York: St John University.

Witz A (1992) *Professions and Patriarchy*. London: Routledge.

Yearly C (2003) Guided reflection as a tool for CPD. *British Journal of Midwifery* **11**(4): 223–226.

20

Clinical Governance: A Framework for improving Quality in Maternity Care

Cathy Rogers

Aim

This chapter provides an introduction to the systems and processes of clinical governance and their application to maternity care.

Learning outcomes

By the end of this chapter you will be able to:

1. demonstrate a sound understanding of the concept and principles of clinical governance and some of the key pillars
2. appreciate some of the current challenges for providing a high-quality maternity service
3. appreciate the inter-relationship between the different components of the clinical governance framework
4. demonstrate an improved understanding of your local frameworks
5. critically discuss your role and responsibilities in relation to the governance framework.

Introduction

An introduction to the systems and processes of clinical governance and their application to maternity care are provided in this chapter. In particular, it focuses on the following key building blocks of clinical governance:

The Student's Guide to Becoming a Midwife, Second Edition. Edited by Ian Peate and Cathy Hamilton.
© 2014 John Wiley & Sons, Ltd. Published 2014 by John Wiley & Sons, Ltd.

- evidence-based practice
- clinical audit
- professional development
- risk management.

Although these are presented as discrete entities, the clinical governance framework requires the integration of all these systems to achieve quality in clinical care and high standards of midwifery practice.

Included in this chapter are activities designed to help you understand and apply the building blocks of clinical governance. Clinical governance systems have evolved in maternity to enable the provision of high-quality maternity care. Quality maternity care is care focused on meeting the needs of women and their families, hence the chapter commences by exploring current concerns about standards for maternity care.

What is clinical governance?

Clinical governance is an umbrella term for systems and processes in NHS organisations that promote excellence in practice (Currie et al. 2004). The report by the Department of Health (DH), *The New NHS: modern, dependable*, states that the NHS 'will have quality at its heart and that every part of the NHS should take responsibility for improving quality' (DH 1997). Clinical governance was promoted as the framework for NHS organisations to focus on the quality of care provided (DH 1997).

Improving the patient's experience is at the heart of the clinical governance framework, and successive directions for the modernisation of the NHS and maternity care have been driven by the need to improve the quality of services offered (DH 1997, 1998, 2000a, 2004a, 2007a, b, 2009, 2012). National bodies which support the implementation of clinical governance throughout the health service include the National Institute for Health and Clinical Excellence (NICE), Health Watch England (HWE), the Care Quality Commission (CQC), Monitor, as well as professional bodies such as the Nursing and Midwifery Council (NMC). Statutory supervision of midwives also provides a framework for promoting quality in midwifery practice (NMC 2012) (see Chapter 19) and there are many similarities between the framework for supervision and the framework for clinical governance.

The central focus of both is the promotion of quality in maternity care. In their review of maternity services at the North West London Hospital's NHS Trust, the NMC concluded that 'the safety of women would be enhanced by cohesive clinical governance systems along with clear lines of reporting that incorporate statutory supervision of midwives' (NMC 2006).

Activity 20.1

Visit www.clinical-governance-toolbox.com/useful-links. This website provides you with lots of information about the background, principles and key pillars of clinical governance.

Current standards for maternity services

Improving women's experience and outcomes of maternity care is the guiding principle of clinical governance and NHS policy on maternity services (DH 2004a, 2007a, b, 2009, 2010, 2012). The National Service Framework (NSF) (DH 2004a), which has had a major impact on current standards for maternity care, specified that women should have access to supportive, high-quality maternity services, designed around their individual needs and those of their babies. These recommendations mirror the recommendations made in previous policy documents as well as current NHS policy. Nevertheless, the evidence indicates that quality of maternity care remains a cause for concern (Care Quality Commission 2012, Health Care Commission 2008, NMC 2012). Whilst overall satisfaction with maternity services is high, concern about the quality of maternity care in many NHS trusts demonstrates the need to ensure that robust mechanisms to promote clinical governance are embedded in practice (Care Quality Commission 2012, Health Care Commission 2008, National Perinatal Epidemiology Unit 2007).

Poor standards of clinical care have been cited by successive Confidential Enquiries into Maternal and Infant Deaths as a major contributing factor in the deaths reported. The most recent Centre for Maternal and Child Enquires (CMACE) (formely known as The Confidential Enquiry into Maternal and Child Health (CEMACH)) report, *Saving Mothers' Lives*, identified that substandard clinical care was present for 70% of direct deaths and 55% of indirect deaths (CMACE 2011).

The CMACE study on women with type 1 and type 2 diabetes found that the majority were poorly prepared for pregnancy and had poor glycaemic control around the time of conception and in early pregnancy. This study also raised serious concerns about the care of these women during pregnancy and labour as well as the care of the baby (CEMACH 2005). The findings of these reports clearly demonstrate the need to strengthen the frameworks for clinical governance in maternity.

The Care Quality Commission (CQC) is responsible to the DH for assessing standards in health and social care, including standards in maternity care. The CQC (previously the Health Care Commission, HCC) has highlighted a number of concerns related to standards of maternity care in the UK (Care Quality Commission 2012, Health Care Commission 2005, 2006, Kennedy 2005). The HCC identified a number of common themes that undermined the safety of mothers and babies.(Kennedy 2005). These include:

- weak risk management structures
- poor working relationships
- inadequate training and supervision
- poor environment, with services isolated geographically or clinically
- shortages of staff
- poor management of temporary employees.

The following activity provides you with the opportunity to reflect on your perceptions of the standards of maternity care within your maternity unit and identify potential gaps in the quality of care. The recommendations in Table 20.1 are drawn from recommendations made in the NICE Quality Standards for antenatal care (2012), caesarean section (2011) and postnatal care (2006a).

Activity 20.2

Reflect on the standards of care in the unit where you have work in relation to the recommendations in Table 20.1.

- In relation to local evidence, identify if each of these standards is met.
- Take one recommendation where you consider the standard is not met, and provide a rationale as to why this standard needs to be met.
- List what you feel should be implemented to support the achievement of this recommendation.

It is likely that you will have identified that these recommendations are based on the recommendations of NICE, and each NHS trust is required to implement them as part of its quality improvement programme.

Table 20.1   NICE recommendations

Recommendations	Met	Not met
1. Pregnant women are supported to access antenatal care, ideally by 10 weeks 0 days		
2. Pregnant women are cared for by a named midwife throughout their pregnancy		
3. Pregnant women with an uncomplicated singleton breech presentation at 36 weeks or later (until labour begins) are offered external cephalic version		
4. Women should be offered one-to-one care by a midwife in established labour		
5. Elective caesarean section should be performed at 39 weeks		
6. A partogram with a 4 hours action line should be used to monitor progress of labour of women in spontaneous labour with an uncomplicated singleton pregnancy at term, because it reduces the likelihood of caesarean section		
7. All women should have an individualised care plan in the postnatal period		

Source: compiled from recommendations from NICE 2006b, 2011, 2012.

Developing action plans to facilitate and monitor the implementation of national standards is an important part of the clinical governance agenda in maternity services. Achieving this involves a range of activities including evidence-based practice, risk management, clinical audit and continued professional development, which are key components of clinical governance. Successful implementation of these systems requires strong leadership and the commitment of the entire organisation.

To facilitate the achievement of quality in maternity care, many maternity units have a clinical governance subgroup. This subgroup is accountable to the trust's clinical governance group for overseeing the promotion of quality in maternity care. Membership of the group includes midwifery and obstetric leads for clinical audit, risk management, evidence-based practice and professional development in addition to a supervisor of midwives. The frequency of meetings is determined by local requirements, but on average the group meets once a month.

Activity 20.3

Find out the local arrangements for clinical governance in your maternity unit.

- Who are the members of this group?
- Discuss with a member of the group the group's overall purpose – this is often referred as the group's terms of reference.
- How does the group relate to the overall clinical governance framework for the trust?
- Identify the key challenges currently facing this group.
- Ask to attend one of their meetings.

You may well discover that the function of the group is to bring together the different components of clinical governance, so that each part is working in harmony with the others to facilitate continuous quality improvement in maternity care. You may also discover that some of the key activities of this group relate to the following:

- evidence-based practice
- clinical audit
- professional development
- risk management.

The following sections will discuss each of these aspects of clinical governance in more depth. However, achieving quality in maternity care requires the integration of all of them.

Evidence-based practice

The development and implementation of evidence-based practice for the care of women throughout their maternity are key components of clinical governance. Evidence-based practice can be defined as 'the conscientious, explicit and judicious use of current best evidence in making decisions about the care of individual patients, based on skills which allow [the practitioner] to evaluate both personal experience and external evidence in a systematic and objective manner' (Sackett et al. 1997).

This definition incorporates knowledge and skills gained from personal experience as well as evidence derived from research (see Chapter 18). The value of individual practitioners' knowledge and skill is also recognised by NICE, which states that although 'clinical guidelines help health professionals in their work, they do not replace their knowledge and skills' (NICE 2006b). Clinical guidelines have been developed to assist practitioners to provide care within an evidence-based framework (Field & Lohr 1990). Guidelines for clinical practice can be developed locally or at a national level by NICE.

The National Institute for Health and Clinical Excellence was established because of concern over disparities in clinical practice between regions and hospitals. Part of the remit of NICE is to develop national clinical guidelines 'on the appropriate treatment and care of people with specific diseases and conditions within the NHS' (NICE 2006b). The group with responsibility for the development of NICE guidelines is drawn from members of all relevant professions as well as user groups. Guidelines in draft form are available on the NICE website and key stakeholders are invited to submit comments and feedback. This is an important part of the production of the guidelines and it is imperative that midwives and other stakeholders are proactive in ensuring that their voice is heard. The Royal College of Midwives, the Consultant Midwives Group and the Independent Midwives Association, amongst others, are registered stakeholders, and individual midwives can have their views represented through these groups. The NICE website provides information on guidance in development, guidance developed and also guidance to be developed, which affect midwifery practice and the standard of maternity care.

The National Institute for Health and Clinical Excellence also produces implementation advice for all clinical guidelines published after October 2005. This offers suggestions on how to implement specific guidance locally, and key drivers to change, as well as potential barriers and strategies to overcome these. Where NICE guidance exists, local guidelines are required to reflect it.

Activity 20.4

Visit the NICE website at www.nice.org.uk.

- List the guidelines that the NICE has produced in relation to maternity care.
- List the guidelines that are in the process of development or review in relation to maternity care.

You will see that NICE has produced a range of guidelines, all of which can be downloaded.

Activity 20.5

- Review two guidelines in your clinical area where NICE guidance is available.
- Review your local guidelines in accordance with the recommendations of the NICE guidelines.
- Consider your responsibilities as a practising midwife if local guidelines do not mirror the recommendations produced by NICE.

The aim of national guidelines and standards is to support equality in clinical standards for all women using maternity services as well as the provision of cost-effective care.

In addition to national guidelines and standards for maternity care, there must be clear local arrangements for the development and implementation of best practice guidelines. The process of developing and implementing guidelines differs among NHS trusts, although the principles underpinning the development and implementation of guidelines are similar.

The Clinical Negligence Scheme for Trusts (CNST) requires each maternity provider to have a systematic framework for the development and implementation of guidelines (NHS Litigation Authority 2012). The overall responsibility for this rests with the executive board of each trust, but each trust division has a structurally identified group whose members include midwives, obstetricians, anaesthetists, paediatricians and risk managers as well as user representatives. The responsibility of this group includes some or all of the following:

- Take the lead to promote the development and implementation of evidence-based practice across the maternity services.
- Ensure that clinical guidelines are appropriately ratified according to trust policies.
- Ensure that guidelines are reviewed in light of NICE recommendations, current evidence as well as recommendations of professional bodies such as the Royal College of Midwives and the Royal College of Obstetricians and Gynaecologists.
- Develop a strategy for the dissemination of the guidelines to all members of the multidisciplinary team.
- Ensure that information to be given to women is evidence based.
- Develop an audit strategy to measure compliance with current guidelines.

The group is also responsible for ensuring that guidelines are reviewed in a timely manner.

Individual practitioners have a duty to practise in accordance with the guidelines, taking into consideration the individual needs of women. The *Midwives' Rules and Standards* specify that a midwife's practice must be based on 'locally agreed evidence-based standards' (NMC 2012). Reasons for non-compliance must be clearly recorded in the woman's records.

Guidelines alone are of limited value in promoting best practice. Therefore, there should be a clear strategy to facilitate their implementation. According to the evidence, multifaceted intervention as opposed to one-off intervention is more successful in embedding guidelines in practice (NICE 2002). Strategies used to support local implementation of evidence-based guidelines include:

- mandatory education programmes
- case study review
- reminders in clinical practice
- reminders in maternity records
- discussion at meetings/handovers
- newsletters
- information to women
- reflective practice forums
- feedback from audit.

As part of the implementation process, barriers to the implementation of evidence-based practice need to be identified, and strategies to overcome these barriers identified (NICE 2002).

Activity 20.6

Identify in this table possible barriers to implementing best practice alongside suggestions for overcoming these.

Barrier	Strategies to overcome this

You may have identified that barriers to successful implementation of guidelines lack of knowledge, fear, lack of resources and lack of ownership, and that strong leadership in practice is critical to overcome these. You may also identify that providing clinicians with feedback on whether the guidelines have been fully implemented is important in promoting compliance. Clinical audit is an important part of the clinical governance framework which aims to achieve this.

Clinical audit

Clinical audit provides a framework for measuring quality in midwifery practice through the systematic analysis of standards and the subsequent implementation of any recommendations to improve the quality of care (NICE 2002). Clinical audit comprises a number of different components, including the identification of audit topics, measuring compliance against agreed standards, and identifying and implementing changes in practice as a result of the audit findings. Further audit is then performed to ensure the successful implementation of recommendations and to monitor effectiveness of the implementation strategy. This process is often referred to as the audit cycle (NICE 2002), the overall aim of which is to improve the quality of care.

Clinical audit is concerned not only with reviewing standards but also implementing the necessary changes to practice resulting from the audit findings (NICE 2002). This ensures that the audit process leads to improvements in practice in line with the aims of clinical governance.

How does audit differ from research?

Many midwives are confused about the differences between research and audit. Although midwifery audit and research have many similarities, the purpose is different. Research is concerned with finding out what we *should be* doing, whereas audit is concerned with what we *are* doing. For example, whilst a midwife researcher might want to find out best practice in the frequency of antenatal visits for women booked for midwifery-led care, the midwife auditor might want to find out if the frequency of visits accords with local guidelines and NICE recommendations.

The audit process facilities the achievement of quality in maternity care by providing feedback on current standards, and improves practice through the implementation of action plans. Therefore, each maternity service should have a multidisciplinary audit strategy that is reviewed annually and is communicated to all members of the multidisciplinary team. Audit leads should include representatives from midwifery practice, supervision of midwives and obstetrics. The role of the audit leads is to ensure that all members of the multidisciplinary team are involved in the development of the audit strategy as well as the audit process.

In order to co-ordinate and lead the audit process, most NHS trusts have audit departments and audit lead personnel who are part of the overall clinical governance team for the trust. Audit facilitators may also be available to provide support for midwives and other clinicians undertaking audit.

Activity 20.7

Provide an example that shows the difference between midwifery audit and research.

Activity 20.8

- Identify the audit leads in your trust for maternity care.
- Discuss with them the support available to undertake audit.
- Identify the audit priorities in your clinical area.
- Find out if there is a local audit strategy for maternity services as well as dates for audit meetings, agendas and minutes for previous meetings.
- Attend an audit meeting.

Doing this will enable you to determine the level of audit activity in your local maternity services.

To reiterate, there are a number of components to the audit process, including:

- identifying of audit topics
- developing and agreeing audit criteria/standards
- measuring performance against the identified standards
- analysing results and practice implications.

The latter stage should include strategies to ensure that audit recommendations are implemented. This includes a date for re-audit to ascertain progress.

Choosing topics for midwifery audit

Topics for audit projects should reflect national and/or local priorities for improving quality in maternity services, such as recommendations from NICE, the Royal College of Midwives and the Royal College of Obstetricians and Gynaecologists.

Activity 20.9

- Write a list of potential topics for audit in midwifery practice.
- Present the rationale for the topics you have suggested.
- Compare your list with the priorities for audit in your NHS trust as you have identified by completing the previous activity.

You may identify a range of midwifery topics covering the care of women in the antenatal, intrapartum and/or postpartum period. The topics you select may be informed by the recommendations from NICE discussed previously.

Defining standards

In order to measure practice, clearly identified standards are required. Standards for midwifery practice can be identified from a number of sources. Box 20.1 shows sources that can be used to identify appropriate standards for midwifery practice and maternity care.

Box 20.1   Useful sources for identifying standards

NICE guidelines
Local guidelines/policies
Literature reviews
Centre for Maternal and Child Enquiries
Royal College of Midwives
Royal College of Obstetricians and Gynaecologists
National Service Frameworks
Local Supervising Authority
Care Quality Commission

For the audit to have an impact on the quality of maternity care, standards to be measured must be valid and based on best practice guidance.

Example of valid audit

The NICE updated guidelines on caesarean section (NICE 2011) recommend that fetal blood sampling (FBS) should be undertaken if technically possible prior to emergency caesarean section for presumed fetal compromise.

This report highlights that this standard was variably met and that the lack of compliance meant that many women were undergoing unnecessary caesarean sections. Given that this standard is a recommendation of NICE (2011) and an important aspect of the quality of maternity care, an audit to measure local compliance is highly appropriate.

Measuring standards

In order to measure the standards identified, careful attention needs to be given to identifying the following.

- What data need to be collected
- Data collection form
- The methods of data collection
- The amount of data that requires collection
- How the data will be analysed

Attention to these areas will ensure the validity of the audit and that only necessary information is collected.

Midwifery wisdom

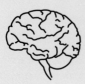

Getting the support of the audit department to help choose which audit tools to use, and the most appropriate methodology to meet the objectives of an audit, is highly recommended.

Activity 20.10

Take the NICE (2011) recommendation on fetal blood sampling prior to emergency caesarean section for presumed fetal compromise and complete the exercise in Table 20.2. Doing this exercise will give you a greater understanding of the complexities involved in choosing the methodology. It also clearly demonstrates that for the results of an audit to be meaningful and accepted, the audit requires careful planning and execution.

The final stage in the audit cycle is the dissemination of the results, and the implementation of any identified recommendations.

Moving practice forward

Audits, like clinical guidelines, have limited value on their own in improving the quality of midwifery care (NICE 2002). For an audit to have an effect on the quality of care, strategies to improve practice need to be identified and implemented. Changing practice requires an understanding of change theory, and in particular how both individual and organisational change can be achieved. For further information on changing practice, see *Principles for Best Practice in Clinical Audit* (NICE 2002).

The results of a local caesarean section audit in one NHS trust showed that FBS was not being offered or performed in accordance with guidelines. Factors that contributed to non-compliance included the expertise of staff, lack of knowledge of the benefits of FBS and the fact that the FBS machine was not working.

In order to begin to address the identified barriers, a multifaceted strategy was implemented to change practice with identified leaders in midwifery and obstetrics. This included:

- dissemination of results in meetings, including multiprofessional audit meetings, unit meetings and staff handovers
- communication of audit findings and recommendations in clinical areas
- regular case reviews held on the labour ward regarding all women who had an emergency caesarean section for presumed fetal compromise
- clinical guidelines displayed in clinical areas
- multidisciplinary workshops held to empower midwives and doctors
- competency assessments of junior doctors, and supportive frameworks to strengthen acquisition of competency in undertaking FBS
- daily checks on FBS machines.

Improving the quality of midwifery practice and sustaining excellence in care are the most challenging and rewarding aspects of the change process and require strong leadership, constant reminders and a great deal of motivation.

Professional development

A fundamental component for promoting and sustaining quality in maternity services and midwifery practice is a commitment by the individual practitioner and the organisation to ongoing professional development. The nature of midwifery practice and the challenges facing practitioners require a

Table 20.2   Choosing your methodology

Question	Consider the following
What data do you need to meet the objective of this audit?	All women who had a caesarean
	Women who had an emergency caesarean section only
	Women who had an emergency caesarean section only for presumed fetal compromise
	Women who had an emergency caesarean section only for presumed fetal compromise and it was technically possible to perform fetal blood sampling in full
	The stage of labour
	Status/experience of midwife/obstetrician providing care
	Was fetal blood sampling discussed, attempted, performed?
	Reason for not performing it/reason for it failing
	Results of fetal blood sampling, number of times performed
	The findings of the fetal heart rate trace
	Experience of professional in decision making to perform
Data collection form	Do you need a pro forma to collect information?
	Can it be obtained from your computer database?
	What information is essential?
How will you collect your data? Will you collect the data prospectively or retrospectively?	Patient records
	Theatre records
	Birth notification
	Computer records
	More than one of these
Sample required	How many women do you need to make sure that the sample is representative?
How the data are analysed and results presented	Who will input information?
	What system will be used to input data?
	Data analysis methods to be used, percentage calculations, statistical methods

commitment to lifelong learning. Continuous professional development (CPD) is mandatory for midwives. The standards for continued eligibility to practise as a midwife are defined in *The PREP Handbook* (NMC 2011). Midwives, like nurses and specialist community public health nurses, are required to renew their registration every 3 years with the NMC. *The PREP Handbook* details what is required from midwives to renew their registration (NMC 2011).

Activity 20.11

- Read *The PREP Handbook*, which can be found the NMC website: www.nmc.org.uk.
- What are the requirements for midwives regarding renewal of their registration?
- What is the aim of this standard?

Public safety is the overall aim of the NMC, and this is achieved through a number of different mechanisms, including setting standards for entry into the profession, as well as standards for continued eligibility to practise. To meet the PREP standard, midwives are required to demonstrate that they have completed 'at least' 35 hours' learning activity in the 3 years prior to the renewal of their registration (NMC 2011). This is the minimum requirement and as a registered midwife, you are accountable for your own practice. Part of that accountability is ensuring that you are up to date with the knowledge and skills to provide appropriate standards of care to women and their families. The *Midwives' Rules* require the practising midwife to have 'the appropriate skills and knowledge to understand, interpret and manage as appropriate, the complex physiological, psychological and social changes a woman or her baby may experience' (NMC 2012). Furthermore, the *Rules* require the midwife to ensure that her practice is up to date and 'tailored to meet the woman's individual needs' (NMC 2012). Continued learning and development are a core requirement for eligibility to practise as a midwife and an essential part of clinical governance. Your responsibility to meet your learning needs is further highlighted in the *Midwives' Rules* – Responsibility and sphere of practice (NMC 2012). To renew your registration every 3 years, you will also be required to provide a signed Notification pf Practice (NoP) declaring that you have met the PREP requirements and are of good health and good character.

Neither *The PREP Handbook* (NMC 2011) nor the *Midwives' Rules and Standards* (NMC 2012) specify what learning activities midwives are required to undertake. As autonomous practitioners, midwives are required to identify their own learning needs and take the necessary steps to achieve them. The supervisor of midwives is available for discussion and support in order to meet professional development needs. You will no doubt include both structured and unstructured learning opportunities, including reflective practice, reading, participating in workshops and study days and attending courses.

Activity 20.12

List different activities you could undertake to meet the PREP standard of 35 hours' learning. Using the format suggested in *The PREP Handbook* (NMC 2011), give an example of a learning opportunity you have undertaken recently.

- Describe the learning activity.
- How did this learning influence your practice?
- What evidence can you provide to demonstrate its impact on your practice?

Most midwives do not find it difficult to identify and describe a range of learning activities. However, providing the evidence to show how that learning has influenced their practice is more challenging.

The government is committed to promoting ongoing learning as an integral part of the modernisation agenda for healthcare, and this is reflected in the publication and implementation of the NHS Knowledge and Skills Framework (KSF) (DH 2004b). The NHS KSF describes the knowledge and skills that all staff working in the NHS need to deliver quality services. It requires all staff to participate in regular reviews with their manager, and an essential part of that review is the identification of a development plan to support each practitioner's attainment of the knowledge and skills required for each particular role (DH 2004b). Like *The PREP Handbook* (NMC 2011), it recognises the different ways in which practitioners can gain new knowledge and skills, but the most important factor is providing evidence to demonstrate how the learning or experience has influenced ongoing practice.

Continuously improving care provided to women and their families requires a commitment to lifelong learning and development, which is a vital part of the clinical governance framework.

Risk management

Risk management is a process that focuses on continuous improvements in the quality of care. This is achieved by taking steps to control actual or potential risks that might adversely affect patient safety or the quality of care (RCOG 2009). There are a number of factors that may adversely affect the quality of care provided to women and their families:

- Lack of access to and provision of robust systems for the implementation of evidence in practice
- Lack of commitment to continuous professional development
- Too few midwives and other staff
- Lack of clinical audit for measuring standards.

Risk management is a framework that aims to identify and then control factors both clinical and non-clinical (i.e. lack of beds, poor standards of cleanliness, health and safety hazards) that pose a threat to overall quality of care. The term 'risk management' is used to describe a logical and systematic method of identifying, analysing, evaluating and reducing risks in a way that facilitates continuous improvements in maternity care.

An Organisation with a Memory, a report published in 2000 by the Department of Health (DH 2000b), raised grave concern over the number of potentially avoidable events that resulted in harm to patients. Box 20.2 provides an overview from this report of some of the key findings that occur annually.

Midwifery wisdom

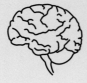

Midwives must continually learn from errors in patient care with the sole intention of ensuring that the care provided to women and their families is safe and effective.

The report also identified that there had been little systematic learning from adverse events and service failures in the NHS in the past. The report proposed that a mandatory system should be introduced to

> **Box 20.2   Key findings of *An Organisation with a Memory* (DH 2000b)**
>
> - 400 people die or are seriously injured in adverse events involving medical devices
> - 10,000 adverse drug reactions are reported
> - 1150 people in recent contact with mental health services commit suicide
> - 28,000 written complaints are received about treatment
> - NHS pays out £400 million per year on clinical negligence claims
> - Potential liability of £2.4 billion
> - 10% of all hospital admissions result in harm to patients due to adverse events
> - The cost to the NHS is £2 billion a year in additional hospital stays alone (i.e. excluding wider costs)
> - Some specific, relatively infrequent, but very serious adverse events happen time and again over a period of years
> - The typical response has been to apportion blame

identify adverse events in healthcare, to gather information as to their causes and to synthesise, learn and act to prevent similar events to reduce risk. The process for the identification, investigation, analysis and subsequent action implementation to minimise adverse events recurring forms the basis of the risk management framework (RCOG 2009).

Risk identification in maternity services

To facilitate the reporting of risks in maternity, many trusts have developed incident trigger lists to prompt staff to report certain types of incidents. Any harm, actual or potential, to childbearing women or their newborn babies will comprise an event trigger. Examples include:

- unexpected poor condition of a baby at birth
- unexpected intrapartum stillbirth
- obstetric emergencies
- third- and fourth-degree lacerations
- staffing and workload difficulties
- equipment shortages and malfunctions
- major obstetric haemorrhage
- maternal collapse/admission to an intensive care unit
- maternal death
- maternal sepsis.

An incident is reported by the member of staff flagging the event by completing an incident report form either by hand or electronically. This is the recognised route within NHS trusts to report actual or near-miss incidents. Incidents are then assessed and given a rating using the scoring mechanism in operation within each trust. Incidents are rated according to:

- actual or potential impact severity on the woman or infant
- impact on service delivery
- impact on the reputation of the maternity services
- financial and legal implications.

The process of incident rating discussed above is commonly undertaken by a senior clinician or midwifery manager. Incidents are rated as low, moderate or high depending on the impact and the likelihood of recurrence.

Incidents that are rated low generally do not require further investigation, but will be recorded and considered as part of trend analysis of maternity services risks. Incidents that are rated moderate to high require investigation. The level of investigation will depend on the severity of the risk or incident, and the actual or potential harm (NPSA 2001). The purpose of the investigation is to identify the contributing factors and to isolate the root cause (NPSA 2001, 2005).

Root cause analysis

All incidents graded high should be the subject of a full root cause analysis (NPSA 2005). Root cause analysis is defined as 'a structured investigation that aims to identify the true cause of the problem, and the actions necessary to eliminate it' (RCOG 2009). The purpose is to provide patients and their families with information and explanation of why things went wrong and to prevent similar events occurring in the future. It is also required because of the potential for a serious complaint or legal claim.

There are a number of models used in root cause analysis (NPSA 2005):

- Five 'why's – a simple questioning technique
- Fishbone diagram for incident analysis
- Gap or change analysis
- Brainshower
- Contributory factors framework.

Further information on these models can be found on the NPSA website: www.npsa.nhs.uk. All the models aim to ascertain, and therefore eliminate or mitigate, the factors that may have contributed to the occurrence of the adverse event in maternity.

Activity 20.13

- Meet your risk manager for maternity.
- Request a copy of an investigation report into an adverse event occurring in maternity.
- Discuss the process used to identify the root causes.
- Review the subsequent action plan(s) arising from the investigation.

Following root cause identification, recommendations and action planning for improvement should be drawn up. This may involve changes in training policies, clinical guidelines and procedures (NPSA 2001). The effects of the improvement strategies will need to be monitored to evaluate whether they produce the intended results (NPSA 2001). Occasionally, particularly in serious incidents, it is important to start implementing improvement strategies before the root cause analysis has been drawn up, as immediate changes may be necessary to reduce immediate and future risk of a similar incident (NPSA 2001). For example, if the preliminary review of the records of a baby born in poor condition showed that the resuscitaire available at the birth was not functioning correctly, this would need to be rectified or replaced immediately, followed by swift communication of the procedural responsibilities of staff regarding responsibility for checking resuscitaires before deliveries.

Status of the incident report and investigation forms

The incident report form and investigation report are confidential and legal documents and so should be kept securely. In the event of legal proceedings, they will be required by all relevant parties. Therefore, in line with all professional records, it is essential that they are completed accurately and factually (DH 2006).

Conclusion

Clinical governance can be defined as a framework by which NHS organisations are accountable for enhancing the quality of their services and safeguarding high standards of care through the creation of an environment in which excellence will flourish. Clinical governance, therefore, provides a framework for all involved in the organisation and provision of maternity care to provide high-quality services designed around the individual needs of women and their families in accordance with the recommenda- tions of the Department of Health.

Providing the best services for women and their families is at the heart of the clinical governance framework and Department of Health policy for the maternity service (DH 2004a, 2007a, b, 2012). The most recent national survey of women's experience of maternity reported that overall satisfaction was high and that maternity care has become more individualised and woman centred (National Perinatal Epidemiology Unit 2010). These findings are encouraging and may reflect the implementation of clinical governance in maternity. According to the NPSA Bulletin 2011, there was an increase of 8.5% in patient safety incidents in England between October 2010 and March 2011 compared to the previous reporting period (1 April 2010 to 30 September 2010).

Midwifery wisdom

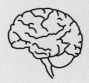

Whilst most women experiencing the maternity services report overall satisfaction, midwives must never rest on their laurels – there is no room for complacency.

The findings of the NPSA, alongside ongoing concerns over the quality of maternity care, support the need for robust frameworks for monitoring and addressing standards of practice. Clinical governance provides a framework for this and is of concern to all of us involved in maternity care. The inter- relationship between clinical audits, risk management, evidence-based practice and continued professional development in promoting a quality maternity service needs to be widely acknowledged. These processes should be a normative part of midwifery and maternity care practice and are the responsibility of every professional.

Quiz

1. Clinical governance is:

    a. a framework to promote quality in maternity care
    b. a system for dealing with clinical incidents in maternity care
    c. a means of regulating midwifery practice.

2. The essence of clinical governance is:

    a. dealing with complaints
    b. promoting best practice
    c. reducing maternity services cost.

2. Clinical governance is primarily concerned with:

    a. clinical audit
    b. women's experiences in maternity care
    c. evidence-based practice
    d. professional development
    e. risk management
    f. all of the above.

2. Which of the following government bodies is responsible for monitoring the standards of maternity care?

    a. National Institute for Health and Clinical Excellence
    b. Care Quality Commission
    c. Nursing and Midwifery Council.

2. The acronym NICE stands for:

    a. National Institute for Health and Clinical Effectiveness
    b. National Institute for Health and Clinical Excellence
    c. National Institute for Clinical Excellence
    d. National Institute for Clinical Effectiveness.

2. The quality of maternity care should be measured by:

    a. women's satisfaction surveys
    b. clinical audit
    c. complaints
    d. all of the above.

2. Woman-centred care means:

    a. care centred on the needs of the organisation
    b. care centred on the needs of the woman
    c. care appropriate to the stage of pregnancy.

8. Clinical incidents should be:

    a. ignored
    b. investigated and those responsible disciplined
    c. investigated and used to improve standards of care.

9. Which of the following activities improves standards of care?:

    a. guidelines
    b. audits
    c. mandatory education
    d. reflective practice sessions
    e. all of the above.

10. Post-registration and Education Practice (PREP) standards require the midwife to:

    a. regularly provide care to women in labour
    b. attend mandatory training every 3 years
    c. notify her intention to practice
    d. undertake 35 hours' learning activity in the 3 years prior to the renewal of her registration.

References

Care Quality Commission (2012) *Investigation Report: University Hospitals of Morecambe Bay NHS Foundation Trust*. London: Care Quality Commission.

Centre for Maternal and Child Enquiries (CMACE) (2011) *Saving Mothers' Lives: reviewing maternal deaths to make motherhood safer: 2006–08*. The Eighth Report on Confidential Enquiries into Maternal Deaths in the United Kingdom. *British Journal of Obstetrics and Gynaecology* **118**(Suppl. 1): 1–203.

Confidential Enquiry into Maternal and Child Health (CEMACH) (2005) *Pregnancy in Women With Type 1 And Type 2 Diabetes 2002–2003*. London: Confidential Enquiry into Maternal and Child Health.

Currie L, Morrell C, Scrivener R (2004) Clinical governance: quality at centre of services. *British Journal of Midwifery* **12**(5): 330–334.

Department of Health (DH) (1997) *The New NHS: modern, dependable*. London: HMSO.

Department of Health (DH) (1998) *A First Class Service. Quality in the new NHS*. London: HMSO.

Department of Health (DH) (2000a) *The NHS Plan. A plan for investment, a plan for reform*. London: HMSO.

Department of Health (DH) (2000b) *An Organisation with a Memory*. London: HMSO.

Department of Health (DH) (2004a) *National Service Framework for Children, Young People and Maternity Service*. London: Stationery Office.

Department of Health (DH) (2004b) *The NHS Knowledge and Skills Framework and the Development Review Process*. London: Stationery Office.

Department of Health (DH) (2006) *Safety First. A report for patients, clinicians and healthcare managers*. London: Stationery Office.

Department of Health (DH) (2007a) *Making It Better for Mother and Baby. Clinical case for change*. Report by Sheila Shribman, National Clinical Director (Read) for Children, Young People and Maternity Services. London: Stationery Office.

Department of Health (DH) (2007b) *Maternity Matters: choice, access and continuity of care in a safe service*. London: Department of Health.

Department of Health (DH) (2009), *Delivering High Quality Midwifery Care: the priorities, opportunities and challenges for midwives*. London: Department of Health.

Department of Health (DH) (2010) *Midwifery 2020: delivering expectations*. London: Department of Health.

Department of Health (DH) (2012) The Health and Social Care Act 2012. London: Department of Health.

Field MJ, Lohr KN (1990) *Clinical Practice Guidelines: directions for a new program*. Washington, DC: National Academy Press.

Health Care Commission (2005) *Review of Maternity Services Provided by North West London Hospitals NHS Trust*. London: Health Care Commission.

Health Care Commission (2006) *Investigation into 10 Maternal Deaths At, or Following Delivery At, Northwick Park Hospital, North West London Hospitals NHS Trust, between April 2002 and April 2005*. London: Health Care Commission.

Health Care Commission (2008) *Towards Better Births. A Review of maternity services in England*. London: Health Care Commission.

Kennedy I (2005) *Kennedy Calls for Improvement in Poor Performing Maternity Services*. Available at: www.onmedica.com/newsarticle.aspx?id=a89a0ce1-b58b-4696-b5f3-da02a0387408 (accessed May 2013).

National Institute for Health and Clinical Excellence (NICE) (2002) *Principles for Best Practice in Clinical Audit*. London: National Institute for Health and Clinical Excellence.

National Institute for Health and Clinical Excellence (NICE) (2006a) *Routine Postnatal Care of Women and Their Babies*. London: National Institute for Health and Clinical Excellence.

National Institute for Health and Clinical Excellence (NICE) (2006b) About clinical guidelines. London: NICE. Available at: www.nice.org.uk/page.aspx?o=202669 (accessed May 2013).

National Institute for Health and Clinical Excellence (NICE) (2011) *Caesarean Section*. London: National Institute for Health and Clinical Excellence.

National Institute for Health and Clinical Excellence (NICE) (2012) *Quality Standard for Antenatal Care*. London: National Institute for Health and Clinical Excellence.

National Patient Safety Agency (NPSA) (2001) *Learning from Experience*. London: National Patient Safety Agency.

National Patient Safety Agency (NPSA) (2005) *Root Cause Analysis Training and Toolkit*. London: National Patient Safety Agency.

National Patient Safety Agency (NPSA) (2011) *Patient Safety Bulletin*. London: National Patient Safety Agency.

National Perinatal Epidemiology Unit (2007) *Recorded Delivery: a national survey of women's experience of maternity care 2006*. Oxford: National Perinatal Epidemiology Unit.

National Perinatal Epidemiology Unit (2010) *Delivered with Care: a national survey of women's experience of maternity care 2010*. Oxford: National Perinatal Epidemiology Unit.

NHS Litigation Authority (2012) *The Clinical Negligence Scheme for Trusts Maternity Clinical Risk Management Standards 2012/13*. London: NHS Litigation Authority.

Nursing and Midwifery Council (NMC) (2006) *Report on the Nursing and Midwifery Council's Review of the North West London Local Supervising Authority*. London: Nursing and Midwifery Council.

Nursing and Midwifery Council (NMC) (2011) *The PREP Handbook*. London: Nursing and Midwifery Council.

Nursing and Midwifery Council (NMC) (2012) *Supervision, Support and Safety: NMC quality assurance of the LSAs 2010–2011*. London: Nursing and Midwifery Council.

Royal College of Obstetricians and Gynaecologists (RCOG) (2009) *Improving Patient Safety: risk management for maternity and gynaecology*. Clinical Governance Advice 2. London: Royal College of Obstetricians and Gynaecologists.

Sackett DL, Rosenberg WM, Haynes BR (1997) *Evidence-based Medicine: how to practise and teach EBM*. London: Churchill Livingstone.

Answers to Quiz Questions

Chapter 1

1. (a) and (e) express sympathy, (c) and (d) deny client feelings, (b) expresses empathy.
2. A good listener pays attention and clarifies and summarises what they have heard: (c) and (e).
3. An active listener looks like they are listening and says little, reflecting back the point so client feels heard: (c).
4. All but (d) and (e) as these are empathic.
5. Reassurance can only come from the client themselves. (f) is most likely to help them. (h) is more traditional authority in control. (g) expresses sympathy. (d) could be helpful when they realise they have to decide.
6. Debriefing is not recommended but clients need to talk to someone who will listen. So often well-wishing relatives will give (a) and (c) as a response. (b) and (d) are empathic. (e) is a leading open question.

Chapter 2

1. Give five reasons why it is important to have a good standard of record keeping in midwifery.
   * Helping to improve accountability.
   * Showing how decisions related to patient care were made.
   * Supporting the delivery of services.
   * Supporting effective clinical judgements and decisions.
   * Supporting patient care and communications.
   * Making continuity of care easier.
   * Providing documentary evidence of services delivered.
   * Promoting better communication and sharing of information between members of the multiprofessional healthcare team.
   * Helping to identify risks, and enabling early detection of complications.
   * Supporting clinical audit, research, allocation of resources and performance planning.
   * Helping to address complaints or legal processes.

The Student's Guide to Becoming a Midwife, Second Edition. Edited by Ian Peate and Cathy Hamilton.
© 2014 John Wiley & Sons, Ltd. Published 2014 by John Wiley & Sons, Ltd.

2. Define the term 'accountability' in relation to record keeping.

'As a professional, you are personally accountable for actions and omissions in your practice and must always be able to justify your decisions' (NMC 2008). If you provide care, then you are accountable for documenting in the records. Should an emergency arise, you may request a 'scribe' but then you should review the records yourself and countersign the entries.

3. Give four statements which apply to the minimum standards of record keeping.

See NMC (2009a), p5 The principles of good record keeping.

4. Give an example(s) of how records could be used in midwifery legislation.

- They can be used by the NMC as evidence to support an allegation of misconduct against a nurse or midwife.
- They can be used to settle a client complaint.

5. We tend to think of records as handwritten clinical notes. List some examples of different records relating to patient care (i.e. documentation on a woman's drug chart).

- Emails
- Letters to and from other health professionals
- Laboratory reports
- X-rays
- Printouts from monitoring equipment (e.g. a CTG recording)
- Incident reports and statements
- Photographs
- Videos
- Tape recordings of telephone conversations
- Text messages

6. Who owns clients' records?

If the midwife is an independent practitioner, she owns the notes. Otherwise, the organisation that employs the midwife owns them. The local supervising authority owns records relating to the statutory supervision of midwives, e.g. supervisory investigations. Ultimately the Secretary of State owns the records. Refer to the NMC circular (NMC 2007) for further information.

7. For how long must records be retained?

All records relating to the care of the woman or baby must be kept for 25 years.

8. Describe what you understand by the term 'contemporaneous' record keeping.

Contemporaneous means that you must complete records as soon as possible after an event has occurred.

9. What would you do if you needed to alter or add to the records after the event?

It is rare that you would need to alter or amend records but if you do, 'you must give your name and job title, and sign and date the original documentation. You should make sure that the alterations you make, and the original record, are clear and auditable' (NMC 2009a, p4).

10. When is it permissible to disclose information about a client in your care?

See NMC (2009a) para 27, p7. Information that can identify a person in your care must not be used or disclosed for purposes other than healthcare without the individual's explicit consent. However, you can release this information if the law requires it, or where there is a wider public interest.

Chapter 3

1. (a)   2. (a)   3. (c)   4. (b)   5. (a)   6. (b)   7. (a)   8. (c)   9. (d)   10. (a)

Chapter 4

1. True: a midwife is the expert in normal birth and a woman can book directly with her.
2. False: it is recommended that the booking visit takes place at around 10–12 weeks' gestation (NICE 2008).
3. False: only women deemed at risk of developing gestational diabetes need to be offered testing.
4. False: women may choose to undertake screening but this is not compulsory.
5. True.
6. True: however, each visit should be structured and purposeful.
7. True.
8. False: her bladder should be empty for comfort and she should avoid being flat on her back to ensure that there is no aortocaval occlusion.
9. True.
10. True: as well as testing for hepatitis B and syphilis.

Chapter 5

1. False: the Birthplace Plus Study (2011) found that low-risk women giving birth in a consultant-led units are more likely to need a casearean section, a forceps birth or perineal suturing than those giving birth in a birth centre.
2. False: IMs are self-employed: however, in the future it may be that the NHS will commisson IMs to give care to women.
3. True.
4. True.
5. False: Walsh & Downe (2004) and the Birthplace Plus Study (2011) both found that women giving birth in a birth centre were more likely to be successful in breastfeeding.
6. False: the safest place for low-risk women to give birth is either at home or in a birth centre.
7. True.
8. False: midwives and specially trained parenthood educators facilitate these classes.
9. False: birth plans are written by the woman to communicate her birth wishes; they can be written in conjunction with the midwife if the woman chooses.
10. False: a couple will usually need to pay for NCT or active birth classes, but there are occasionally subsidies offered for those on very low incomes. The NHS parenting classes are free.

Chapter 6

1. health and wellbeing
2. professions, collaboration, quality of care
3. As appropriate
4. Forming, storming, norming and performing.
5. Storming – now the individuals in the team are likely to compete with each other for their positions within the team and subgroups are likely to form. Team members are likely to be distracted from the goal and the team's functioning is likely to be poor during this phase.
6. Nine.
7. The completer-finisher is the person who has an eye for detail and is likely to spot mistakes and gaps. This preference for keeping an eye on detail will highlight the quality of the work.
8. **E**very **R**eally **C**aring **I**ndividual **F**eels **R**ewarded: **e**ye contact; **r**eally listen; **c**larify; (don't) **i**nterrupt; **f**eedback; **r**espect.

367

9. Non-verbal communication can be interpreted in a number of ways; a useful strategy is to consider both the situation and the verbal communication. Active listening will support you in interpreting behaviour accurately.

10. Where health is considered as the absence of disease, and where understanding of the human body is broken down into specific areas, e.g. anatomy and physiology.

Chapter 7

1. True. It is suggested that adrenocorticotrophic hormone (ACTH) is released from the fetal pituitary gland which causes the woman's hormone progesterone to be converted to oestrogen. This increases the sensitivity of the uterus to prostaglandins and oxytocin, which are produced by both the mother and the fetus.

2. True; see NICE (2008).

3. False. NICE (2007) recommends Syntocinon 10 international units administered intramuscularly. This is due to the side-effects experienced by many woman after being given syntometrine.

4. True.

5. False. Opioid drugs (such as pethdine and diamorphine) do cross the placenta and may affect the baby's behaviour and respiratory rate at birth.

6. False. The Valsalva manoeuvre is when the woman is encouraged to take a deep breath and hold it while pushing during the second stage of labour.

7. True. This is confirmed by research studies.

8. False. Research shows that this line does exist and has a medium positive correlation to cervical dilation and the station of the fetal head.

9. True.

10. False. The latest recommendation is that the cord is left for 2–3 min in order for the baby to receive extra blood. There is an associated risk of jaundice requiring phototherapy but the benefits of the practice are believed to outweigh the risks.

11. True. The epidural usually gives a high degree of pain relief but research shows that it prolongs the second stage of labour, increases the incidence of fetal malposition, increases the need for oxytocin augmentation of labour and leads to an increased number of instrumental deliveries.

12. True, as stipulated in the *Midwives' Rules and Standards* (NMC 2012).

Chapter 8

1. (b)   2. (b)   3. (c)   4. (c)   5. (b)   6. (c)   7. (b)   8. (a)   9. (c)   10. (b)

Chapter 9

Across
2. Pseudomenstruation
4. Subconjunctival
5. Epstein's pearls
7. Hypoglycaemia
9. Polydactyly
11. Talipes
12. Moro
13. Trisomy 21
14. Apgar
5. Hypothermia

Down
1. Caput succedaneum
3. Occipitofrontal

6. Hypospadias
7. Hip stability
8. Glucose
10. Brown fat

Chapter 10

Answers to quiz:
1. False
2. True
3. True
4. True
5. False
6. True
7. False
8. False

Answers to word search:
Wide open mouth
Lower lip curled out
Swallowing heard
Wet and dirty nappies
Rhythmical sucking
Pain free

Chapter 11

1. False: pethidine is a controlled drug and under current legislation a student is unable to administer this even with a qualified midwife in attendance.
2. True: the NMC (2007) recommends that this term is no longer used and that drugs are administered as patient group directions instead.
3. False: a midwife may give a drug included on midwives' exemptions without a prescription chart. Patient group directions do not require a prescription chart.
4. False: it is not a legal requirement for two healthcare professionals to check a drug prior to administration but it is considered best practice. It is also recommended when a controlled drug is being administered in a hospital setting (NMC 2007).
5. True.
6. False: midwives' exemptions are a list of drugs which a midwife can administer on her own initiative in the course of her professional practice, without a prescription.
7. False: a student midwife should be observed by her midwife mentor at all times and through every step in the process of drug checking and administration.
8. True.
9. False: a woman should be informed as soon as possible of any drug error.
10. False: this injection is given into the area beneath the skin containing connective tissue and fat.

Chapter 12

1. Your answers might include some of the following:

- The midwife is able to prevent ill health, so that a woman is fitter and healthier after her pregnancy than she was before.
- The midwife can help women reduce weight and improve diet, through dietary advice and appropriate exercise and support.

- The midwife can promote better lifestyles, for example by reducing the number of women who are smoking and/or misusing drugs.
- The midwife can make a real difference to a woman's life by enabling her to escape from violent relationships by facilitating access to resources to help her.
- The midwife has access to a wide range of resources – information and other healthcare professionals which can help women in a number of different ways to improve their well-being, such as immunisation programmes, screening programmes, etc.

2.

- Poor-quality housing (e.g. overcrowded, damp, difficult to heat) affects adult and infant health by facilitating the spread of infection.
- Low income affects domestic budgets for food, leading to poorer nutrition.
- Deprivation is stressful and may lead to harmful stress reduction strategies such as smoking or use of drugs or alcohol.
- Work may be difficult to find and any available work may expose the individual to workplace-related risks such as unsafe practices or exposure to pollutants.

3. Each maternity service should have guidelines for staff.

- If none exist it is worth investigating why not.
- The local refuge may cover a wide area but it is important that you know where it is and contact details.
- The Women's Aid website www.womensaid.org.uk has lists of domestic violence services across the UK.

4.

- Screening may be offered via the hospital genitourinary medicine clinics.
- It may be offered within local sexual health services or young people's clinics.
- Major supermarkets may also offer free screening to under-25s.
- Chlamydia screening is offered to all women undergoing termination of pregnancy or evacuation of retained products of conception after a partial miscarriage.
- Pregnant women should be informed about chlamydia at booking but screening is not part of routine care.

5. Your answers might include some of the following.

- Birthplace and locality
- Employment within the household – economics of the household
- Exposure to violence/living in an unsafe environment
- Poor housing and diet
- Limited access to healthcare
- Substance misuse and smoking
- Education
- Environmental pollutants
- Immigrant status can have a negative impact on health and well-being

6.

- Sepsis, in particular genital tract infection
- Pre-eclampsia and eclampsia
- Thrombosis and thromboembolism
- Amniotic fluid embolism
- Early pregnancy deaths, including ectopic pregnancy, spontaneous miscarriage and legal termination of pregnancy

7. Your answers might include some of the following.

   - Pre-eclampsia
   - Miscarriage
   - Haemorrhage
   - Caesarean section
   - Wound infection

8.

   - Do you feel safe at home?
   - Can you tell me why you smoke?
   - Have you ever considered giving up/changing your diet/changing your habit? What do you think might be hindering you?

   If a woman chooses not to accept your advice and help (e.g. says she cannot give up smoking despite the apparent risks to her and her unborn child or says she cannot leave her partner, even though she lives in a violent relationship), how will that affect your attitude to her? And will you persist in trying to help her change her mind?

9. You could choose any from the list of 10, because they have been devised to improve maternal health as a whole, but from the midwife's point of view you might have chosen:

   - promote gender equality and empower women
   - improve maternal health.

10. (a): Midwives are the first point of professional contact and are ideally suited to have positive relationships and impacts on women's health.

371

Chapter 14

1. The exact date changes every year. Muslims must abstain from all food, food preparation, drink and tobacco from dawn to dusk for a period of 30 days.
2. They take the names of both parents.
3. It is to do with phases of the moon. Start with the equinox, usually 20th March, then wait for the first full moon and Easter falls on the next Sunday.
4. Sikhs are defined by the 5 Ks, which are:

   - Kesh – long hair
   - Kangha – comb to keep hair in order
   - Kara – steel bangle (worn on left hand)
   - Kirpan – dagger or small sword (Sikhs are a warrior race)
   - Kachera – undergarment like boxer shorts (both men and women wear these).

   These symbols are important and should never be removed.

5. Blood-free meat.
6. A pagan festival celebrated on the eve before All Saints Day.
7. Hinduism.
8. Islam.
9. Hindi (English is the second most widely spoken language)
10. Christianity, Islam, Rastafarianism.

11. Urdu.
12. Jamaica.
13. Patron saint of travellers.
14. Jewish ceremony for 13-year-old boys.
15. Religion and culture (now a protected group).
16. Spirituality is central to Rastafarianism. Recognising the dignity of each individual, the assertion of self and the importance of humility and peace come through strongly in their beliefs and attitude. Natural food that is as whole and pure as possible is highly valued. Breastfeeding is strongly encouraged. Where bottle feeding is necessary, women will want to know the brand and will avoid those containing animal products.
17. They have to pray five times facing Mecca. Beforehand, they must wash hands, feet, face, top of head and nose.
18. Buddhist equivalent to Heaven. The aim of the Buddhist is to achieve Nirvana.
19. South East Asia.
20. Vegetables.
21. They can choose for themselves.

Chapter 15

Gillick competence
Bolam test
Documentation
White Paper
Statutory Instruments
Common law
Crown Court
Human Rights Act
Consent
Incapacity
Advanced directive
Freebirthing

Chapter 16

1. (c)   2. (b)   3. (b)   4. (d)   5. (b)   6. (d)   7. (e)   8. (d)   9. (e)   10. (c)

Chapter 17

1. Look for any hazards; decide who might be harmed and how; evaluate the risks and decide whether the existing precautions are adequate or whether more should be done; record your findings; review your assessment, revising if necessary.
2. The answer includes the following: boring or repetitive work; too little to do; too much to do or not enough time to do it in; inadequate or excessive work-based training; uncertainty about roles within the team; having responsibility for others; lack of flexible work schedules; the threat of violence; poor working conditions; lack of control over work activities; lack of communication between managers and staff; a negative culture or lack of developmental support.
3. Stress will lead to the following: increase in sickness and other absences; poor time-keeping; poor performance; increased intake of alcohol, drugs, tobacco or caffeine; social withdrawal; frequent headaches and blackouts; indecisiveness and poor decision making.

4. Exercise regularly; make sure you bend at knees and hips (rather than stooping over); hold heavy objects close to you when you lift and carry them; use rucksacks instead of over-the-shoulder bags; if you smoke, stopping will help increase the blood supply to the discs (smoking is believed to reduce the blood supply and cause degeneration of the discs); ensure that you maintain a healthy weight, excessive weight will put more of a strain on your back; maintain a good posture at all times; when you are sitting, make sure that your back is well supported in a chair with a backrest, placing your feet firmly on the floor; make sure that your bed suits your age, height and sleeping position; avoid twisting and lifting at the same time.

5. Identify exits when entering a building; ensure that you can handle all your equipment safely; do not work alone if you have a medical condition that would make it dangerous or impractical to do so; consider which tasks can be carried out on your own and which require assistance; undertake any training offered; seek advice from a manager as and when necessary; maintain regular contact with colleagues; ensure that someone (e.g. a colleague) knows where you are due to go each day; use your judgement, walk away if you feel threatened; consider whether you need to take a colleague with you; consider whether you are the most suitable person; ensure that you have the equipment necessary to deal with emergency situations; check in with colleagues when you return to your base site or home; an alarm system should be used which will send an alert out when you have had periods of inactivity.

Chapter 18

1. (e) 2. (c) 3. (a, b, d) 4. (d) 5. (d) 6. (d) 7. (a, b, c, d) 8. (a, b, c, d)
9. (a) 10. (a)

Chapter 19

1. (b) 2. (c) 3. (d) 4. (c) 5. (b) 6. (d) 7. (c) 8. (b) 9. (c) 10. (c)

Chapter 20

1. (a) 2. (b) 3. (f) 4. (b) 5. (b) 6. (d) 7. (b) 8. (c) 9. (e) 10. (d)

Glossary

Accountability	An individual is aware of, understands and has the ability to take responsibility for their actions
Active listening	A technique where the listener repeats back to the speaker what they have heard as a way of making sure both speaker and listener have the same understanding of the conversation
Analgesia	Relief from pain
Antenatal care	Care given to a pregnant woman during pregnancy. If the pregnancy is low risk and 'normal' all care will be delivered by her midwife
Anticoagulant	A drug or substance used to prevent/slow down coagulation (clotting) of blood
Assessment	A means to check on physical and emotional well-being and may cover areas such as routine observations and checking the growth of the fetus by regular visits in the antenatal period
Autonomy	The ability of a person to make an independent decision based on their own knowledge and understanding
Bartholin's glands	Two glands situated in the labia majora which have ducts opening into the vagina just external to the hymen. The secretion lubricates the vulva
Body Mass Index (BMI)	A measure of a person's weight relative to their height that was introduced as a statistic to view populations
Booking visit	The first visit that a woman will have with her midwife when she is pregnant. In this visit a number of physical and emotional 'baselines' will be assessed as well as this being an opportunity for information giving
Candida albicans	A diploid fungus that grows as both yeast and filamentous cells and is a causal agent of opportunistic oral, skin and genital infections in humans

The Student's Guide to Becoming a Midwife, Second Edition. Edited by Ian Peate and Cathy Hamilton.
© 2014 John Wiley & Sons, Ltd. Published 2014 by John Wiley & Sons, Ltd.

Canthus	The angle at the inner (medial) and outer (lateral) margins of the eye. Also known as the inner and outer commissure
Cardiotocograph	The strip of paper showing the continuous record of the fetal heart rate and/or maternal uterine activities. More commonly known as the CTG or CTG trace or the fetal heart trace
Care pathway	A tool introduced to decrease variability in quality and improve outcomes of healthcare by standardising processes
Cervix	The neck of the uterus
Collaboration	Teams working together towards a common goal, using awareness of communication and behaviour patterns to increase the likelihood of success
Communication	A general term that describes transmission of information, by various methods, such as speech, writing, behaviour or images
Communication skills	Expert ways in which we deliver information with sensitivity using our listening and non-verbal skills
Complex	Something that is composed of intricate, mutually related parts
Congenital adrenal hyperplasia (CAH)	A condition caused by an enzyme defect which interferes with the synthesis of cortisol in the adrenal glands. Often the first indication of this condition may be the presence of ambiguous genitalia or dehydration (with 'salt' crisis). There may be a history of CAH or unexplained neonatal death
Congenital heart malformation	Any defect in the structure of the heart and/or great vessels which is present at birth
Controlled cord traction	Used during active management of the third stage of labour. The umbilical cord is pulled downwards, following the administration of an oxytocic drug, in order to facilitate delivery of the placenta
Controlled drug	Medicine which may be misused or sold illegally, so there are stricter legal controls on its supply and administration
Coroner	A coroner is an independent official who investigates cause of death in cases where the cause is unclear. They are usually doctors or lawyers
Crepitus	The sound of two fractured bone surfaces rubbing together or the clicking sound sometimes caused when moving skeletal joints. Crepitus is also the name given to flatulence or the noisy discharge of fetid gas from the intestine through the anus
Diabetes	A group of metabolic diseases that are the result of a body tissue's response to insulin when not enough insulin is produced
Discipline	A specific branch or area of knowledge, usually relating to a profession
Drug	A substance used to modify a chemical process in the body with the intention of treating a disease, relieving a symptom, enhancing performance or altering a state of mind
Dysplasia	An abnormal development of the tissues or organs

375

Effective	When the achieved result is both expected and desirable
Engagement	Movement of the widest presenting part of the fetus through the pelvic brim
Epidural anaesthesia	The introduction of local anaesthetic into the epidural space to block selected spinal nerves
Epispadias	When the urethral opening is found on the dorsal (upper) surface of the penis
Epstein's pearls	Tiny whitish-yellow protein-filled cysts that form on the gums and roof of the mouth in a newborn baby. The condition is harmless
Ethics	This generally refers to a written code of value principles that are used in the research context. A code of research ethics is required to ensure that there are agreed standards of acceptable behaviour for researchers, which protect participants' moral and legal rights
Ethnography	A qualitative research method for the purpose of investigating cultures that involves data collection, description and analysis of the data to develop a theory of cultural behaviour
Fetal anomaly	An anomaly is a deviation from normal development of the fetus. This includes structural anomalies, for example cardiac abnormalities, or may be related to chromosomal defects such as Down's syndrome
Fetal alcohol spectrum disorder	This refers to a range of fetal effects which result from maternal alcohol consumption in pregnancy. These may relate to physical appearance, behavioural or cognitive disorders
Fistula	An abnormal opening between two cavities such as the rectum and vagina, or between a cavity and the skin surface
Frenulum	A longitudinal fold of mucous membrane connecting the underside of the tongue to the floor of the mouth
Fundus	The upper part of the uterus
General sales list medicines	These can be obtained by members of the public from supermarkets or other retail outlets
Group	A number of objects or people with some commonality with each other
Habitus	The general appearance, in terms of size and shape, of a body
Haemorrhage	Excessive blood loss
Health promotion	A process, often directed by public policy, to support people to increase control over their own health
Hierarchy	An arrangement which indicates more or less value to the individual parts, with items placed in order of value
Hydrocephalus	An extremely serious pathological condition characterised by an abnormal collection of cerebrospinal fluid. Usually this causes an increase in cerebrospinal fluid pressure with related dilation of the ventricles within the cranial vault. The congenital condition is usually demonstrated by a rapid increase in the size of the occipitofrontal diameter. Signs and symptoms

	directly relate to the amount of pressure and trauma caused to the brain and brainstem
Hymen	The fold of mucous membrane, skin and fibrous tissue that covers the introitus of the vagina. The hymen can be absent, small, pliant or occasionally so tough and dense that it completely occludes the introitus
Hypospadias	When the urethral opening is located on the ventral (underside) surface of the penis
Hypothesis	A tentative answer to a research question; it is a statement about the factors that the researcher is studying
Incidence	Incidence is the number of individuals within a population affected by a disease or condition
Infibulation	Infibulation is the most extreme form of female genital mutilation and usually involves the removal of the clitoris, much of the labia majora and labia minora, with the construction of a small vulval orifice to permit the escape of urine and menstrual blood
Jargon	Part of language that is specific to people who work in a particular area or who have the same area of expertise, recognised as excluding those from outside the area
Malposition	Where the occiput is in one or other posterior quadrant of the pelvis
Malpresentation	Any presentation other than the vertex
Maternal mortality	Death of a woman while pregnant or within 42 days of termination of pregnancy
Medicinal product	Substance prescribed as a remedy for a disease or ailment.
Medicines and Healthcare products Regulatory Authority	The government agency which is responsible for ensuring that medicines and medical devices work and are acceptably safe
Microcephaly	A congenital anomaly characterised by an abnormally small head in relation to the rest of the body. Resulting mental retardation is caused by under-development of the brain
Midwives' exemptions	A list of drugs which can be supplied and administered by a qualified midwife on her own initiative and during her professional practice for which no prescription is required
Millennium Development Goals	United Nations-devised aspirations to improve the health of the global population, including reducing maternal mortality and infant death.
Morbidity	Morbidity is a state of disease or ill health. Maternal morbidity refers to ill health as a result of pregnancy or childbirth
Mortality	Mortality refers to deaths associated with particular events. Statistical information on deaths associated with, for example, childbirth or surgery is useful for monitoring the standard of care and acts as a baseline for improvement initiatives

Multiagency	When a number of representatives from different agencies come together to share information and make decisions together
Multidisciplinary team	A unit that crosses traditional boundaries to work together
Multipara/multiparous	A woman who has been pregnant or given birth more than once
Myocardial infarction	A 'heart attack', resulting from the interruption of blood supply to a part of the heart, causing heart cells to die
Neonatal jaundice	Jaundice or yellow discoloration of the skin occurs in the newborn infant due to high level of bilirubin in the blood (i.e. hyperbilirubinaemia)
Nursing and Midwifery Council	Professional body set up by Parliament to protect the public by ensuring that nurses and midwives provide high standards of care to their patients and clients
Occipitoposterior	The fetal occiput lying towards the back of the pelvis
Occiput	The bone at the back of the head
Oedema	Excessive amounts of fluid in the tissues
Oestrogen	A female sex hormone
Operculum	The plug of mucus contained in the cervical canal
Osteogenesis imperfecta (brittle bones)	An autosomal dominant genetic disorder caused by a defective development of the connective tissue. May be suspected on late ultrasound scans. At birth, the condition is known as osteogenesis imperfecta type II, with the newborn baby suffering multiple fractures that have occurred *in utero*. The baby's appearance will be deformed due to imperfect formation and mineralisation after bone fractures. Duration of life may be limited if head trauma has occurred
Ovulation	The release of an ovum from the ovary during the menstrual cycle
Oxytocin	A hormone released by the posterior pituitary gland which is involved in contraction of the uterus
Palpation	Examination by touch
Palsy	An abnormal condition characterised by paralysis, such as Erb's palsy
Partogram	A tool used to assess the progress of labour
Paternalism	A paternalistic system attempts to control behaviour by offering limited choice. The provision of limited care options restricts the individual's freedom by offering only those choices approved by the service. The behaviour mimics that of a parent–child relationship, where choices are made for another on the assumption that the midwife or doctor knows best
Patient group directions	These make it legal for medicines to be given to groups of patients without individual prescriptions having to be written for each person
Patient-specific directions	Used once a patient has been assessed by the prescriber, who then asks another healthcare professional to give a drug to the patient

Perinatal mortality	Death of a fetus (i.e. stillbirth) or neonate. This is the basis used to calculate the perinatal mortality rate
Pharmacy-only medicines	These can only be bought from a registered pharmacy provided that the pharmacist supervises the sale
Phenomenology	This provides an examination of an individual's experience. It is therefore a descriptive and introspective study of how individuals see and understand their world. In other words, it is the study of an individual's 'lived experience' in relation to the topic being studied
Phimosis	Constriction of the orifice of the prepuce so that it cannot be drawn back over the glans penis.
Pilot study	A smaller version of a proposed study which is conducted to develop or refine the methodology of a research study, such as treatment, instruments or the data collection process to be used in a larger study
Placenta	The structure in the uterus responsible for fetal respiration, excretion and nutrition
Positivism	Deals with positive facts and observable phenomena. This type of research is associated with the 'scientific method'. Its goals are prediction, explanation and description
Postpartum haemorrhage	Blood loss of greater than 500 mL following vaginal delivery, or 1000 mL following caesarean section
Preauricular sinus	A sinus located anterior to the auricle (external ear or pinna) of the ear
Pre-eclampsia	A serious hypertensive disorder occurring only in pregnancy, which may be fatal in its outcome for both mother and fetus. The disease includes hypertension, proteinuria and damage to organs and tissues throughout the body
Prescription-only medicines	These can only be supplied and given to a client on the instruction of an appropriate practitioner (for example, a doctor or dentist)
Preventive healthcare	Healthcare that is designed to prevent the occurrence of diseases
Primigravida	A woman who is pregnant for the first time or has been pregnant one time
Profession	A vocational role that is based on specialised education and provides a unique service that is essential for the well-being of society
Prospective study	This type of study takes place over a period of time in which the participants are followed to see what will happen to them
Prostaglandin	A hormone associated with the initiation of labour.
Proteinuria	Protein detected in the urine
Randomisation	The allocation of participants to treatment conditions in a random manner; that is, the allocation is determined by chance only
Reductionist	This procedure explains complex behaviour in terms of simple principles, reducing it to its smaller individual parts

379

Rehabilitation	A service from a number of professions designed to support an individual in improving function following traumatic injury or disease
Retrospective study	A type of study that uses past information about the participants to look at what happens to them in order to draw conclusions
Screening	Tests that may give an indication of whether the fetus is at risk of having certain genetic and chromosomal conditions. Tests are also applied to the woman, assessing for certain conditions such as gestational diabetes, and help to ascertain risk
Shoulder dystocia	Difficulty delivering the fetal shoulders as they fail to enter the pelvic brim
Sudden infant death syndrome	The unexpected death of an infant, for which no cause can be found
Syntocinon	A synthetic form of oxytocin
Syntometrine	An oxytocin drug or artificial hormone used to contract the uterus after the delivery of the baby, in conjunction with the active management of the third stage of labour
Tachypnoea	In babies under 6 months of age, this is usually defined as a respiratory rate persistently above 55
Team	A group of people with a common purpose
Theorem	A belief or truth that is accepted because of previously proven or established truths
Thromboprophylaxis	The prevention of deep vein thrombosis, and the associated risk of pulmonary embolism
Torsion	Twisting of the spermatic cord that can cut off the blood supply to structures such as the testicle and epididymis. Partial loss of circulation may result in atrophy and complete ischaemia for approximately 6 hours may result in gangrene of the testis
Trimester	In childbearing, this refers to a third part of a pregnancy. For example, the first trimester is usually taken to be up to 12 weeks' gestation, the second trimester is usually taken to be from 13 to 28 weeks and the third trimester runs from 29 weeks to term, or delivery of the baby
Umbilical cord	The temporary structure carrying blood from the placenta to the fetus
Urinalysis	Analysis of constituents of urine
Ventouse / Kiwi Extraction	A method of assisting vaginal delivery of a baby using a suction cap attached to the baby's head and then applying traction
Vertex (of skull)	The part of the fetal skull surrounding the posterior fontanelle which presents first in a fully flexed fetus

Index

Page numbers in *italics* denote figures, those in **bold** denote tables.

The Student's Guide to Becoming a Midwife, Second Edition. Edited by Ian Peate and Cathy Hamilton.
© 2014 John Wiley & Sons, Ltd. Published 2014 by John Wiley & Sons, Ltd.

389